RECENT ADVANCES IN
ANIMAL NUTRITION — 2008

Recent Advances in Animal Nutrition

2008

P.C. Garnsworthy, PhD
J. Wiseman, PhD
University of Nottingham

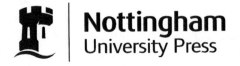
Nottingham
University Press

Nottingham University Press
Manor Farm, Main Street, Thrumpton
Nottingham, NG11 0AX, United Kingdom

NOTTINGHAM

First published 2009
© The several contributors names in the list of contents 2009

British Library Cataloguing in Publication Data
Recent Advances in Animal Nutrition — 2008:
University of Nottingham Feed Manufacturers
Conference (42nd, 2008, Nottingham)
I. Garnsworthy, Philip C. II. Wiseman, J.

ISBN 978-1-904761-04-4

Disclaimer

Every reasonable effort has been made to ensure that the material in this book is true, correct, complete and appropriate at the time of writing. Nevertheless the publishers, the editors and the authors do not accept responsibility for any omission or error, or for any injury, damage, loss or financial consequences arising from the use of the book.

Typeset by Nottingham University Press, Nottingham
Printed and bound by the MPG Books Group in the UK

PREFACE

The 42nd University of Nottingham Feed Conference was held at the School of Biosciences, Sutton Bonington Campus, 2nd – 4th September 2008. As usual, the Conference was divided into themed sessions that grouped papers into areas of topical interest to the animal feed industry. These sessions were Ruminants, Biosecurity and Food Safety, Developments in the Industry, Non-ruminants and Biofuels.

The theme of the Ruminant session was improvement of production efficiency through advances in nutrition, health and genetics. The first paper reports recent studies on the relationships between nutrition, metabolism and reproductive efficiency in both dairy and beef cattle, highlighting the multiple common mechanisms that explain a large part of the lower reproductive performance in both types of cow. One of the limitations for improving reproduction and health of dairy cows is lack of sub-clinical information about the status of individual cows. The second paper reports a pilot study that uses online monitoring to provide early detection of diseases and reproductive status, which has the potential to improve cow welfare and reproductive efficiency. Increasing feed costs and environmental regulations emphasise the role of home grown forages in overall feed efficiency. The third paper reviews advances in plant genetics that aim to increase the efficiency of nitrogen and energy use by ruminants. Animal genetics has always played a major role in determining production efficiency of cattle, historically through selection on milk yield and growth traits. More recently, attention has focussed on improved feed efficiency as a desirable genetic goal. The fourth paper defines residual feed intake and discusses the potential benefits of including this trait in breeding programmes.

The session on Biosecurity and Food Safety comprised three papers that addressed topics of considerable importance to producers and consumers. The first paper outlines the prevalence of food-borne infections, approaches to Biosecurity on farms, and challenges faced by livestock producers and the feed industry. Campylobacter infection from chicken products is the most common cause of bacterial food-borne disease in the world. The second paper reports a large study designed to identify the main risk areas and to develop strategies to control campylobacter infection on farms. The third paper discusses the potential of bacteriophage, a relatively new technology in Western countries that was exploited in the former Soviet Block for many years, for reducing campylobacter contamination of poultry.

The session on Developments in the Industry took a global perspective. The first paper discusses recent global trends in supply and demand for agricultural commodities that are having dramatic effects on World markets in animal feeds. The second paper continues the series of papers looking at animal production in different countries by describing developments in the Russian livestock industry and their implications for the European feed industry.

The non-ruminant session consisted of three papers concerned with aspects of pig nutrition, environmental impact and health. To reduce the environmental impact of pig production, it is desirable to reduce nitrogen and phosphorus excretion. The first paper uses practical examples to illustrate how feed formulation software can be used to achieve this aim. Gut health is of vital importance for maintenance of pig performance and efficiency. The second paper in this session looks at the interactions between the gut bacteria and development of immunity in the host. The third paper continues the theme and discusses the role of fibre in maintaining a healthy gut and its implications for reducing the incidence of diseases.

The Biofuels session took a detailed view of the implications for the animal feed industry of this rapidly growing technology. Manufacture of biofuels is generally considered as a threat to the food supply chain through increased demand for raw materials, particularly cereals, and greater pressure on land to grow these crops. The first paper, however, critically assesses the arguments and concludes that when the increased supply of protein concentrates from co-products is taken into account, there is little if any requirement for new land. Furthermore, the paper shows how Europe could meet its targets for biofuels from indigenous cereal production whilst reducing imports of protein from tropical countries. The anticipated availability of co-products is significant and information is required about how they can be included in formulations and likely responses in animal performance. The second paper in this session presents details of the nutritional and economic value of co-products from biofuel production. The third paper reports experiences from Canada on coping with the large variation in quality of co-products so that they can be used effectively to achieve predictable animal performance. The fourth paper discusses practical aspects of feeding distillers grains to pigs under commercial conditions. The fifth paper reviews the potential use of enzymes to improve the nutritive value of co-products. The sixth paper outlines some of the potential negative effects on carcass quality, particularly on fatty acid profile, of feeding high levels of distillers grains to pigs.

We would like to thank all speakers for their presentations and written papers, which have maintained the high standards and international standing of the Nottingham Feed Conference. We are grateful to all members of the Programme Committee (see the List of Participants) for their significant inputs into designing and arranging the conference programme. We would also like to acknowledge the input of those who helped us to chair sessions (Mike Bedford and Mike Varley) and the administrative (managed by Sue Golds), catering and support staff who ensure the smooth running of the conference. Finally we would like to thank the delegates who made valuable contributions both to the discussion sessions and the general atmosphere of the meeting.

The 2009 event will be held at the University of Nottingham Sutton Bonington Campus 8th – 10th September.

P.C. Garnsworthy
J. Wiseman

CONTENTS

1

IMPACT OF ENERGY BALANCE ON METABOLIC CHANGES AND REPRODUCTIVE TISSUES; CONSEQUENCES FOR OVARIAN ACTIVITY AND FERTILITY IN DAIRY AND BEEF CATTLE

P. HUMBLOT[1], B. GRIMARD[2], S. FRERET[3], G. CHARPIGNY[4] A.A. PONTER[2], H. SEEGERS[5] AND C, PONSART[1]

[1] UNCEIA R&D, 13 rue Jouet, 94704, Maisons Alfort, France
[2] UMR INRA-ENVA Biologie du Développement et Reproduction, 94704, Maisons Alfort, France
[3] INRA-PRC, 37380 Nouzilly, France
[4] INRA, Biologie du Développement et Reproduction, 78350, Jouy en Josas, France
[5] UMR 708 INRA-ENVN, Gestion de la Santé Animale, 44307, Nantes, France

Introduction

Dairy and beef cows are affected by Negative Energy balance (NEB) during early lactation. The magnitude and duration of NEB depend on body condition score at calving, post partum feed supply, milk yield and genetic origin (Chilliard *et al.*, 1998; Vila Godoy *et al.*, 1998; Tillard *et al.*, 2008). NEB is associated with metabolic changes which in turn affect the reproductive potential of high yielding dairy cows and beef cows. Especially in the dairy cow, genetic selection for milk production and the induced changes in key metabolic hormones (Garnsworthy *et al.*, 2008) have been associated in many countries with a reduction in reproductive potential, including delayed resumption and increased irregularities of ovarian cyclicity and lower conception rates (Humblot 2001, Royal *et al.*, 2002, Barbat *et al.*, 2005, Grimard *et al.*, 2006). Similar observations have been reported in underfed beef cows following calving (Grimard *et al.*, 1995). Various mechanisms are involved, including central effects that affect gonadotrophin secretion and effects on the ovary and genital tract. There is now evidence that the metabolic changes that impair reproductive function may be initiated during the end of pregnancy (Wathes *et al.*, 2008, Tillard *et al.*, 2008). This chapter aims to integrate the corresponding information and some of the strategies which have been used to limit NEB and its unfavourable effects on reproductive function will be discussed.

Metabolic and BCS changes around calving and Negative Energy Balance

The homeostatic controls of blood glucose are of a critical importance in post partum cows because of the major use of glucose for synthesis of lactose which in turn determines milk yield. Insulin plays a major role in glucose homeostasis as it stimulates glucose uptake by tissues, promotes protein synthesis and increases lipogenesis (Garnsworthy *et al.*, 2008). Some changes occur in the regulation of nutrient partitioning and in glucose metabolism, both at the end of pregnancy and during early lactation that make the post partum cow likely to suffer from NEB. At the end of pregnancy, the dam provides adequate nutrients for the final stages of foetal growth. This is achieved by development of peripheral insulin resistance which leaves more nutrients available for placental transfer (Bell, 1995). The shift in adipose tissue metabolism in favour of mobilisation to provide nutrients for foetal growth results in a pre-partum rise in Non Esterified Fatty Acids (NEFA) and initiates a loss of Body Condition Score (BCS) that continues after calving (Wathes *et al.*, 2007). This rise in NEFA contributes to insulin resistance in the dam as lipid accumulation inhibits phosphorylation of insulin receptors (Wathes *et al.*, 2008). A similar and even more pronounced mechanism is observed during lactation as fewer nutrients are directed towards body fat reserves following a meal and more nutrients are taken-up by the mammary gland to support milk synthesis because of altered response to insulin (Bauman 2000, Ponter *et al.*, 1997). The low glucose availability before calving and during the early post partum period is associated with low plasma insulin and cholesterol concentrations, in addition to higher NEFA concentrations which characterise NEB (Tillard *et al.*, 2007, 2008). A similar situation (low blood glucose, tissue mobilisation and elevated NEFA) leading to insulin resistance has been reported in underfed beef cows during the post-partum period (Grimard *et al.*, 1995, Ponter *et al.*, 1997, Ponsart *et al.*, 1999). In this experiment, beef cows progressively adapted themselves to underfeeding and their metabolic status was the same as controls by 10 weeks post partum (Figure 1).

NEB and the IGF system

Insulin and the Insulin-like Growth Factors (IGF-I and IGF-II) are metabolic hormones that initiate mitogenic, metabolic, differentiation and survival responses in many tissues (Wathes *et al.*, 2008). IGF-I is synthesised primarily in the liver in response to Growth Hormone (GH). IGF receptors are found in most tissues, but IGF availability for target tissues is mainly under the control of 6 high affinity binding proteins (IGFBP). In both beef and dairy cows, especially in cases of

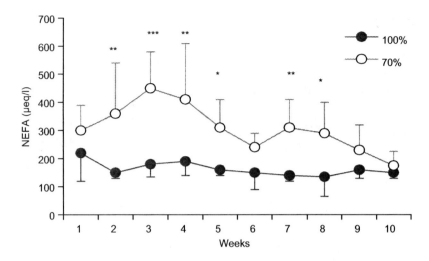

Figure 1. Blood NEFA concentrations in post-partum Charolais beef cows that received either 100% or 70% of dietary energy requirements (from Grimard *et al.*, 1995).

severe NEB (underfeeding in beef cows , high milk production in dairy cows), GH receptors in the liver are down regulated during early lactation and IGF-I concentrations are dramatically reduced despite elevated GH concentrations (Butler *et al.*, 2003, Garnsworthy *et al.*, 2008). These changes can contribute to reinforced insulin resistance because IGF-I can bind to insulin receptors and stimulate glucose uptake. IGF-I also appears necessary for normal insulin sensitivity (Wathes *et al.*, 2008).

Leptin also has a regulatory role in these processes by acting as an indicator of body fatness and it is part of a feedback mechanism that controls feed intake. On going effects of leptin signalling may contribute to reduce feed intake in cows with high BCS before calving making them even more susceptible to NEB and likely to lose excessive amounts of BCS during early lactation. This may explain, at least in part, why in many studies, an increase in BCS at calving was associated with greater BCS losses in early lactation (Garnsworthy 2008, Tillard *et al.*, 2007, Ponsart *et al.*, 2008; Figure 2).

This trend has also been observed during the pre-partum period. In a study involving 234 multiparous Prim'Holstein cows (Ponsart *et al,,* 2008), more than 60 % of the cows had a BCS between 2.5 and 3.5 at start of the dry period and of those, 72 % had a similar score at time of calving. Depending on herds, 6 to 32 % of the cows had a lower BCS at time of calving when compared to 60 days before, whereas the proportions of cows that increased their BCS ranged from 8 to 50 %. These BCS changes before calving were related to the ante partum score. In cows that were lean at 60 days ante partum, 37.5% increased BCS and 8.3% decreased BCS, whereas in cows that had high BCS at 60 days ante partum, 0 increased BCS and 11.4% decreased ($p<0.01$).

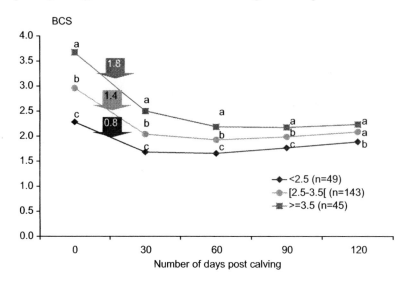

Figure 2. Post Partum BCS changes according to BCS status 60 days before calving (<2.5 ◆ ; 2.5 to 3.5 ● ; ≥ 3.5 ■ ; ⬦ mean BCS loss between 0 and 60 days postpartum; From Ponsart *et al.*, 2008).

There is evidence that both dairy and beef cows adjust their feed intake to regulate body fatness and lipid mobilisation over the first 3 months of lactation. However, for a given BCS at time of calving, the intensity of post-partum loss shows large individual variations. In both types of cattle, the changes described above during the pre and post partum period in metabolism, BCS and alterations in growth hormone, IGF, insulin and leptin (Garnsworthy *et al.*, 2008) are observed. They are associated with lipid mobilisation, high NEFA, peripheral insulin resistance and major alterations in insulin-like growth factor (IGF) that interact with re-establishment of ovarian activity, and ability for an ovum to be fertilized and for a normal pregnancy to be sustained.

Relationships between BCS/metabolic changes and re-establishment of ovarian activity

Many studies have shown that the events underlying follicular growth (growth of antral follicles, dominance, oestradiol secretion, restoration of LH pulsatility), which are prerequisites for first post-partum ovulation, are influenced by diet, especially by energy supply. It is clear that gonadotrophin secretion, especially LH which is stimulated in a pulsatile manner by GnRH, can be influenced by a number of metabolic hormones and growth factors (glucose, fatty acids, insulin, IGF-I;

Sinclair and Webb 2005). NEB together with low insulin, glucose and IGF-I, have been shown to be often associated with reduced LH pulse frequency (Butler, 2003). This was observed also in post partum beef cows fed diets with differing energy levels (either 100% or 70% of energy requirements); LH pulsatility was impaired in the underfed group (Grimard *et al.*, 1995). This was observed by 30 days post partum, but the response to diet was related to individual metabolic status and the reduction in pulsatility was observed mainly in cows that presented elevated NEFA concentrations by that time. Such changes were associated also with differences in terms of follicular growth, with fewer follicles growing and a reduction in the size of the largest follicle in the 70% energy group.

A large number of *in vitro* studies have demonstrated the direct action of metabolic factors on granulosa and theca cells (Webb *et al.*, 1999a,b, Lucy, 2000, Spicer *et al.*, 2002) and many experiments have also illustrated direct effects of diet on follicular variables during a normal cycle or following superovulation. Guttierez *et al.*, 1997, Garnsworthy and Webb 1999, Gong *et al.*, 2002, have shown for instance that short term changes in plane of nutrition affect follicular recruitment resulting in a larger number of ovulations following a gonadotrophin challenge.

The roles of the IGF system and insulin appear particularly critical. Increased energy decreases IGFBP2 and IGFBP4 expression in small follicles. IGFBP2 has been shown to inhibit the actions of IGF in different cell lines and is present at high concentrations during the post partum period (Hoeflich *et al.*, 1998, McGuire *et al.*, 1995, Vleurick *et al.*, 2000). Lowered IGFBP2 may in turn increase bioavailability of systematically derived IGF-I and locally produced IGF-II in these follicles. On the contrary, in cases of strong NEB, Wathes *et al.* (2008) reported increased expression of IGFBP2 in the liver, whereas transcripts for IGFBP3 to 6 were down regulated. Together with the reduced IGF-I production, these changes are likely to lower IGF-I availability and receptivity for follicular cells, leading to impaired follicular growth.

There is evidence that insulin may be one of the key metabolic factors regulating follicular growth and ovulation during the post partum period through its action on the IGF system. Low insulin concentrations were associated with a delay in first ovulation and resumption of ovarian cycles in cows selected for high genetic merit (HGM; Guttierez *et al.*, 2006, Gong *et al.*, 2002a). Despite no difference being observed in terms of gonadotrophin secretion and follicular growth, feeding an isoenergetic diet designed to increase insulin concentrations led to an earlier first post partum ovulation. This indicates that insulin signalling may really be one of the first signals necessary for resumption of normal cyclicity. These results may be explained by the fact that increased insulin may be important to restore GH signalling during early lactation (Butler *et al.*, 2003, Jiang and Lucy, 2001) which could in turn stimulate IGF-I transcription in the liver whose control is under GH receptor signal transduction.

This striking role of insulin has been documented also in studies in which high energy supply, and more especially insulin status, was associated with increased incidence and improved characteristics of ovarian cycles. It has been shown for example that increasing circulating insulin concentrations can enhance follicular growth together with detrimental effects on the developmental competence of the oocyte (Garnsworthy *et al.*, 2008). This is consistent with the metabolic changes and reproductive results observed (increased follicular growth and lower early embryonic development) following superovulation obtained with increased energy diets in dairy heifers expressing high growth rates (Freret *et al.*, 2006).

Taken together, results from these experiments may explain the strong relationships between markers of energy balance (both from BCS and milk measurements) and re-establishment of ovarian cycles found from recent epidemiological studies (Table 1).

Table 1. Relationships between individual markers of energy balance (BCS*) and milk production (MP) and milk variables (PC; Protein Content, FC; Fat Content) by 30 days post partum and reestablishment of ovarian activity.

Study	Marker	Effects on reproductive performance
Seegers *et al.*, unpublished) (ENVN, KEENAN, VET TEL, UNCEIA)	BCS loss 0-30 d PP ≥ 1 pt	↑ anoestrus by 45 days PP ↑ interval calving – 1st AI
Ponsart *et al.*, 2007	BCS < 2, 30 d PP	↑ irregular cyclicity
Dubois *et al.*, 2006	High MP, 30 d PP PC/FC < 0.7, 30 d PP	↑ irregular cyclicity
Ponsart *et al.*, 2006b	BCS loss 0-30 d PP ≥ 1 pt	↓ oestrus expression at 1st heat
Ponsart *et al.*, 2006a	minimum PC < 26 g/kg	↓ oestrus expression at 1st heat
Ponsart *et al.*, 2006a	PC/FC < 0.7 30 d PP	↑ anœstrus
Seegers *et al.*, unpublished	Low PC	↑ anœstrus by 45 days PP

* for BCS and BCS changes the scale is always from 1 to 5

Relationships between BCS/metabolic changes and fertility

All of the above mentioned changes affecting follicular growth can potentially impair fertility as the quality of the oocyte and its ability to be fertilized and develop into a normal embryo are largely dependant on its development within the follicle and duration of maturation time within the follicle (Mihm *et al.*, 1994). More specifically, development of the early embryo until the blastocyst stage relies mainly on the expression of mRNA accumulated during the pre-ovulatory stages (Burns *et al.*, 2003, Wu *et al.*, 2003).

The above mentioned relationship between low IGF-I and high IGF-BP2 expression and follicular growth reported by Wathes *et al.* (2008) has also been related to fertility (Ponter *et al.*, 2005, Remy *et al.*, 2005). In this experiment lower plasma IGF-I concentrations were found through to 80 days post-partum in unfertile cows (non-pregnant after 2 AIs) than in fertile dairy cows ($p<0.05$) and at 70 days post partum, IGF-I mRNA expression in the liver tended to be reduced and IGF-BP2 mRNA expression tended to be higher in unfertile cows than in fertile cows.

Direct negative effects of NEB on fertility may also be related to metabolic changes in follicular fluid that may be detrimental to the quality of the oocyte and its surrounding cumulus cells (Leroy *et al.*, 2008). Several *in vitro* studies have shown relationships between nutrient intake, the environment of the oocyte and its developmental competence. In the case of NEB, it has been shown that changes in glucose, insulin and NEFA observed in serum are more or less reflected in the follicular fluid of the dominant follicle (Leroy *et al.*, 2008). Some buffering capacity of the follicle when compared to changes observed in serum was demonstrated for glucose and NEFA, but not for urea and ß-OHB. Despite this buffering mechanism, low glucose and high NEFA were observed in the microenvironment of the oocyte. In addition to elevated NEFA concentrations, it has been reported that the composition of the fatty acids present in follicular fluid is changed with NEB, the 3 most abundant ones being oleic, palmitic and stearic acids. Even a short direct exposure for 24 hours of oocytes to concentrations of palmitic or stearic acid, such as those found in follicular fluid during the previous experiments, resulted in a dramatic reduction in maturation, fertilization and early cleavage rates. Cumulus expansion was also affected. A similar result was observed when oocytes were exposed to low glucose. Leroy *et al.* (2008) reported that high NEFA and low glucose concentrations in the microenvironment of pre-ovulatory oocytes are associated with lower developmental competence/early embryonic development and reduced tolerance to cryopreservation. Direct effects on embryo quality have been observed also at later stages of development following fertilisation (Leroy *et al.*, 2008).

Since all these detrimental effects were observed after a short period of exposure of oocytes to low glucose and high NEFA, it may be hypothesized that these effects may be even more pronounced for oocytes produced during NEB, when cows experience a longer time of exposure to an unfavourable metabolic environment.

These results are in full agreement with those from recent studies performed in high yielding cows demonstrating low development rates from oocytes collected from cows in NEB, and poor quality of the associated COCs collected during the early post-partum period (Charpigny *et al.*, unpublished).

Apart from direct effects on reproductive tissues, there is evidence that alterations due to NEB of other functions, such as the immune system, may impair reproductive performance. Specific detrimental effects of severe NEB on the immune system were illustrated by Wathes *et al.* (2008). These included reduced white blood cell count, lymphocyte number and platelet count. Negative correlations were found between white blood cell count, lymphocyte number and NEFA, whereas platelet count was positively correlated with IGF-I and glucose. In addition, a complementary approach aiming to identify gene networks that would be significantly affected by NEB revealed many differences in gene expression in cows expressing severe NEB. The state of NEB significantly affected signalling pathways and networks associated with oxidative stress. These changes may contribute to a prolonged state of inflammation within the uterus making it more susceptible to uterine disease/incomplete involution.

Taken together, results from these experiments may explain the strong relationships between markers of energy balance (both from BCS and milk measurements) and fertility found in recent epidemiological studies (Table 2).

Table 2. Relationships between markers of energy balance (BCS*), milk production (MP) and milk variables (PC; Protein Content, FC; Fat Content) by 30 days post partum and fertility.

Study	Marker	Effects on reproductive performances
Seegers *et al*, 2005	PC/FC < 0.64	↓ fertility
NEC+REPRO Ponsart *et al.*, 2006a	PC/FC < 0.7 30 d PP	↑ culling for infertility
UNCEIA/FERTILIA (unpublished)	minimum PC < 28 g/kg	↓ fertility
Ponsart *et al.*, 2007	High MP , 30 d PP PC/FC < 0.7, 30 d PP BCS loss 0-30 d PP ≥ 1	↑ culling for infertility
Tillard *et al.*, 2008	Low glucose at calving** BCS loss 0-30 d PP ≥ 1.5	↓ fertility

* For BCS and BCS changes the scale is always from 1 to 5
** Associated with high milk production during the previous lactation

Strategies to reduce NEB

In most epidemiological studies, nutritional disorders and factors are often cited as the main source of infertility (Tillard *et al.* 2008, Ponsart *et al.*, 2008b). All the above mentioned unfavourable changes due to NEB on reproductive function have led to development of strategies to minimize NEB through manipulation of the dry period and/or use of specific dietary and management regimes (Grummer *et al.*, 2008, Mee *et al.*, 2008, Ponsart *et al.*, 2008). Shortening the dry period results in earlier post partum ovulation and higher pregnancy rate, especially in multiparous cows. However, in these studies different regimes given during the dry period did not induce a significant improvement in post partum reproductive efficiency if lactation management was not also changed (Grummer *et al.*, 2008, Ponsart *et al.*, 2008). For cows in seasonal pastoral management systems, Mee *et al.* (2008) showed that offering grass silage or grass alone during the dry period improved reproductive performance, whereas poor reproductive performance in high genetic merit cows was not improved by supplementation with higher levels of concentrate or maize silage pre or post partum. In this system, an alternative management strategy aiming to lower NEB through reduction of milk production by once daily milking resulted in earlier ovarian activity and better reproductive performance.

There is evidence from these studies that NEB is susceptible to modulation by shortening the dry period and by better control of pre-partum energy supply, which reduce milk production with subsequent positive effects on reproductive function. These results tend to show that it is probably more effective to improve reproductive efficiency by modifying feeding and management to slightly lower milk production in such a way that genetic potential is not completely expressed and/or peak milk yield is lower, than to maximise feeding to obtain as much milk as possible.

Conclusion

The impact of NEB on reproductive function in high producing dairy cows and in beef cows involves multiple common mechanisms that, when taken together, may explain a large part of the lower reproductive performance observed in both types of cows. The relative importance of nutritional factors and of the different mechanisms involved in specific events, such as early or late embryonic mortality during pregnancy, remains to be studied in more detail. In beef cows, control of energy balance during the post partum period appears less critical when adequate feed resources are available pre and post partum. The situation may be different in high producing dairy cows, for which changes in the management of lactation started during the pre-partum period for a better control of energy reserves may lead to a greater improvement in reproductive efficiency (and probably to a better general health status) than nutritional practices aimed at maximizing feed intake and milk production. Further work is needed to evaluate the real technical and economic impacts of specific changes that slightly limit milk production in the early post partum period and their effect on reproductive efficiency.

References

Barbat A., Druet T., Bonaïti B., Guillaume F., Colleau J.-J. and Boichard D. (2005) Bilan phénotypique de la fertilité à l'insémination artificielle dans les trois principales races laitières françaises. *Renc. Rech. Rum.* **12**: 137-140.

Bauman D.E. (2000) Regulation of nutrient partitioning during early lactation: homeostasis and homeorhesis revisited. In: *Ruminant physiology: digestion, metabolism, growth and reproduction* (ed PB Cronje), pp 329-351. CABI Publishing, Wallingford, UK.

Bell A.W. (1995) Regulation of organic nutrient metabolism during transition from pregnancy to early lactation. *J. Anim. Sci.*, **73**: 2804-2819.

Burns K.H., Viveiros M.M., Ren Y., Wang P., DeMayo F.J., Frail D.E., Eppig J.J. and Matzuk M.M. (2003) Roles of NPM2 in chromatin and nucleolar organization in oocytes and embryos. *Science*, **300**:633-6.

Butler W.R. (2003) Energy balance relationships with follicular development, ovulation and fertility in post partum dairy cows. *Livestock Production Science*, **83**:211-218.

Butler S.T., Marr A.L., Pelton S.H., Radcliff R.P., Lucy M.C. and Butler W.R. (2003) Insulin restores GH responsiveness during lactation induced negative energy balance in dairy cattle; effects on expression of IGF-I and GH receptor 1A. *Journal of Endocrinology*, **176**:205-217.

Chilliard Y, Bocquier F. and Doreau M. (1998) Digestive and metabolic adaptations of ruminants to undernutrition and consequences on reproduction. *Reprod. Nutr. Dev.* **38**: 131-152.

Dubois P., Fréret S., Charbonnier G., Humblot P. and Ponsart C. (2006) Influence des paramètres laitiers sur la régularité de cyclicité post-partum et les performances de reproduction en race Prim' Holstein. [Influence of milk parameters on the regularity of post-partum cyclicity and performances of reproduction in Holstein cows]. In: *Renc. Rech. Rum.*, Paris. **13**:295.

Freret S., Grimard B., Ponter A.A., Joly C., Ponsart C. and Humblot P. (2006) Reduction of body weight gain enhances in vitro production in overfed superovulated dairy heifers. *Reproduction*, **131**:783-794.

Garnsworthy P.C. and Webb R. (1999) The influence of nutrition on fertility in dairy cows. In *Recent Advances in Animal Nutrition*. (Eds Garnsworthy and Wiseman), pp 39-57. Nottingham University Press, Nottingham UK.

Garnsworthy P.C., Sinclair K.D. and Webb R. (2008) Integration of physiological mechanisms that influence fertility in dairy cows. *Animal*, **2**:1144-1152.

Gong J.G., Armstrong D.G., Baxter G., Hogg C.O., Garnsworthy P.C. and Webb R. (2002a) The effect of increased dietary intake on superovulatory response to FSH in heifers. *Theriogenology*, **57**:1591-1602.

Gong J.G., Lee W.J., Garnsworthy P.C. and Webb R. (2002b) The effect of dietary induced increases in circulating insulin concentrations during the early post partum period on reproductive function in dairy cows. *Reproduction*, **123**:419-427.

Grimard B., Humblot P., Ponter A.A., Mialot J.P., Sauvant D. and Thibier M. (1995) Influence of post partum energy restriction on energy status, plasma LH and oestradiol secretion and follicular development in suckled beef cows. *J Reproduction and Fertility*, **104**:173-179.

Grimard B., Freret S., Chevallier A., Pinto A., Ponsart C. and Humblot P. (2006) Genetic and environmental factors influencing first service conception rate and late embryonic/foetal mortality in low fertility dairy herds. *Anim. Reprod. Sci.*, **91**, 31-44.

Grummer R., Watters R., Wiltbank M., Silva del Rio N. and Fricke P. (2008) Manipulating the dry period and regimes to minimize NEB. Consequences on milk production and reproductive activity. In *proceedings of the 25th World Buiatrics Congress*. Factors affecting reproductive performance in the cow. O Szenci and Bajcsy Ed. pp 204-210.

Guttierez C.G., Campbell B.K. and Webb R. (1997) Development of a long term bovine granulosa cell culture system: induction and maintenance of oestradiol production, response to follicle stimulating hormone and morphological characteristics. *Biology of Reproduction,* **56**:608-616.

Guttierez C.G., Gong J.G., Bramley T.A. and Webb R. (2006) Selection on predicted breeding values for milk production delays ovulation independently of changes in follicular development, milk production and body weight. *Animal Reproduction Science*, **95**:193-205.

Jiang H. and Lucy M.C. (2001) Involvement of hepatocyte nuclear factor-4 in the expression of the growth hormone receptor 1A messenger ribonucleic acid in bovine liver. *Mol. Endocrinol.*, **15**:1023-1034.

Hoeflich A., Lahm H., Blum W., Kolb H. and Wolf E. (1998) Insulin-like growth factor-binding protein-2 inhibits proliferation of human embryonic kidney fibroblasts and of IGF-responsive colon carcinoma cell lines. *FEBS Lett.*, **434**:329-334.

Humblot P. (2001) Use of pregnancy specific proteins and progesterone assays to monitor pregnancy and determine the timing, frequencies and sources of embryonic mortality in ruminants. *Theriogenology,* **56**:1417-1433.

Leroy J. Van Soom A. Opsomer G. and Bols P. (2008) The interaction between metaboloism and fertility at the level of the oocyte. In *proceedings of the 25th World Buiatrics Congress*. Factors affecting reproductive performance in the cow. O Szenci and Bajcsy Ed. pp172-181.

Lucy M.P. (2000) Regulation of ovarian follicular growth by somatotropin and Insulin growth factors in cattle. *Journal of Dairy Science*, **83**: 1635-1647.

McGuire M.A., Bauman D.E., Dwyer D.A. and Cohick W.S. (1995) Nutritional modulation of the somatotropin/insulin-like growth factor system: response to feed deprivation in lactating cows. *J. Nutr.*, **125**:493-502.

Mee J.F. (2008) Reproductive performance and energy balance of dairy cows in seasonal pastoral management systems. In *proceedings of the 25th World Buiatrics Congress*. Factors affecting reproductive performance in the cow. O Szenci and Bajcsy Ed. pp182-192.

Mihm M., Baguisi A., Boland M.P. and Roche J. (1994) Association between the duration of the dominance of the ovulatory follicle and pregnancy rate in beef heifers. *Journal of Reproduction and Fertility*, **102**:123-130.

Ponsart C., Ponter A.A, Khirredine B., Humblot P., Sauvant D., Mialot J.P. and Grimard B. (1999) A period of energy supplementation but not the type of supplement influences the insulin response to exogenous glucose in food restricted post-partum suckled beef cows. *Anim. Sci.*, **68**:749-761.

Ponsart C., Fréret S., Charbonnier G., Giroud O., Dubois P. and Humblot P. (2006a) Description des signes de chaleurs et modalités de détection entre le vêlage et la première insémination chez la vache laitière. *Renc. Rech. Rum.*, Paris. **13**:273-276.

Ponsart C., Léger T., Dubois P., Charbonnier G., Fréret S. and Humblot P. (2006b) Identification de profils de note d'état caractérisant des primipares et des multipares de race Prim'Holstein et relations avec le délai de mise à la reproduction [Identification of body condition profiles in primiparous and multiparous Holstein cows and relationship with the time interval between calving and first insemination]. In : *Renc. Rech. Rum.*, Paris.**13**:288.

Ponsart C., Dubois P., Charbonnier G., Léger T., Fréret S. and Humblot P. (2007) Evolution de l'état corporel entre 0 et 120 jours de lactation et reproduction des vaches laitières hautes productrices. In: *Journées Nationales GTV*, 2007. Nantes, 347-354.

Ponsart C., Freret S., Seegers H., Paccard P. and Humblot P. (2008a) Epidemiological approach of nutritional factors influencing dairy cow fertility during the dry and post partum periods. In *proceedings of the 25th World Buiatrics Congress*. Factors affecting reproductive performance in the cow. O Szenci and Bajcsy Ed. pp 194-203.

Ponsart C., Frappat B., Barbat A., Le Mezec P., Freret S., Seegers H., Paccard P. and Humblot P. (2008b) A wide range of tools to improve reproduction in dairy cows. In *proceedings of the 25th World Buiatrics Congress*. Factors affecting reproductive performance in the cow. O Szenci and Bajcsy Ed. pp 76-87.

Ponter A.A., Grimard B., Humblot P., Novak N., Khireddine B., Sauvant D., Thibier M. and Mialot J.P. (1997) Parity influences the utilization of exogenous glucose in suckled anoestrous Charolais beef cows. *Animal Science*, **65**: 183-192.

Ponter A.A., Remy D., Richard C., Marquant-Leguienne B., Humblot P. and Grimard B. (2005) Energy metabolism between calving and 80d postpartum is related to fertility after 80d in dairy cows. 9th Annual Conference of The European Society for Domestic Animal Reproduction. 1-3 September, Murcia, Spain.

Remy D., Ponter A.A., Charpigny G., Grimard B. and Nuttinck F. (2005) Expression des ARN du système IGF dans le foie en début de lactation en relation avec la fertilité chez la vache laitière Prim'Holstein. *Renc. Rech. Rum.*, Paris. **12**:175.

Royal M.D., Wooliams J.A. and Flint A.F.P. (2002) Genetic and phenotypic relationships among endocrine and traditional fertility traits and production traits in Holstein Friesian dairy cows. *Journal of Dairy Science,* **85**: 958-967.

Seegers H., Beaudeau F., Blosse A., Ponsart C. and Humblot P. (2005) Performances de reproduction aux inséminations de rangs 1 et 2 dans les troupeaux Prim'Holstein. *Renc. Rech. Rum.*, Paris. **12**:141-144.

Sinclair K.D. and Webb R. (2005) Fertility in the modern dairy heifer. In *Calf and heifer rearing: principles of rearing the modern dairy heifer from calf to calving* (Ed PC Garnsworthy), pp 277-306. Nottingham University Press, Nottingham UK.

Spicer L.J., Chamberlain C.S. and Maciel S.M. (2002) Influence of gonadotropins on insulin and insulin growth factor-I (IGF-I) induced steroid production by bovine granulosa cells. *Domestic Animal Endocrinology*, **22**:237-254.

Tillard E., Humblot P., Faye B., Lecomte P., Dohoo I. and Bocquier F. (2007) Precalving factors affecting conception risk in Holstein dairy cows in tropical and sub-tropical conditions. *Theriogenology*, **68**:567-581.

Tillard E., Humblot P., Faye B., Lecomte P., Dohoo I. and Bocquier F. (2008) Postcalving factors affecting conception risk in Holstein dairy cows in tropical and sub-tropical conditions. *Theriogenology*, **69**:443-457.

Villa Godoy A., Hughes T.L., Emery R.S., Chapin L.T. and Fogwell R.L. (1988) Association between energy balance and luteal function in lactating dairy cows. *J. Dairy Sci.*, **71**:1063-1072.

Vleurick L., Renaville R., VandeHaar M., Hornick JL., Istasse L., Parmentier I., Bertozzi C., Van Eenaeme C. and Portetelle D. (2000) A homologous radioimmunoassay for quantification of insulin-like growth factor-binding protein-2 in blood from cattle. *J. Dairy Sci.*, **83**:452-458.

Wathes D.C., Cheng Z., Bourne N., Taylor V.J. and Coffey M.P. (2007) Multiple correlation analyses of metabolic and endocrine profiles with fertility in primiparous and multiparous cows. *J. Dairy Sci.*, **90**:1310-1325.

Wathes D.C., Fenwick M.A., Liewellyn S., Cheng Z., Fitzpatrick R., McCarthy S.D., Morris D.G., Patton J. and Murphy J.J. (2008) Influence of energy balance on gene expression in the liver and reproductive tract of lactating cows and consequent effects on fertility. In *proceedings of the 25ᵗʰ World Buiatrics Congress*. Factors affecting reproductive performance in the cow. O Szenci and Bajcsy Ed. pp158-171.

Webb R., Campbell B.K., Garverick H.A., Gong J.G., Gutierrez C.G. and Armstrong D.G. (1999a) Molecular mechanisms regulating follicular recruitment and selection. *Journal of Reproduction and Fertility*, Supplement **54**: 33-48.

Webb R., Gosden R.G. and Moor R.M. (1999b) Factors affecting folliculogenesis in ruminants. *Animal Science*, **68**:257-284.

Wu X., Viveiros M.M., Eppig J.J., Bai Y., Fitzpatrick S.L. and Matzuk M.M. (2003) Zygote arrest 1 (Zar1) is a novel maternal-effect gene critical for the oocyte-to-embryo transition. *Nat Genet.* **33**:187-191.

2

OPPORTUNITIES FOR ONLINE MONITORING OF HEALTH AND PERFORMANCE IN DAIRY COWS

PETER LØVENDAHL AND NIC FRIGGENS
Dept. Genetics and Biotechnology, Faculty of Agricultural Sciences, University of Aarhus, Denmark

Automatic monitoring based on indicators in milk

The basis for good dairy herd management is reliable information about each cow's current production and health combined with a systematic way of handling the data. With growing herd sizes the demand for automated and computerised solutions has increased. This has created a business opportunity for manufacturers of complete dairy herd management systems and a range of subcontractors developing sensors, software and consumables. A scientific input is also needed in order to combine available biological, chemical and statistical knowledge into workable solutions and to ensure further improvements.

This chapter aims to describe the potential of this kind of solution using as an example the HerdNavigator® system, which has just been introduced commercially as an on-farm management system. This system is unique as it integrates information about production, health and reproduction, and exchanges data with existing advisory systems and national databases. Yet, it is possible to use it as a "stand-alone" system.

Elements of the HerdNavigator

Management systems have already been developed to handle production data in dairy herds and several commercial versions are available (e.g. AlproWin, DeLaval, Tumba, Sweden). HerdNavigator adds facilities for detection of health status, fertility status and metabolic status using supplementary measurements in milk. It combines collection of production data from every milking with sensor based measurements in the milk. Milk data is furthermore combined with recorded

15

events (health disorders and treatments) as well as standard background data for each cow (ID, calving, etc.).

As fresh data are collected at every milking, there is a need for filtering noise out of the data and for frequent update of all decision parameters. This is achieved first by a time-series-model module and then by a "biological-model" making inferences from filtered data. The output is presented to the herd manager through a graphical user interface. The elements and data streams are illustrated in Figure 1.

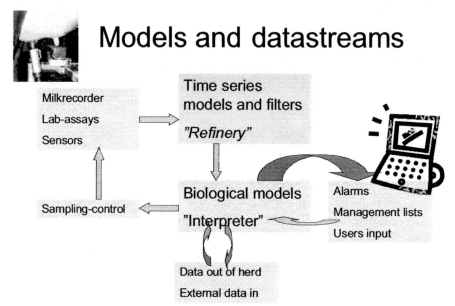

Figure 1. The main modules of the HerdNavigator system and data streams between these. At each milking yield data are acquired from milk recorders and the sensors for L-Lactate dehydrogenase, ß-hydroxybutyrate, Progesterone and Urea. Data are filtered and standardised in the time-series model, and interpreted by bio-models to suggest actions. Suggested actions taken or overruled by the farmer are recorded. Data are exchanged with external databases. Sampling intensity is controlled through a feedback loop from the bio-models.

Time series analysis and filtering of data

A time series model approach was taken for isolation of systematic changes over time from measurement noise. This approach focuses on one cow at a time, and initially analyses one trait at a time. Statistics for time-series are based on the Kalman filter which is also referred to as a "state-space-model" (Korsgaard and Løvendahl, 2002). The "state-space model" observes an object at various points in time. The object is assumed to follow a systematic orbit or curve in time and space. For this case, imagine the object is somatic cells in milk from cow number 161, call her "Nora", and call the cell count Y_t when recorded at time point t. However, Y could also be milk yield, progesterone, or L-Lactate dehydrogenase

(LDH) as is used in place of somatic cells by HerdNavigator (Figure 2), (Chagunda and Friggens, 2006b).

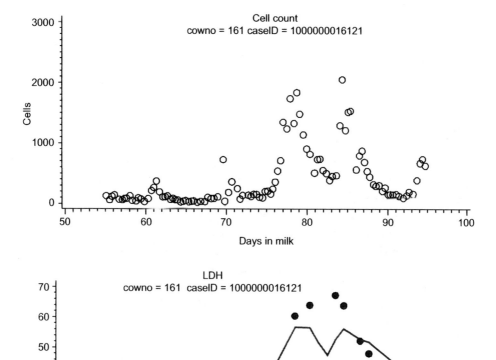

Figure 2. Somatic cells (upper) and L-Lactate dehydrogenase (LDH; lower) in single milk samples from cow 161, having a clinical mastitis in her 2nd lactation at 85 days in milk. Smoothed values for LDH are shown as the solid line.

The expected value of Y_t at the present time point t is roughly given by its value at time $t\text{-}1$, plus some systematic change plus some measurement error. At the observed time points measurements have some random error, but the curve is assumed to follow the systematic curve or be in steady-state. If deviations from the predicted curve happen at more than one time point, this indicates that the systematic curve is changing its shape. The idea behind the model is now to split the model into two parts, one describing the systematic part and another describing the noise part. This can be formulated as two equations, for an observation of Y at time point t:

Observation equation $Y_t = \theta_t + v_t$

System equation $\theta_t = G\,\theta_{t-1} + \omega_t$

The observation equation contains the systematic level θ_t and a measurement error v_t with variance σ^2_v. The systematic level θ_t is a linear function G of its value in the previous step $t-1$ and a deviation ω_t with variance $\sigma^2\omega$.

Having these equations as a base model, different states were described by four models differing in G and their base parameters for variances. In "steady state" (Model 1) the measurement variance and the systematic variance are both small. In a constant level change (Model 2) the slope of a growth curve is constant, so the systematic variance is increased, but the measurement noise remains small. A case where the slope changes is similar (Model 3). Finally, in cases where abrupt changes occur, these could be due to an extreme observation or outlier (Model 4) and the observation variance increases. By having all four models operating at the same time, four probabilities are provided (Prob1 – Prob4) to describe the state of the cow, and they sum to unity (Figure 3).

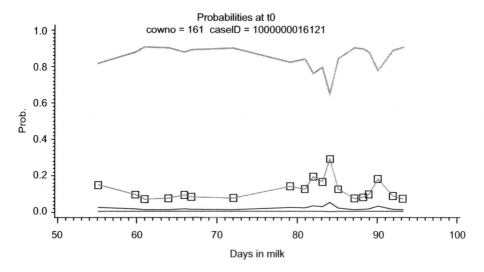

Figure 3. Probabilities (posterior) obtained at time t for the four models. The upper line represents the "normal or steady state". Outliers are shown by the line with square symbols; Level is shown by the lower (fluctuating) solid line and Slope is the lowest (flat) solid line. Clinical mastitis was treated at 85 days in milk in this example cow (ID number 161).

When a new data point is recorded and included, probabilities for this new point are calculated. However, a step called "back smoothing" recalculates probabilities for the models in the previous step, given the new data. By doing so it becomes clear if a previous point was an outlier, or if it was the beginning of a systematic change. This will be reflected in increased probabilities for the level and the slope models (M2 and M3). Technically, a second step of back smoothing can also be calculated, and this is effective in discriminating between changes in level and changes in slope. Although back smoothing is effective in obtaining better probability estimates, these relate to previous time points, hence they become less important for acute decisions. The effects of back smoothing are shown on Figure 4.

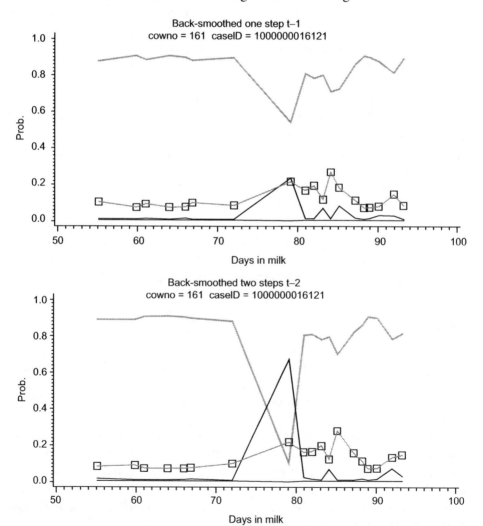

Figure 4. Estimates of probabilities for a one-step (upper) and two-step (lower) back smoothing based on somatic cell count for a cow (161) with clinical mastitis at day 85.

The models also provide smoothed estimates of level and slope for the trait, at time t and as back smoothed values for $t-1$ and $t-2$. In cases where the probability of an outlier (Prob 4) gets high, the situation can only be resolved by obtaining fresh data. This signal is therefore used as trigger for the "days to next sampling" function described below for the "biological models".

The development of time series models was initiated using somatic cell count data and validated with a closely controlled dataset (Korsgaard *et al.* 2005). Estimates of sensitivity and specificity are highly dependent on threshold settings for alarms. However, both parameters could reach values around 0.90 or better at the same time.

The application of the mixture models to LDH required little modification, as LDH changes almost in parallel to somatic cell count (Chagunda *et al.* 2006a,b).

Previously, time series models have been fitted to mastitis indicator traits such as somatic cell counts, and to electric conductivity (de Mol *et al.*, 1999; de Mol and Ouweltjes, 2001).

Although the time series models are highly effective in supplying probabilities for relevant deviations from normal steady state, they still require interpretation. Thus, we have chosen to combine them with rule-based biological models as described below. A similar approach was taken by de Mol and Ouweltjes (2001) using fuzzy-logic methods for decision support.

The models as implemented in HerdNavigator use a single indicator trait as input. However, the theory and algorithms can accept data from different sensors describing a common underlying biological trait. For reproduction, work is ongoing to combine progesterone in milk with activity monitoring data (O'Connell *et al.* 2008). Among the complications are that data from different sources arrive at different times and with different recording frequencies.

Biological elements

Four main biological elements are addressed in HerdNavigator: Health as mastitis; Metabolism as ketosis; Reproduction; and Urea status. Each element has a sub-module in the statistical as well as in the bio-module. These will be described in detail below.

In general, the bio-models consist of a part interpreting the indicator trait in terms of smoothed levels and slopes, with associated probabilities giving the acute changes, and another part with additional risks. The additional risks are factors predisposing the given animal to elevated risk of disease, but without direct impact on the indicator trait. Therefore, the two types of risk are additive and their sum give the best prediction of the total acute risk.

An important function built into the biological models is the calculation of days to next sample. Indications of large or unexpected changes in indicators prompt closer examination of the trait, which require more data coming from more frequently taken samples. After the animal has returned to steady state, sampling frequency is again lowered in order to avoid excessive sampling and assaying.

Health Model concept – degree of infection or health

It is difficult to say precisely if a cow has mastitis or not, mainly because the definition is not clear. It gets even worse when "sub-clinical" cases are considered. For the same reason, it is difficult to say if a cow is completely healthy or not. Most cows may in fact be somewhere in between these two categories. A more realistic representation is that disease status is on a continuum from 100 % healthy to full blown sick (Figure 5). The degree of infection concept, and the parallel term degree of risk, have been suggested by Detilleux *et al.* (2006) and was implemented for mastitis (Chagunda *et al.*, 2006 a,b; Friggens *et al.*, 2007) and for ketosis (Nielsen *et al.*, 2005). However, using a continuous way of describing disease causes problems in applying the traditional test parameters sensitivity and specificity.

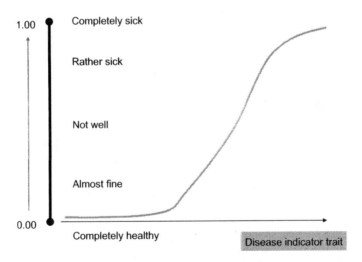

Figure 5. Hypothetical model of health and sickness seen as a continuum between 0 and 100%, and a calibration curve towards an associated indicator trait.

Another issue in testing is to have a reference or gold standard of sufficient quality. For mastitis and ketosis, this becomes a problem because the indicators used are similar to the reference methods; e.g. ketosis is defined as high levels of ketone bodies, and our test measures ketone bodies in the form of ß-hydroxybutyrate (BOHB). Details of ketosis and mastitis detection and testing of the models are in the following sections.

Metabolism: Ketosis in early lactation

Ketosis occurs mostly in early lactation, and mostly in cows in second or later lactations (Nielsen *et al.* 2003). There is evidence for ketosis being more frequent in high yielding cows, and there is some hereditary predisposition (Mantysaari *et al.* 1991). With feeding regimes of the *ad lib* TMR type, ketosis usually has low incidence compared with other regimes. But, even at low incidence of clinical level ketosis, there may be a substantial number of cows having milder degrees, which could still affect milk production. These cows may benefit from some treatment that will enable them to overcome the ketosis and be back on track instead of continuing to a clinical level.

During ketosis, elevated levels of ketone bodies are found in blood, breath, and milk. Ketone bodies can be acetone, aceto-acetate or butyrate. Of these, acetone is itself volatile and aceto-acetate easily turns into acetone, which complicates assaying. On the other hand, BOHB is stable in milk (and blood), assaying samples is possible with high accuracy (Larsen and Nielsen, 2005), and BOHB a good indicator of ketosis (Nielsen *et al.*, 2003). Furthermore, cows fed TMR show little diurnal variation in BOHB (Nielsen *et al.*, 2003).

INDICATOR BASED RISK

In order to turn measurements of BOHB into an indicator for ketosis status, data were first taken through the time series filter described above. This produces four probabilities of which two are used here, one for the change in level and one for the change in curve slope. The interpretation of probabilities depends on the direction of the changes. That is, if the level increases, a high probability means increased risk of ketosis, but if the level decreases a high probability means that the cow is recovering! It should be noted that "risk" is used here in its common sense rather than as a formal statistical term. At this step, probabilities are adjusted to a 0 to 1 scale using a function of slope:

$$Risk\_Slope\_BOHB = \frac{Slope \times (1 + sign\_Slope \times P\_Slope)}{Max\_Slope}$$

Similarly for level change:

$$Risk\_Level\_BOHB = \frac{(Level - baseline) \times (1 + sign\_Level \times P\_Level)}{Max\_Level}$$

Finally, the two risk components are added together to give the *indicator based risk* for ketosis:

$$Risk\_Indicator\_BOHB = Risk\_Slope\_BOHB + Risk\_Level\_BOHB$$

ADDITIONAL RISK FACTORS

If information is not available to calculate additional risk, the model will still run, but the 25% of information from the additional risk will be ignored. This has special relevance for animals bought into the herd, and during the start up phase.

The predisposition risk for ketosis has elements which are not directly reflected in BOHB, but are known or assumed to impose an additional risk for ketosis. These elements include the acceleration in milk yield, diseases in current lactation, lifetime number of ketosis incidences and body condition at calving.

The *acceleration in milk yield* is the slope of the milk yield curve, which is regarded as a trait describing the change in physiological demands of the cow in early lactation (Ingvartsen *et al.* 2003; Hansen *et al.*, 2006). As cows with high yield are also cows with large acceleration, this factor takes yield as such into account.

The *current lactation disease history* includes incidences which disrupt voluntary feed intake. Specifically, incidences of right or left displaced abomasum, milk fever, metritis, retained placenta and mastitis are taken into account. The added risk associated with each disease is assumed to roll off over a number of days. Also, the severity of each case is included as three categories. To avoid double counting, only the disease with the greatest risk is used for the calculation. This approach is supported by epidemiological literature (e.g. Gröhn *et al*, 1989; Rajala and Gröhn, 1998; Rasmussen *et al.*, 1999).

The *lifetime number of ketosis incidences* accounts for genetic effects where estimates of heritability between 0.03 and 0.16 were found (e.g. Mäntysaari *et al.* 1991; Gröhn *et al.*, 1986). Also, repeatable animal effects have been found, so incidences in one lactation severely (factor 4 to 12) increase the risk in following lactations (e.g. Rasmussen *et al.*, 1999).

Excessive *body fatness at calving* is first of all a risk by itself (Rasmussen *et al.* 1999) for body condition scores above 2.8, so that at 3.5 the risk is doubled compared with the risk at 2.0. Secondly, the indicator based risk may not be available in the first days after calving because colostrum is often not assayed and the number samples assayed is small. However, especially during the very early lactation the ketosis risk is high, so additional risk factors are important as the only available information. However, the effect is faded out so that it is only seen as an additional risk over the first 8 days after calving.

The total additional risk factor is found by simply adding the four element factors. Finally, the indicator based risk and the additional risk are added with a weight of 1.00 to 0.25 to produce a *total ketosis risk*.

A *feedback loop requesting a new sample* changes the default sampling settings (4-d interval) in cases where a statistical outlier is encountered, or in cases when the risk of ketosis is increased. The purpose is partly to verify measurements and partly to follow the ketosis development more closely, not least to follow the response to any treatment. The function calculates the ideal days to next sampling and by coming out with a zero estimate sampling will happen at the first available milking.

EXPERIENCES FROM DEVELOPMENT AND INITIAL VALIDATION OF THE KETOSIS MODEL

Model development was reported in detail by Nielsen *et al.* (2005). Formal and global testing requires large numbers of herds, preferably in several climate zones and using different feeding strategies. This has of course not been possible, and preliminary results are based on a few clinical cases seen in the research herd.

An illustration of the time-course of a ketosis case is given in Figure 6. The level of BOHB started to increase soon after parturition and then steadily increased until 21 DIM, when there were some days with lower levels, and then increased again until the ketosis became clinical and was treated at 37 DIM. The risk for ketosis is seen to increase, especially after 20 DIM, and reaches a peak at 37 DIM, followed by a steady decline. Clear indications of ketosis were therefore available several days before treatment was given.

Another case of a cow encountering ketosis in her second parity and getting treated at 32 DIM is shown in Figure 7. This cow had shown elevated risk of ketosis in her first lactation, but was not treated in that parity. However, the high risk in the early part of first lactation demonstrates that the repeatable nature of ketosis occurrence previously described by Mäntysaari *et al.* (1991), is also expressed through monitoring of risk.

Mastitis

The most common disease problem for dairy cows (and their owners) is mastitis. It is assumed that early detection of mastitis will allow more efficient treatments

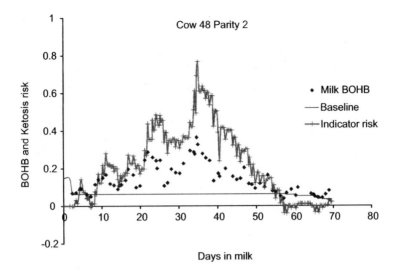

Figure 6. Example cow with elevated levels of BOHB and consequently increased risk of ketosis. This cow was treated at 37 DIM. The baseline represents the individual low level of BOHB used as reference in risk calculations.

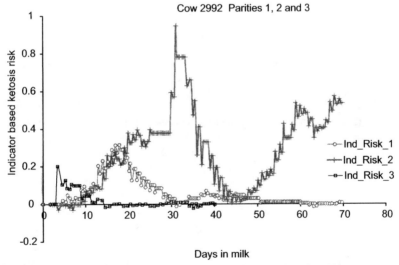

Figure 7. Example of cow with repeated cases of high ketosis risk in early lactation. This cow was treated at 32 DIM in second parity, but cured herself in first parity.

and therefore less suffering for the cow. In turn, infection pressure may be reduced with fewer and less severe infections.

Somatic cell count has proved an efficient sensor for changes in mammary gland health. Along with somatic cells, a number of enzymes are released into milk during infected states. Of these, the activity of NAG-ase (N-acetyl-ß-Dglucosaminidase) and LDH (Lactate-DeHydrogenase) have been studied and introduced as alternatives to somatic cell count for mastitis detection (Chagunda *et al.* 2006 b). This has allowed for simpler chemical measurements (Larsen, 2005) without loss of detection efficiency, in comparison to detection based on cell count (Chagunda *et al.* 2006 b). An example mastitis case, assayed for both cell count and LDH activity, shows the similarity in response profile of the two (Figure 8). This particular cow (ID 157) had a mastitis case treated at 20 DIM. Other, yet simpler indicators (electrical conductivity) of mastitis have been studied but found to have lower sensitivity and specificity than cell count (e.g. Norberg *et al.* 2004).

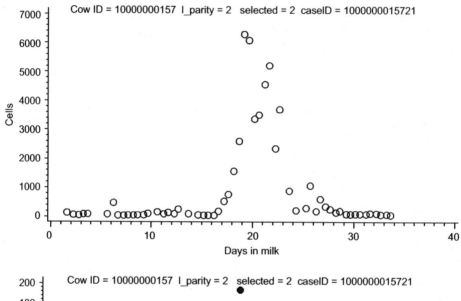

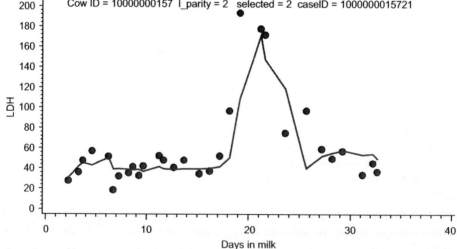

Figure 8. LDH concentrations and somatic cell count at a mastitis case (Cow 157, Parity 2).

CALCULATION OF ACUTE MASTITIS RISK

The basic input for the mastitis model comes from the time series of LDH measurements. This is called the "indicator based risk" (IBR) and roughly is the sum of probabilities for "level" and "slope" changes in the model, similar to the ketosis model. However, the mastitis model differs from the ketosis model by assessing changes in LDH relative to a 7-day moving average. Thus, the model primarily indicates acute cases, whereas chronic cases are reflected in the 7-day average.

The mastitis model modifies the indicator based risk using an "additional risk", and adding the two gives the total mastitis risk. The added risk elements are herd and animal-specific effects, which are not acting on LDH. Also, these are readily available and require no further measurements except for what is basic in a modern dairy herd. The traits are direct measures or derivatives of milk yield, milking duration, udder characteristics, herd mastitis level, current lactation disease history and quarter level electrical conductivity.

Although milk yield itself is not seen as a risk factor, the time derivative, milk yield acceleration is seen as an indicator of metabolic stress (Ingvartsen *et al.* 2003) in early lactation where the frequency of mastitis is also highest. The duration of each milking is another risk because long milkings are stressful to teat tissue and allow pathogens to be transmitted and dispersed within the udder. Other udder characteristics are considered to be heritable traits and thereby preset the individual cows' mastitis risk. If these are measured they are assumed to remain constant over time. Peak flow rate during milkings is obtainable from electronic milk recorders, and is a useful proxy for other morphological measures, such as teat canal dimensions. This set of animal-level risk factors is collectively named "udder risk".

Herd-level risk comes from the additional risk of getting infected when several other cows in the herd are infected (e.g. Østergaard *et al.* 2005). An environmental seasonal effect arising from annual cyclic change in climate is modelled as a sine function of the day in the year.

The history of previous infections, especially in the current lactation, has in other studies been shown to predispose to re-infection, thus increasing the potential risk of new acute mastitis. Other diseases may also predispose to mastitis (Hillerton *et al.* 1995; Chagunda *et al.* 2006b).

Although quarter-level electrical conductivity is by itself not as efficient as somatic cell counts in detection of mastitis, it has the advantage of being inexpensive and already a standard part of modern milking equipment. A further advantage comes from its ability to indicate which quarter is infected, as sensors provide signals from each teat separately. This allows calculation of inter-quarter ratios, where healthy quarters are used as reference, a method that is effective in adjusting for individual animal differences leading to improved detection efficiency (Norberg *et al*. 2004). Data from electrical conductivity are pre-processed in a time series biometric model and risk estimates conveyed to the mastitis model as an added risk (Chagunda *et al*. 2006b).

Each of the additional risk factors is scaled using various functions before they are summed to a single added risk factor. The total risk of acute mastitis is calculated by weighting the indicator based risk with the added risk factor at a 1.00 to 0.25 ratio.

In addition to the risk of acute mastitis, the model also gives an indication of chronic mastitis using the same information.

When the biometric model finds LDH values differing from expected values, this can either be an outlier or a true change. Although the back smoothing function will resolve this, it will only do so when new data are available. Hence, it is important to get a new sample as soon as possible. If the interval to next sample is long, and it could be several days for a healthy cow, the interval must be shortened to nil. After a new sample has been assayed, the model will run an update to confirm or override the previous result.

MASTITIS MODEL EFFICIENCY

Testing the mastitis model in commercial applications must await sufficient number of herds and cows. Meanwhile, a test based on intensive research station data was reported (Friggens *et al*. 2007), and is presented here in a condensed form. Having accepted the concept of "degree of mastitis" as the model output, a panel of tests was carried out. First, a comparison between cows which were diagnosed and treated for mastitis by a veterinarian with 1 to 3 herd mates of similar age, lactation state, breed and milk production that were not treated and so were defined as healthy (Figure 9). Second, a comparison of time for detection between clinical treatments and significant changes in model based mastitis risk (Figure 10); third, a comparison between the model-based mastitis risk and somatic cell count as the gold standard defining degree of mastitis (Figure 11).

Figures 9-11 show that cases of mastitis are not necessarily treated on the day where the mastitis risk is greatest. However, the model-based risk was significantly elevated from 4 days before veterinary treatment (Figure 9). The elevated risk becomes much clearer after alignment according to time of maximum risk (Figure 10). Using this alignment, there is a concurrent rise in somatic cell score (Figure 11). Also, a significant drop in milk yield was observed some time before mastitis was detected and treated (Friggens *et al*., 2007). In conclusion, the mastitis model based on LDH measured in milk is an efficient way of assigning udder health status to cows.

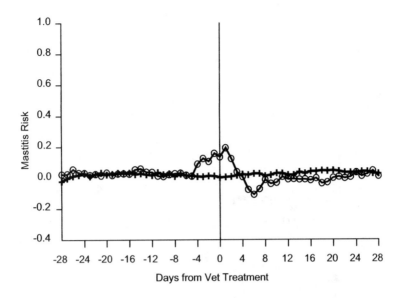

Figure 9. Model estimates of risk in truly healthy cows (line and +) versus cows treated for mastitis (line and circles), aligned to day of veterinary treatment (Friggens *et al.*, 2007).

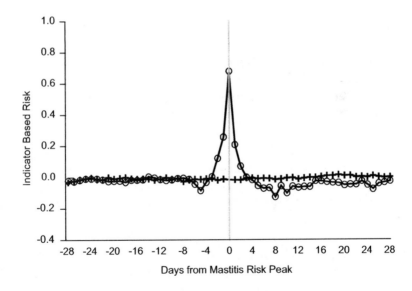

Figure 10. Model estimates of risk in truly healthy cows (line and +) versus cows treated for mastitis (line and circles), aligned to day of maximum estimated risk (Friggens *et al.*, 2007).

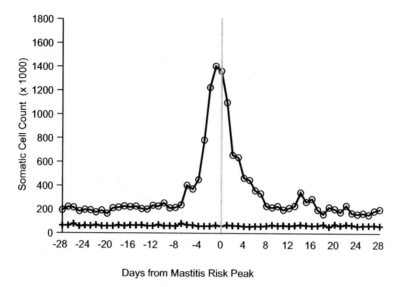

Figure 11. Somatic cell count in truly healthy cows (line and +) versus cows treated for mastitis (line and circles), aligned to day of maximum estimated risk (Friggens *et al.*, 2007).

Reproduction: Detection of oestrus and reproductive status

The gold standard for detection of reproductive cyclic activity is progesterone measurement in blood or milk, and other states of the reproduction cycle can be assigned from knowledge about present and prior progesterone concentrations. The biological interpretation model was described in detail by Friggens and Chagunda (2005), and was tested further by Friggens *et al.* (2008) following minor modifications. The model will be briefly described, along with validation results obtained by Friggens *et al.* (2008) using data from a research herd.

Cow status assignment. Starting from day of calving, the cow is assumed to be in postpartum anoestrus (Status=0). Status changes to cycling (Status=1) when two consecutive smoothed progesterone measurements exceed 4 ng/ml. A further shift to potentially pregnant (Status=2) is caused by progesterone again decreasing below 4 ng/ml (model cow in Figure 12). However, the cow may shift back to status 1 if AI is not performed within 5 days, or remain at status 2 if AI is performed and the model does not detect a new oestrus. The fixed 4 ng/ml threshold was found to be too restrictive, so modifications were introduced based on analysis of pregnancies established even when the threshold was not reached. The modification takes care of an unwanted effect of the smoothing algorithm, and effects of individual animal variation as well as bias due to assay variance. The relaxed threshold was set at 6 ng/ml, but is only used if a concentration greater than 15 ng/ml had been recorded previously.

At each detected oestrus, cow-status is set to 1, and a likelihood of success for AI is calculated as a guide for decisions (Friggens & Chagunda, 2005). During cow-status 2, the likelihood of pregnancy is continuously recalculated. If this likelihood falls below a certain threshold, the cow is deemed no longer pregnant, and returns to status 1. For cows more than 30 days pregnant, two consecutive low likelihood of pregnancy values are required to trigger a change in status.

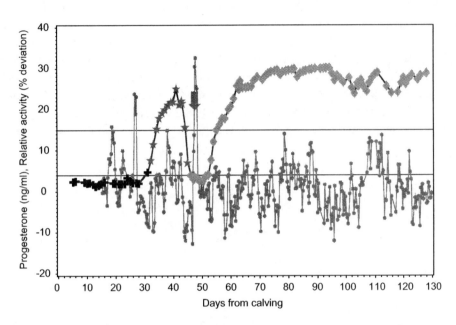

Figure 12. Progesterone profile (bold line) for an individual cow relative to days from calving. This cow was inseminated on day 46 (broad arrow). The symbols on the progesterone profile indicate the model determined reproductive status: postpartum anoestrus (+), oestrus cycling (star), and potentially pregnant (♦). (From Friggens and Løvendahl, 2008)

Performance measures and gold standards. The ability of the model to detect oestrus was tested in two ways, both having certain drawbacks in defining the gold standard against which they could be tested. However, results from the evaluation study by Friggens *et al.*, (2008) are briefly presented below.

First, successful pregnancies were used in form of AI's performed that resulted in a calf within expected time (274 to 294 d). For ongoing pregnancies not yet finished, palpation was used to confirm pregnancy. Together these were totalled and referred to as "confirmed pregnancies" (N = 121 pregnancies). The model detected 120 of these.

Secondly, progesterone profiles from around time of AI for the 121 pregnancies were used as a template against which other oestrus events were evaluated. The degree of similarity between profiles was evaluated using "Mahalanobis distance" for which a statistical test exists. A total of 587 oestrus events were detected by the Mahalanobis distance approach, of which 528 were detected also by the model. Depending on the type of evaluation chosen, the performance of the progesterone-based reproduction model is far better or at least as good as previously presented methods of oestrus detection based on progesterone or activity metering (review by Firk *et al.* 2002).

Effects of dynamic sampling scheme: Days to Next Sampling. Samples were obtained daily, which is more frequent than regarded as necessary for routine use. A facility of the model produces a request for a new sample according to various rules described in detail by Friggens and Chagunda (2005). Briefly, statistical outliers will trigger a new sample request. Other deviations from expected values will have the same effect. The efficiency of the DNS function was tested against fixed default settings of full 1-d, 2-d, 3-d, 4-d, and 5-d sampling intervals by sub-sampling the original data and re-running the model on sub-samples (Friggens *et al.* 2008).

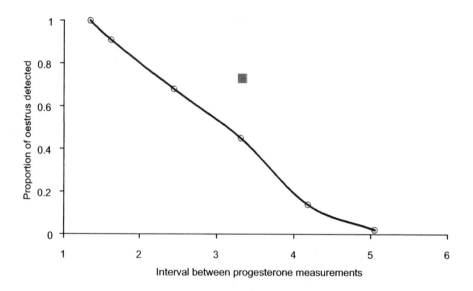

Figure 13. Reduction in efficiency as a function of sampling intensity with equidistant sampling (solid line and circles) or from using dynamic request for new samples (solid square) via the DNS function.

Generally, extending intervals between samples will reduce the detection efficiency. This effect was partly counteracted by the DNS function that optimizes the time to next sample given the information obtained up to now, so that sampling intervals are not equidistant. In fact, by using DNS the efficiency at an average of 3.3 days was similar to that of 2.3 days using equidistant sampling interval.

POSSIBLE ADVANTAGES OF COMBINING PROGESTERONE AND ACTIVITY MONITORING

Although the HerdNavigator is fully competent at detecting oestrus in milked cows, it is not able to monitor non-lactating heifers. This can be achieved using activity monitors. Activity monitors are used on many farms for both cows and heifers, and they show a reasonably good agreement with progesterone in detected oestrus cases (Figure 14).

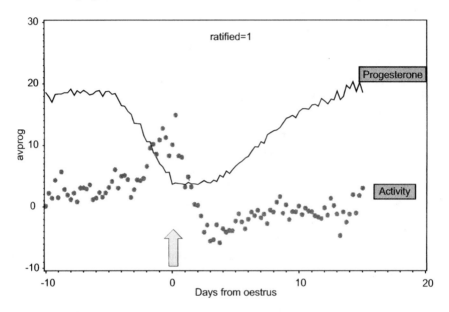

Figure 14. Average progesterone (thin line) and relative activity profiles (dots) from 10 days before to 15 days after oestrus (arrow) (From Friggens & Løvendahl, 2008).

Although both types of equipment are costly, it may still be beneficial to combine them as they can complement each other (Friggens and Løvendahl, *in press*; Løvendahl *et al.*, 2008). The progesterone model is designed to allow input of other external oestrus detection signals (e.g. activity). Progesterone is efficient for describing the exact cow status and can pick up irregularities. Progesterone is weak, however, in detecting the correct time for AI, whereas activity monitored at shorter intervals (1 or 2 h) provides better estimates for ideal timing. Also, as stated previously, activity can work in young stock not yet milking. Finally, activity measures may help to provide information equivalent to a higher progesterone sampling rate.

Potential of the system for research and in genetic selection

The online methods presented here offer an opportunity to have accurate day to day status of large numbers of cows. This is efficient for quantifying health at subclinical levels and thus to develop and evaluate treatment strategies. Because the models are based on objective measurements, it is possible to distinguish biological effects from management decisions. The untangling of biological events from management decisions is helpful also in genetic selection for traits with low heritability, such as fertility.

A clear negative genetic correlation between milk yield and days to first oestrus has been found in several studies (e.g. Royal *et al.* 2002). Consequently the higher yields in modern dairy cows have led to later expression of oestrus, both as an endocrine trait and as prolonged calving intervals (e.g. Royal *et al.* 2002). This has prompted an interest in direct genetic selection for improved fertility and consequently, fertility traits are included in the selection in numerous countries (Philipsson and Lindhe 2003; Miglior *et al.* 2005). However, traditional AI-service derived fertility traits suffer from low heritability hampering genetic improvement. Alternative methods based on progesterone in milk have been suggested and been successful in pilot experiments (e.g. Petersson *et al.* 2007). Another possibility is to use oestrus traits detected from activity monitors. As activity monitors are widely used, they could provide data from several herds already, if data could be collated. The value of using either progesterone or activity based information in genetic selection was recently reported by Løvendahl *et al.* (2008) who found that both methods give fertility measures with moderate heritability ($h^2 \sim 0.2$). Furthermore, both traits are objective and thus not affected by possible bias from farmers' decisions on when to start the AI programme for a given cow.

Simulated estimates of benefit

The commercial interest in developing the HerdNavigator stems from a belief that health and reproduction can be improved effectively in herds implementing the system. Direct assessment of economic benefits was initially not possible, but was estimated using SimHerd software. SimHerd provides stochastic simulations of herd events over time and is therefore able to determine the average long term effects as well as variance of effects. Details were reported by Østergaard *et al.* (2005a) and Østergaard *et al* (2005b). For mastitis, benefits were obtained mainly from a lowered incidence of mastitis at the clinical and subclincal level; seen as reduced severity and reduced loss of milk, including withdrawn milk. Similarly, improved reproduction was obtained especially for herds with a bad current reproduction performance. The achievable economic benefits were in both cases highly dependent on the present herd level and the changes realised.

Conclusion

A large amount of biological knowledge has been formulated into operational algorithms that are able to automatically detect a cow's status with respect to metabolism, health and reproduction, based on sensor measurements in milk. Although initially rule-based, the system is self adjusting and has functions to correct common errors in data, using time series statistical procedures. The system is open for communication with relevant external databases and advisory services. Because the system enables earlier detection of diseases, possibilities for cure are enhanced and welfare of cows may improve. Large field-studies for evaluating the economic benefits to farmers have not been performed, but simulation studies give encouraging results.

Acknowledgement

We are grateful to the many colleagues within the BIOSENS project portfolio groups who have contributed to this work. The work was supported by the BIOSENS project portfolio, which is supported by the Danish Ministry of Food, Fisheries and Agriculture, The Danish Cattle Association, and the company behind HerdNavigator Lattec (Hillerød, Denmark).

References

Chagunda, M.G.G., Friggens, N.C., Rasmussen, M.D. and Larsen T. (2006a) A model for detection of individual cow mastitis based on an indicator measured in milk. *Journal of Dairy Science*. 89:2980-2998.

Chagunda, M.G.G., Larsen, T., Bjerring, M. and Ingvartsen, K.L. (2006b) L-Lactate dehydrogenase and N-acetyl- -D-glucosamininidase activities in bovine milk as indicators of non-specific mastitis. *Journal of Dairy Research*. 73:431-440.

de Mol, R. M., Keen, A., Kroeze, G. H. and Achten, J. M. F. H. (1999). Description of a detectionmodel for oestrus and diseases in dairy cattle based on time series analysis combined with a Kalman filter. *Computers and Electronics in Agriculture*. 22:171–185.

de Mol, R. M., and Ouweltjes, W. (2001). Detection model for mastitis in cows milked in an automatic milking system. *Preventive Veterinary Medicine*. 49:71–82.

de Mol, R. M., and Woldt, W. E. (2001). Application of fuzzy logic in automated cow status monitoring. *Journal of Dairy Science*. 84:400–410.

Detilleux, J., Vangroenweghe, F. and Burvenich, C. (2006) Mathematical model of the acute inflammatory response to *Escherichia coli* in intramammary challenge. *Journal of Dairy Science* 89:3455–3465.

Firk, R., Stamer, E., Junge, W., and Krieter, J. (2002). Automation of estrus detection in dairy cows: a review. *Livestock Production Science* 75:219-232.

Friggens, N.C. and Chagunda, M.G.G. (2005) Prediction of the reproductive status of cattle on the basis of milk progesterone measures: model description. *Theriogenology* 64:155-190.

Friggens, N.C., Chagunda, M.G.G., Bjerring, M., Ridder, C., Højsgaard, S. and Larsen, T. (2007) Estimating degree of mastitis from time-series measurements in milk: A test of a model based on lactate dehydrogenase measurements. *Journal of Dairy Science* 90:5415-5427.

Friggens N.C., Bjerring, M., Ridder, C., Højsgaard, S. and Larsen, T. (2008) Improved detection of reproductive status in dairy cows using milk progesterone measurements. *Reproduction in Domestic Animals* 43(Suppl. 2), 113-121.

Gröhn, Y.T., Erb, H.N., McCulloch, C.E. and Saloniemi, H.S. (1989) Epidemiology of metabolic disorders in dairy cattle: association among host characteristics, disease and production. *Journal of Dairy Science* 72:1876-1885.

Hansen, J.V., Friggens, N.C. and Højsgaard, S. (2006) The influence of breed and parity on milk yield, and milk yield acceleration curves. *Livestock Science* 104:53-62.

Hillerton, J. E., Bramley, A. J., Staker, R. T. and McKinnon, C. H. (1995) Patterns of intramammary infection and clinical mastitis over a 5-year period in a closely monitored herd applying mastitis control measures. *Journal of Dairy Research* 62:39–50.

Ingvartsen, K.L., Dewhurst, R. and Friggens, N. (2003) On the relationship between lactational performance and health: is it yield or metabolic imbalance that cause production diseases in dairy cattle? A position paper. *Livestock Production Science* 83:277-308.

Korsgaard, I.R. and Løvendahl, P. (2002) An introduction to multiprocess class II mixture models. In: *Proceedings 7th WCGALP*, CD-rom Communication No 16-13. pp. 185-188.

Korsgaard, I.R., Løvendahl, P. and Sloth, K.H. (2005) Monitoring daily measurements of somatic cell count –automatic and on-line detection of mastitis. *Proc. of the 4th IDF International Mastitis Conference. Mastitis in dairy production*. Current knowledge and future solutions (ed. H. Hogeveen). Wageningen Academic Publishers (ISBN 9076998701).

Larsen, T. (2005). Determination of lactate dehydrogenase (LDH) activity in milk by a fluorometric assay. *Journal of Dairy Research* 72:209-216.

Larsen, T. and Nielsen, N.I. (2005). Fluorometric determination of (D-β-OH-butyrate in milk and blood plasma. *Journal of Dairy Science* 88:2004-2009.

Løvendahl, P. and Chagunda, M.G.G. (2006) Assessment of fertility in dairy cows based on electronic monitoring of their physical activity. *Proceedings of the 8th World Congress on Genetics Applied to Livestock Production*, August 13-18, 2006, Belo Horizonte, MG, Brasil. 18:496-500.

Løvendahl, P., Chagunda, M.G.G., O'Connell, J. and Friggens, N.C. (2008) Genetics of fertility indicators based on behaviour and progesterone in milk. *Cattle Practice* (*in press*).

Mäntysaari, E.A., Gröhn, Y.T. and Quaas, R.L. (1991) Clinical ketosis: Phenotypic and genetic correlations between occurrences and with milk yield. *Journal of Dairy Science* 74:3985-3993.

Miglior, F., Muir, B.L., and Van Doormaal, B.J. (2005) Selection indices in Holstein cattle in various countries. *Journal of Dairy Science* 88:1255-1263.

Nielsen, N. I., Friggens, N. C., Chagunda, M.G.G. and Ingvartsen, K.L. (2005) Predicting Risk of Ketosis in Dairy Cows Using In-Line Measurements of β-Hydroxybutyrate: A Biological Model. *Journal of Dairy Science* 88:2441–2453.

Norberg, E., Hogeveen, H., Korsgaard, I.R. Friggens, N.C., Sloth, K.H.M.N. and Løvendahl, P. (2004) Electrical conductivity in milk: ability to predict mastitis. *Journal of Dairy Science* 87:1099-1107.

Petersson, K.-J., Berglund, B., Strandberg, E., Gustafsson, H., Flint, A.F.P., Woolliams, J.A. and Royal. M.D. (2007) Genetic analysis of postpartum measures of luteal activity in dairy cows. *Journal of Dairy Science* 90:427-434.

Philipsson, J., and Lindhe. B. (2003) Experiences of including reproduction and health traits in Scandinavian dairy breeding programmes. *Livestock Production Science* 83:99-112.

O'Connell, J., Tøgersen, F.A., Friggens, N. and Løvendahl, P. (2008) Hidden semi-Markov models for detecting reproductive status in cattle, *XXIVth International Biometric Conference*, July 13 - July 18, 2008, University College Dublin, Ireland

Østergaard, S., Chagunda, M.G.G., Friggens, N.C., Bennedsgaard, T.W. and Klaas, I.C. (2005a) A stochastic model simulating pathogen-specific mastitis control in a dairy herd. *Journal of Dairy Science* 88:4243-4257.

Østergaard, S., Friggens, N.C. and Chagunda, MG.G. (2005b) Technical and economic effects of an inline progesterone indicator in a dairy herd estimated by stochastic simulation. *Theriogenology* 64:819-843.

Rajala, P. J., and Gröhn, Y. T. (1998) Disease occurrence and risk factor analysis in Finnish Ayrshire cows. *Acta Veterinaria Scandinavica* 39:1–13.

Rasmussen, L.K., Nielsen, B.L., Pryce, J.E., Mottram, T.T. and Veerkamp, R.F. (1999) Risk factors associated with the incidence of ketosis in dairy cows.

Animal Science 68:379-386.

Royal, M.D., Flint, A.F.P. and Woolliams, J.A. (2002) Genetic and phenotypic relationships among endocrine and traditional fertility traits and production traits in Holstein-Friesian dairy cows. *Journal of Dairy Science* 51:7-14.

Smith, A. F. M. and West, M. (1983) Monitoring renal transplants: An application of the multiprocess Kalman filter. *Biometrics* 39:867–878.

Veerkamp, R.F., Oldenbroek, J.K., van der Gaast, H.J. and van der Werf. J.H.J. (2000) Genetic correlation between days until start of luteal activity and milk yield, energy balance, and live weights. *Journal of Dairy Science* 83:577-583.

Wall, E., Brotherstone, S., Woolliams, J.A., Banos, G. and Coffey, M.P. 2003. Genetic evaluation of fertility using direct and correlated traits. *Journal of Dairy Science* 86:4093–4102.

3

IMPROVEMENT OF FORAGES TO INCREASE THE EFFICIENCY OF NITROGEN AND ENERGY USE BY RUMINANTS

J. M. MOORBY, A. H. KINGSTON-SMITH, M. T. ABBERTON, M. O. HUMPHREYS AND M. K. THEODOROU
Institute of Biological, Environmental and Rural Sciences, Aberystwyth University, Gogerddan, Aberystwyth, SY23 3EB United Kingdom

Introduction

Home grown forages offer the livestock farmer high quality and traceable feeds for his or her animals. As animal genetics change to give faster growth rates and higher milk yields, the genetics of forage crops also need to improve to match animal requirements. Breeding is essentially a process of exploitation of genetic variation. This has to be either selected or created and then incorporated into genetic stock that already contains a number of desirable characteristics, combining new genes while maintaining other required traits. For forage improvement, this genetic variation must then be fixed into new plant varieties. This is a more complex task in out-breeding species that have incompatibility mechanisms, such as most forage grasses and legumes, compared with inbreeding species such as most cereal crops.

Until relatively recently, increased efficiency of utilisation of feed nutrients was largely viewed as a way of increasing the output of animal products. In the last few years the impact of farming on the environment has become much more apparent and a focus of national and international policy development. Thus, reduced excretion of nitrogen (N) and energy-rich substances is a major goal not only because of the loss of productivity but also because of the release of greenhouse gases and other potential pollutants such as ammonia. Indeed, agricultural processes contribute significantly to emissions of the greenhouse gases methane (CH_4) and nitrous oxide (N_2O), globally accounting for approximately 50% of CH_4 and 60% of N_2O emissions from anthropogenic sources (Smith, Martino, Cai, Gwary, Janzen, Kumar, McCarl, Ogle, O'Mara, Rice, Scholes and Sirotenko, 2007). Livestock and livestock-related activities contribute approximately a third of CH_4 emissions (Beauchemin, Kreuzer, O'Mara and McAllister, 2008) and half of N_2O emissions (de Klein and Eckard, 2008), although these can be reduced with increased efficiency of use of nitrogenous and energy-yielding components of the diet. An increased efficiency of nutrient utilisation to promote productivity and reduced excretion are mutually compatible objectives, and the improvement of forage crops has a substantial role to play in these objectives.

The ruminant animal has evolved to maximise digestion of roughage through its symbiotic relationship with the rumen microbial population (Mackie, 2002). Ruminant tissue physiology is adapted to utilising volatile fatty acids produced during fermentation of feeds. However, although energy is efficiently extracted from forages, proteins are typically used inefficiently, with a large proportion of dietary N being excreted (typically as much as 70-80% of dietary intakes in dairy cows). The key to understanding how to improve efficiency of forage utilisation through improvement programmes is understanding the processes of rumen fermentation and how these can be manipulated, providing breeding targets for novel forage varieties.

Based on our increasing understanding of genetics and genes, new prospects for plant breeding have emerged. Both forward and reverse genetic approaches and techniques such as marker assisted selection (MAS) and introgression, mutation breeding and transformation, are increasingly available. Increased precision in genetic manipulation promotes the application of more targeted breeding strategies to a wider range of traits serving a broader range of objectives. Given well defined targets and a combination of traditional and modern plant breeding tools, plant breeders are now able to create new varieties of crop plants at an unprecedented rate. Although modern plant breeding makes use of molecular breeding methodologies, it is also increasingly reliant upon an enhanced appreciation of the mechanisms and inheritance of complex traits and a significant understanding of their phenotypic expression and environmental influences. Terms such as "designer breeding" and "breeder's toolkits" have been used to describe new approaches in plant breeding (Thomas, Humphreys and King, 2001). Polymorphic molecular markers that are tightly linked to traits of interest can be used to speed up selection in breeding programmes.

Initial focus has been on disease and pest resistance, reflecting the generally simple inheritance of genes conferring these traits. However, examples are beginning to emerge of traits associated with abiotic stress tolerance which are important to cope with climate change. Cahill and Schmidt (2004) listed a wide range of marker-trait associations in crop plant species. Markers have been used to improve downy mildew resistance and drought tolerance in pearl millet (Serraj, Hash, Rizvi, Sharma, Yadav and Bidinger, 2005). Other genes linked to drought-tolerance traits are listed in Duncan and Carrow (1999).

NITROGEN USE EFFICIENCY WITHIN THE RUMEN

The rapid breakdown of herbage proteins in the rumen and inefficient incorporation of herbage nitrogen by the rumen microbial population are major determinants of N loss and environmental pollution in pasture-based agriculture (Dewhurst, Mitton, Offer and Thomas, 1996; Siddons, Paradine, Gale and Evans, 1985). Ruminant nutritionists have known for some time of these fundamental problems associated with microbial fermentation of dietary components in the rumen. Indeed, over the last 50 years, many feeding strategies have been devised (including use of ruminal by-pass mechanisms) for enhancing the conversion of dietary proteins into microbial proteins in order to increase the delivery of amino acids for absorption in the small intestine and hence for growth and/or milk production.

In temperate parts of the world where livestock production is based on pastoral grassland systems, sustainable agriculture is encouraging the use of minimal fertiliser and strategic (limited) concentrate feeding. Therefore, the emerging challenge for forage breeding will be to deliver ways in which the basic forage can be altered in order to increase the efficiency of incorporation of forage proteins into meat and milk and thereby reduce environmental-N pollution. In order to consider possible mechanisms for enhancing N-conversion efficiency in the forage fed ruminant, it is first necessary to understand some of the emerging concepts associated with the digestion of plant proteins in the rumen.

Grazing ruminants ingest large quantities of living plant biomass, and the degradation of plant proteins is carried out by a combination of plant and microbial proteases (Kingston-Smith, Bollard, Humphreys and Theodorou, 2002; Kingston-Smith, Bollard, Thomas, Brooks and Theodorou, 2003; Kingston-Smith, Merry, Leemans, Thomas and Theodorou, 2005; Kingston-Smith and Theodorou, 2000; Zhu, Kingston-Smith, Troncoso, Merry, Davies, Pichard, Thomas and Theodorou, 1999). The processes of initial plant cell death following ingestion, protein degradation and plant material colonisation are being investigated further in order to find novel traits for forage breeding programmes.

After freshly grazed plant material enters the rumen, and prior to significant plant cell wall degradation, there is often a phase of rapid proteolysis which we believe is mediated by plant proteases. This liberates peptides and amino acids to the colonising rumen microbial population, but can exceed that needed to maintain the microbes. Although the mechanisms(s) that control and direct these plant-microbe interactions have yet to be determined, it is clear that the microbial population uses liberated forage protein breakdown products to synthesise microbial protein, from which much of the meat and milk protein is ultimately derived. A source of energy is needed to drive this microbial synthesis, but when protein breakdown products are present in abundance the colonising microbial population is likely to be energy limited due to the much slower rates of degradation of their main energy yielding substrates, the structural carbohydrates, cellulose and hemicellulose. Thus, it is possible that the microbial population uses protein breakdown products during initial colonisation of freshly ingested herbage both as the building blocks for new microbial biomass and as an energy source to drive microbial maintenance and synthesis. Where amino acids are used to produce energy, ammonia is produced as a waste product. Alternatively, scarcity of readily available energy during time of maximal protein degradation restricts microbial protein synthesis and only a modest proportion of the available N released from forage protein is incorporated into microbial protein. In the two cases outlined above, ammonia accumulates and, if it is not incorporated into microbial proteins, is absorbed from the rumen. It is subsequently converted to urea in the liver (Lobley, Connell, Lomax, Brown, Milne, Calder and Farningham, 1995) and is either recycled back to the rumen or excreted as waste nitrogen in urine. This imbalance in the timing (or asynchrony) of nitrogen and energy sources in the rumen has long been considered (Johnson, 1976), and improving the synchrony of availability of nitrogen and energy in the rumen should theoretically improve nitrogen utilisation and reduce its excretion.

Figure 1 demonstrates an asynchronous – and unbalanced – supply of energy and protein to the rumen. Proteins in fresh forages are typically quickly fermentable, but energy provided by cell wall components takes much longer to liberate. Consideration of Figure 2 suggests two possible strategies for increasing the efficiency of conversion of forage-N to microbial-N. One strategy is to increase the amount of readily available energy accessible during the early part of the fermentation to match quickly available nitrogen sources. The second strategy is to provide a level of protection to the forage proteins, thereby reducing the rate at which their breakdown products are made available to the colonising microbial population.

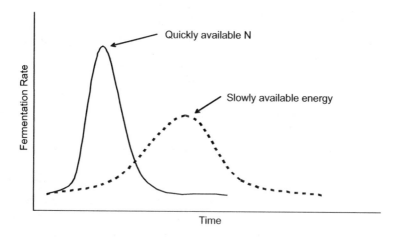

Figure 1. Schematic representation of the asynchrony principle in the rumen, in which forage nitrogen is quickly available but energy comes from slowly fermented sources such as cell walls. The efficiency of utilisation of rumen available nitrogen by the microbial population is therefore low (after Johnson, 1976).

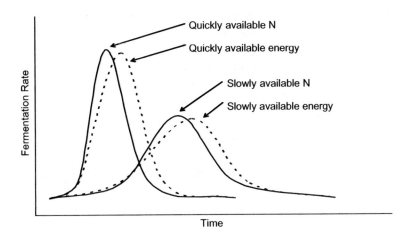

Figure 2. Schematic representation of matching availability of nitrogen and energy in the rumen to optimise the efficiency of feed utilisation.

ENERGY USE EFFICIENCY WITHIN THE RUMEN

The energy supplied by a feed is directly related to its digestibility. A major target for plant breeding strategies has traditionally been to increase dry matter digestibility (Kingston-Smith and Thomas, 2003). Increased digestibility, to a point that still enables normal gut function, is a major approach to increasing feed energy use efficiency. More recently, however, as discussed in the previous section other factors are becoming increasingly important. Although ruminants are efficient at extracting energy from plant cell walls compared with monogastric animals, it has been known for a long time that production of methane as a product of rumen fermentation is an inefficiency in the use of feed energy (Beijer, 1952). Up to 0.15 as a proportion of gross energy intake can be lost as a result of methane production (Van Nevel and Demeyer, 1996). A number of authors have recently reviewed the effects of nutrition on methane emissions from ruminants (Beauchemin *et al.*, 2008; Boadi, Benchaar, Chiquette and Masse, 2004; Kebreab, Clark, Wagner-Riddle and France, 2006; Monteny, Bannink and Chadwick, 2006). Increasing the proportion of concentrate in the ruminant's diet is a major factor in decreasing the emissions of methane (Blaxter and Clapperton, 1965) which is driven by the chemistry of methane production by the methanogenic microbial population in the rumen and a change in the fermented substrate from fibre in forages to starch in concentrate feeds. Increasing the concentration of starch in forage diets can be achieved using whole-crop cereals, such as maize silage and whole-crop wheat silage, although the effects of starch from ensiled cereals on methane emissions may not be as great as the effect of feeding concentrate sources (e.g. Cammell, Sutton, Beever, Humphries and Phipps, 2000). Feeding fat has long been known to reduce methane emissions (Czerkawski, Blaxter and Wainman, 1966), and more recently a number of plant secondary products such as saponins and tannins have been shown to be effective at reducing methane by altering the rumen microbial population (Carulla, Kreuzer, Machmuller and Hess, 2005; Hess, Kreuzer, Diaz, Lascano, Carulla, Soliva and Machmuller, 2003; Ramírez-Restrepo and Barry, 2005).

Manipulation of forage characteristics for improved efficiency

WATER SOLUBLE CARBOHYDRATES IN GRASSES

According to the asynchrony principle, rapid availability of protein degradation products is not balanced with an appropriate supply of readily available energy for microbial growth. As a consequence ammonia is absorbed by the animal rather than being captured in the rumen through microbial protein synthesis.

The rapidly available energy in forages comes mainly from soluble carbohydrates and over recent years we have demonstrated improvements in live-weight gain (Lee, Jones, Moorby, Humphreys, Theodorou, MacRae and Scollan, 2001), milk production, and particularly nitrogen partition away from urinary excretion (Miller, Moorby, Davies, Humphreys, Scollan, MacRae and Theodorou, 2001; Miller, Theodorou, MacRae, Evans, Humphreys, Scollan and Moorby, 2000; Moorby, Evans, Scollan, MacRae and Theodorou, 2006) when animals have been fed ryegrasses bred specifically for higher concentrations of water soluble carbohydrates. These production gains are most likely due to increased feed intake, whereas the reductions in the proportion of dietary nitrogen excreted in urine come from reduced ammonia absorption with greater incorporation of microbial nitrogen in the rumen (Merry, Lee, Davies, Dewhurst, Moorby, Scollan and Theodorou, 2006). Rumen ammonia concentrations are more stable throughout the day with increased water soluble carbohydrates in grass (Lee, Harris, Moorby, Humphreys, Theodorou, MacRae and Scollan, 2002). Importantly, even though production responses to increased water soluble carbohydrates have been variable (Miller *et al.*, 2001; Moorby *et al.*, 2006; Tas, Taweel, Smit, Elgersma, Dijkstra and Tamminga, 2006a; Tas, Taweel, Smit, Elgersma, Dijkstra and Tamminga, 2006b; Taweel, Tas, Smit, Elgersma, Dijkstra and Tamminga, 2005) there have been reductions in excretion of nitrogen in urine in dairy cow studies (Figure 3).

Edwards, Parsons and Rasmussen (2007) showed that apparent inconsistencies in the literature about responses to increased water soluble carbohydrates in ryegrass varieties can be explained by the ratio of water soluble carbohydrates to crude protein in the forage. Optimum ryegrass growth is achieved at rates of nitrogen

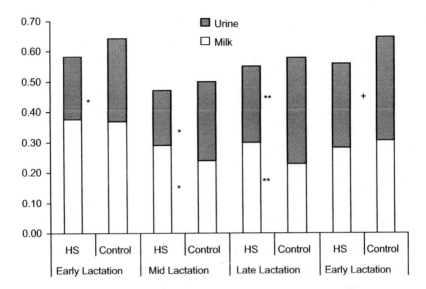

Figure 3. Secretion of nitrogen in milk and excretion in urine expressed as a proportion of nitrogen intake in dairy cows zero-grazed fresh ryegrass in early- (Moorby *et al.*, 2006), mid- (Miller *et al.*, 2000), late- (Miller *et al.*, 2001), and early-lactation (J.M. Moorby, unpublished results). The two grass varieties were HS - bred to contain a high water soluble carbohydrate concentration – and Control - a standard variety. Characters between columns indicate level of statistical significance within each group (+ = $P < 0.1$; * = $P < 0.05$; ** = $P < 0.01$).

fertiliser application that maximise light-harvesting protein concentrations. This is approximately 40 g N/kg of DM in the plant material, which equates to about 250 g crude protein/kg DM. However, at high concentrations of plant protein, the amount of soluble carbohydrates required to achieve the ratio for optimum utilisation efficiency is probably unachievable in practice. Therefore, in order to manipulate the nitrogen to soluble carbohydrate ratio that is available to the rumen microbial population, a number of options can be considered. Lower rates of N fertiliser application to grass pastures is one, although this will probably result in reduced grass yield. Another is to alter rumen degradability of the forage protein to reduce its availability to rumen microbes, matching the availability of soluble carbohydrates present.

PROTEIN MOBILISATION AND PLANT CELL DEATH

Animals grazing pasture consume large portions of leafy tissue containing numerous intact cells (Baumont, 1996; Wilson and Mertens, 1995). These cells are subject to a number of simultaneous stresses including elevated temperature, oxygen deficiency, constant darkness and the presence of an invasive microbial population. Plants contain a wide array of proteases for a variety of functions including dissolution of storage proteins during seed germination, protein turnover, degradation of damaged or mis-formed proteins, and for remobilisation and conservation of nitrogen during senescence. Plant cells contain proteases in lytic vacuoles (Matile, 1997) and in chloroplasts (Andersson and Aro, 1997). Proteases and peptidases are present in significant quantities in mature leaves and are further induced during stress and senescence (Kingston-Smith and Theodorou, 2000). Leaf cells therefore possess the intrinsic capacity to degrade their own proteins prior to invasion by cellulolytic and other rumen micro-organisms and it is reasonable to expect that plant cell death, in response to ruminal stresses, influences protein turn-over rate.

Many articles have been published exploring the mechanisms of cell death in plants as they relate to molecular, cellular and whole-organ processes such as senescence, disease resistance, the hypersensitive response, herbivore protection mechanisms, and the formation of morphological features (del Pozo and Lam, 1998; Drew, He and Morgan, 2000; Mittler, Lam, Shulaev and Cohen, 1999; Ryerson and Heath, 1996). These have been added to by the proposition that proteolysis and plant cell death are important in determining the efficiency with which grazing ruminants use nitrogen ingested in feed (Kingston-Smith, Davies, Edwards and Theodorou, 2008; Kingston-Smith and Theodorou, 2000; Theodorou, Merry and Thomas, 1996). It has been shown, for example, that grass incubated for several hours in the presence of an active population of rumen micro-organisms has a similar complement of degraded plant proteins (polypeptides) to that observed after incubations in which micro-organisms are excluded (Zhu *et al.*, 1999). Studies in the laboratory have also provided evidence that a microbial population is not needed under rumen-like conditions for rapid and extensive degradation of plant proteins (Figure 4). In these studies, loss of foliar protein was accompanied by significant increases in free amino acids accumulating in both the incubation medium and the leaves. Studies by Kingston-Smith *et al.* (2005), aimed at differentiating between the proteolytic activities of plants and micro-organisms during incubation of grass in the rumen of cattle, also concluded that plant proteases were responsible for degradation of proteins in freshly ingested herbage.

Grass leaves incubated anaerobically at 39°C showed substantial protein breakdown over a period of just a few hours (Beha, Theodorou, Thomas and Kingston-Smith, 2002). Rubisco, which is the most abundant protein in leaves, appeared to be highly susceptible to protein breakdown under rumen-like conditions. Both large and small subunits of rubisco were confined to the chloroplasts and absent from other areas of the cell, indicating *in situ* degradation. In cells subjected to rumen-like stress, extensive protein degradation was observed that substantially preceded any detectable nuclear degradation. This suggests that grass cells in the rumen may not undergo an uncontrolled, necrotic-type of cell death but remain metabolically active for a considerable time. Hence, it is necessary to understand the metabolic and molecular processes occurring within newly ingested cells during herbivory-induced cell death in ruminants in order to identify and devise putative control strategies that involve plant breeding.

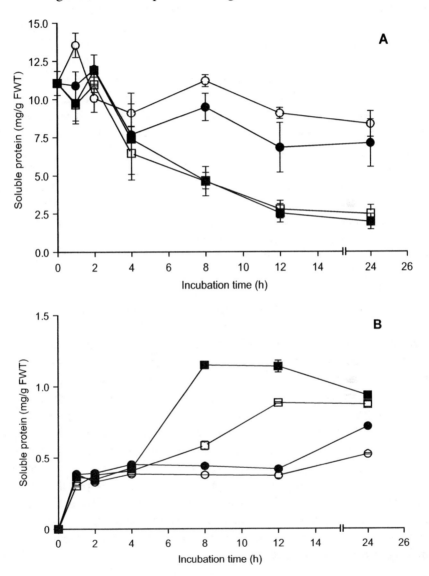

Figure 4. Protein content of leaf blades and corresponding incubation buffers during aerobic and anaerobic incubations in the absence of rumen micro-organisms (Beha *et al.*, 2002).

(A) Foliar protein; (B) protein in incubation buffer under; ○, aerobic 25°C; ●, anaerobic 25°C; □, aerobic 39°C; ■, anaerobic 39°C. Error bars represent SEM where n=3.

PROTEIN PROTECTION USING THE STAY-GREEN PHENOTYPE

Typically, plant senescence is accompanied by leaf yellowing as chlorophyll is degraded (Matile, Hortensteiner and Thomas, 1999). Many crop plants exhibit variation in, or absence of, normal senescence processes (Thomas and Smart, 1993), and are often termed 'stay-green' because they retain chlorophyll. Retention of chlorophyll in senescing leaves of a stay-green mutant of meadow fescue (*Festuca pratensis*) was associated with the persistence of several chlorophyll binding proteins (Thomas, 1987; Thomas, Ougham and Davies, 1992). Through conventional breeding, the *sid* gene has been transferred to forage and amenity grasses to produce stay-green varieties of ryegrass (*Lolium perenne*) and darnel (*Lolium temulentum*) (Thomas, Evans, Thomas, Humphreys, Morgan, Hauck and Donnison, 1997; Thomas, Morgan, Thomas and Ougham, 1999; Thorogood, 1996).

Kingston-Smith *et al.* (2002) investigated the stay-green phenotype to determine its potential to provide a nutritional advantage to grazing or hay-fed ruminants. This possibility arises because stay-green leaves undergoing normal senescence retain light-harvesting protein of photosystem II (LHCPII), which in the rumen may lead to smaller losses of protein. These authors tested their hypothesis, that the stay-green mutant will preserve protein, under three contrasting conditions: (1) in a standing crop similar to that used for grazing, (2) in hay making, and (3) during incubation of fresh and dried leaves under rumen-like conditions. From the field data, Kingston-Smith *et al.* (2002) found very little evidence of an advantage of the trait in terms of protein concentrations or rate of protein degradation in the living standing crop or when the crop was cut and conserved as hay. However, an advantage of the stay-green phenotype, in terms of increased protein content in leaves, was seen in un-defoliated plants after extended natural senescence. This suggests that advantage could be gained from the stay-green phenotype in field situations where a standing crop of largely senescing leaf material is used as a forage source for livestock. For example, stay-green could be exploited to maximise nutritional quality of dead and dried sorghum leaves used as 'strip-feeding' fodder for livestock in the semi-arid tropics. The stay-green phenotype could also be exploited to decrease the environmental impact of methods currently employed to prevent protein losses during preparation of standing hay in Australia (Dove, Wood, Simpson, Leury, Ciavarella, Gatford and Siever-Kelly, 1999; Gatford, Simpson, Siever-Kelly, Leury, Dove and Ciavarella, 1999; Leury, Siever-Kelly, Gatford, Simpson and Dove, 1999; Siever-Kelly, Leury, Gatford, Simpson and Dove, 1999).

PROTEIN PROTECTION AND REDUCED METHANE EMISSIONS WITH TANNINS

The benefits of protecting proteins from degradation in the rumen have been known for some time and are relatively easy to demonstrate. Thus, freezing of forage (which reduces plant protein breakdown by as much as 0.50; MacRae, Campbell and Eadie, 1975) leads to increased synthesis of microbial protein (1.25 times) and increased absorption of amino acids from the small intestine (1.15 times; see MacRae, 1976). Similarly, comparisons of duodenal nitrogen flow per unit nitrogen intake in animals fed forages containing different levels of condensed tannin indicate a dose-responsive increase in efficiency of capture of microbial protein (Barry and McNabb, 1999). This protection can be reduced if polyethylene glycol (PEG) is infused into the rumen, because PEG competitively binds to the tannin making it less effective in terms of protecting the forage protein. However, to date, attempts to manipulate the plant chemistry of the main forages in order to introduce polyphenolics into commercial varieties has proved to be difficult.

A viable strategy for improving microbial efficiency in animals given forages would be to protect proteins in order to reduce the rate at which they become degraded to ammonia. The phenylpropanoid pathway in plants gives rise to many of the bioactive secondary metabolites involved in plant defence and symbioses. Of these, condensed tannins have both positive and negative effects on animal nutrition, often through interactions with proteins and bacteria in the rumen (Min, Barry, Attwood and McNabb, 2003). Depending on their concentration and structure, condensed tannins are able to protect proteins from degradation and to improve the efficiency of conversion of plant protein to animal protein, but they can also be anti-nutritional (Barahona, Lascano, Narvaez, Owen, Morris and Theodorou, 2003; Barry and McNabb, 1999). A significant proportion of ruminant production in tropical and sub-tropical regions relies on grazing of native and introduced grasses growing in acidic, low fertility soils. Under these conditions, especially during the dry season, the poor quality and low availability of forage limits animal production. Introduction of forage and browse legumes into these grazing systems is intended to alleviate this problem. However, many of the forage legumes that have good agronomic performance when placed on low-fertility soils (e.g. *Desmodium ovalifolium, Calliandra calothyrsus, Flemingia macrophylla*) are of limited feeding value and are poorly accepted by livestock. According to Barahona *et al.* (2003) this is because of high concentrations of condensed tannins in these plants. In general, their results suggest that tannins from different legumes have different nutritional effects, even where tannin concentrations are similar. This could be due to differences in tannin chemistry (i.e. molecular size and monomer composition) affecting the strength of interaction of tannins with dietary proteins.

Tannin-rich species also have the potential to reduce methane emissions from ruminant livestock. As with protein protection, the effectiveness depends on the species used, because methane emissions can be reduced by using tannins of some plants (e.g. *Acacia mearnsii*; Carulla *et al.*, 2005) but not those of others (e.g. quebracho; Beauchemin, McGinn, Martinez and McAllister, 2007). Ramírez-Restrepo and Barry (2005) reviewed the ability of temperate grazed forage crops to reduce methane emissions, and concluded that although condensed tannins in crops such as birdsfoot trefoil (*Lotus corniculatus*) reduce methane output, the agronomic characteristics (yield and persistency in particular) need to be improved. It has also been shown that environmental conditions influence tannin chemistry within the same species of legume (Carter, Theodorou and Morris, 1997; Carter, Theodorou and Morris, 1999). Thus, translation of the use of natural condensed tannin protection, through the protein-binding affinity of condensed tannins and reductions in methane output by grazing ruminants, into commercial practice has so far proved to be difficult and the application of this approach has been restricted to strategic use of crops such as lotus and sainfoin species which naturally contain tannins (Min *et al.*, 2003).

Future studies with tanniniferous legumes should attempt to quantify differences in tannin chemistry and relate them to environmental conditions and forage quality. This is a prerequisite to selection and breeding of tanniniferous forages and browse species for tropical and sub-tropical regions.

PROTEIN PROTECTION USING THE POLYPHENOL OXIDASE MECHANISM

Polyphenol oxidase (PPO) enzymes catalyse aerobic conversion of monophenols to o-diphenols and subsequently to o-quinones (Macheix, Sapis and Fleurit, 1991). Rapid polymerisation of quinones produces black, brown or red pigments that are characteristic of browning (which can be desirable or undesirable) in food such as apples, tea and cocoa. As a consequence, PPO in food crops has been extensively studied and applications include breeding of fruit crops with low levels of PPO activity.

Until recently, no nutritional or environmental significance had been attributed to PPO in forage crops. High levels of the enzyme are present and active in red clover leaves when cut or crushed and exposed to air (Jones, Muck and Hatfield, 1995; Winters, Minchin, Merry and Morris, 2003). The o-quinoines generated by PPO are highly reactive electrophilic molecules that covalently modify and cross-link a variety of nucleophilic cellular constituents, including proteins (Brown, 1983). These addition products may be further oxidised to their respective quinines and a second addition may occur resulting in the formation of a cross-linked protein complex. It has been demonstrated that such protein-phenol complexes are resistant to enzymatic digestion by proteases including trypsin, -chymotrypsin and pepsin (Kroll and Rawel, 2001). Lee *et al.* (Lee, Olmos Colmenero, Winters, Scollan and Minchin, 2006; Lee, Winters, Scollan, Dewhurst, Theodorou and Minchin, 2004) have shown that the PPO enzyme can reduce the extent of both plant mediated proteolysis and lipolysis in red clover and cocksfoot (*Dactylis glomerata*). They hypothesized that this may be due to complexing of phenols with plant proteins/polar membrane lipids and/or denaturing of plant proteases/lipases. The concept that protein protection may be provided via denaturation of plant enzymes is intriguing and requires further investigation, not just in relation to PPO activity, but also in relation to the mode of action of condensed tannins. According to Broderick, Walgenbach and Maignan (2001), the PPO mechanism effectively reduced protein breakdown and resulted in over 80% of red clover silage protein being retained as 'true protein', providing improved nitrogen use efficiency and product quality when fed to dairy cows.

Although the inhibitory effect on proteolysis and lipolysis of red clover PPO activity in ensiled forage is recognized (Broderick *et al.*, 2001; Winters and Minchin, 2002), it has yet to be established if the enzyme can scavenge sufficient oxygen from the ruminant feed bolus to permit protein protection in the rumen (Theodorou, Kingston-Smith, Winters, Lee, Minchin, Morris and MacRae, 2006). For PPO to be active in a grazing context requires damage to plant tissues and an adequate supply of molecular oxygen. Mastication during initial chewing will damage plant cells and, although the rumen is generally anaerobic, Hillman, Lloyd and Williams (1985) measured decreasing levels of dissolved oxygen in the rumen of sheep for up to 30 minutes post ingestion of herbage. More recently, Lee, Tweed, Minchin and Winters (2008) measured dissolved oxygen concentrations in consumed boluses of red clover, and found them to be depleted within just 2-3 minutes.

Another recently discovered source of PPO activity is that found in forage grasses (Table 1; Lee *et al.*, 2006). These enzymes in monocotyledonous plants have several properties and are generally more labile then red clover PPO (Winters *et al.*, 2003). With the exception of cocksfoot, in which activity levels are equivalent to those found in red clover, PPO activity in production grasses is substantially lower than in red clover. Nevertheless, protein complexing, reduced proteolysis and reduced lipolysis can be demonstrated with grass leaf extracts (Lee *et al.*, 2006). The inhibitory effect of PPO activity on proteolysis and lipolysis adds support for a strategy to breed forages with increased PPO activity. Despite cocksfoot's limited agricultural importance in temperate pastoral systems, transfer of genetic material between cocksfoot and other production grasses may provide a protein protection mechanism that can be extensively exploited. The opportunity of transferring the cocksfoot PPO system to a high water soluble carbohydrate containing-forage is an intriguing possibility and offers considerable potential.

Table 1. Polyphenol oxidase (PPO) activity (U/g fresh weight) of a range of grass genotypes (Lee et al., 2006).

Grass	PPO activity	SEM	No. of cultivars	n
Tall fescue (*Festuca arundinacea*)	6.5a	0.41	2	6
Timothy (*Phelum pratense*)	16.3a	0.11	3	9
Perennial ryegrass (*Lolium perenne*)	119.0b	6.52	6	18
Italian ryegrass (*Lolium multiflorum*)	213c	15.95	2	6
Hybrid ryegrass (*L. perenne* x *L. multiflorum*)	291.9d	31.88	1	3
Cocksfoot (*Dactylis glomerata*)	740.6e	53.84	3	9
SED	30.36			
Overall significance	***			

Values followed by different letters are significantly different within the column. SED, standard error of the differences; SEM, standard error of the mean; *** P< 0.001.

Improving genotypes

Conventional breeding relies on two fundamental principles. The first is to generate a breeding population with high variation in traits that are agriculturally interesting. This usually involves crossing parent plants with complementary traits to generate various combinations of traits in their offspring. The second principle is selection of progeny that combine the best traits with the fewest shortcomings. Modern breeding techniques essentially increase the speed with which traits can be introduced into, and selected from, a breeding population of forage plants.

MARKER ASSISTED SELECTION

Marker assisted selection (MAS) is the most promising emerging genetic technology to have an immediate impact on forage breeding. It depends on detection of DNA variation among individuals using a variety of established molecular techniques, including restriction fragment length polymorphisms (RFLPs), random-amplified polymorphic DNA (RAPDs), simple sequence repeats (SSRs - microsatellites), expressed sequence tags (ESTs) and amplified fragment length polymorphisms

(AFLPs) (Henry, 2001). Successful breeding using MAS depends on understanding the genetic architecture of relevant traits. Traditionally, major gene and polygenic variation has been analysed in different ways, but the techniques of quantitative trait locus (QTL) analysis now allows a more integrated approach in dissecting complex traits and assessing gene effects. Examples of QTL associated with valuable traits are increasing in a wide range of crops including rice, wheat, maize, sorghum, barley, forage and turf grasses, brassicas, soyabean, pea, alfalfa, beans, tomato, beet and potato (Cahill and Schmidt, 2004; Duncan and Carrow, 1999; McCouch and Doerge, 1995; Mohan, Nair, Bhagwat, Krishna, Yano, Bhatia and Sasaki, 1997). QTL analysis can be used to determine the location or locations of variation for a complex trait directly onto the genetic map of a particular species. At the same time, the density of markers on these maps has increased dramatically, associated with the use of the DNA markers described above.

Although research associated with identification of QTLs is expanding rapidly, examples of the application of MAS methodology in breeding programmes are still relatively limited. Resistance to the environmental influences of abiotic and biotic stresses are the most popular targets for MAS so far. Despite the promising potential of MAS, however, poor precision in locating QTL, bias of individual gene effects, and risks of identifying 'false-positive' associations have generated disappointing responses (Kearsey and Farquhar, 1998). More work is required on the practical use of MAS in breeding programmes and the value of specific markers. Marker assisted selection should be more efficient than conventional phenotypic selection when traits are difficult, time-consuming or expensive to measure. In future, it is likely that many applications of MAS in forage species will utilise markers within the genes of interest rather than associated with them. Such single nucleotide polymorphisms (SNPs) are currently being developed for a range of forage species.

The use of molecular markers offers considerable potential advantages for breeding perennial species where evaluation of advanced lines in plots takes several years and where studies involving animals or impacts on the environment are time consuming and expensive. Progress has been slow relative to other crops, not just because of poor funding of such studies on a global level, but also because of the out-breeding, and in some cases polyploid, nature of the species concerned.

Marker assisted selection in forage grasses

Based on initial work to produce genetic linkage maps for perennial ryegrass (Armstead, Harper, Turner, Skøt, King, Humphreys, Morgan, Thomas and Roderick, 2006; Jones, Mahoney, Hayward, Armstead, Jones, Humphreys, King, Kishida, Yamada, Balfourier, Charmet and Forster, 2002), there has been rapid progress identifying QTLs for a range of traits and initiating MAS for traits including nitrogen use efficiency (van Loo, Dolstra, Humphreys, Wolters, Luessink, de Riek and Bark, 2003) and water soluble carbohydrate content (Turner, Cairns, Armstead, Ashton, Skot, Whittaker and Humphreys, 2006; Turner, Cairns, Armstead, Thomas, Humphreys and Humphreys, 2008).

As mentioned above, resistance to pests and diseases has provided well-defined targets for improvement using MAS in a wide range of species including forage crops and turfgrasses (Humphreys, Zwierzykowski, Collin, Rogers, Zare and Lesniewska, 2001). Identification of QTLs and closely linked molecular markers for specific resistant genes can facilitate the pyramiding of resistance genes into breeding lines in order to increase durability against pathogen attack in cultivars. For example, genetic markers have been used to assist the introgression of crown rust (*Puccinia coronata*) resistance from meadow fescue (*Festuca pratensis*) into Italian ryegrass (*Lolium multiflorum*) (Armstead *et al.*, 2006).

Exploiting genetic variation in stay-green characteristics of plants has been a major objective of turfgrass breeding at IBERS and there is considerable quantitative variation within perennial ryegrass that is inherited independently of the *sid* gene introgressed from meadow fescue. Analysis of leaf pigment loss in detached leaves, measured as reduction in reflected hue angle, in a perennial ryegrass mapping family has revealed 6 large QTLs (Thorogood and Laroche, 2001). The stay-green phenotype and its associated genetics may also confer considerable advantages for ruminant production systems in the tropics and sub-tropics, as discussed previously.

Marker assisted selection in forage legumes

Progress and targets with respect to forage legume breeding, particularly clovers, have been reviewed recently for different parts of the world (Abberton and Marshall, 2005; Taylor, 2008; Williams, Easton and Jones, 2007). Application of molecular approaches in forage legume breeding was reviewed by Bowley (1997) and the potential of genomic methods by Spangenberg, Kalla, Lidgett, Sawbridge, Ong and John (2001) and Dixon (2004). Lucerne (or alfalfa; *Medicago sativa*) is one of the most important temperate forage legumes. It is an outbreeding tetraploid with tetrasomic inheritance and current cultivars are heterogeneous synthetics. In North America, all of these cultivars are derived from intercrossing between nine original accessions. Tetrasomic inheritance causes difficulties for breeders and accordingly there is considerable focus on haploid production leading to development of cultivated alfalfa at the diploid level. In terms of genetic analysis, accessions and breeding populations have been characterised in terms of genetic diversity by RAPDs and RFLPs, and linkage maps have been produced at the diploid level based on different populations (Brummer, Bouton and Kochert, 1993; Echt, Kidwell, Knapp, Osborn and Mccoy, 1994; Kiss, Csanadi, Kalman, Kalo and Okresz, 1993).

White clover (*Trifolium repens*) is an important perennial forage legume in Northern Europe, New Zealand and parts of Australia. The first white clover map has been developed in collaboration between the UK and Australia. The map was constructed using a cross between self-compatible inbred lines with AFLP and SSR markers technologies (Jones, Hughes, Drayton, Abberton, Michaelson-Yeates, Bowen and Forster, 2003). Targets for MAS based on the white clover map include disease resistance (Humphreys *et al.*, 2001) together with environmental, agronomic, physiological and quality traits (Webb and Abberton, 1999; Webb, Abberton and Young, 2004).

There has been a resurgence of interest in red clover (*Trifolium pratense*), a crop more suited to monoculture cultivation, in the UK in recent years. From the research perspective, red clover is interesting because of its PPO protein protection mechanism, discussed earlier. A genomic map of red clover has been developed recently (Isobe, Klimenko, Ivashuta, Gau and Kozlov, 2003) and QTL analysis in this species is now being carried out at IBERS (Aberystwyth). Targets for MAS in this species include yield, persistency, and resistance to pest and diseases. Developments in white and red clover are being aided by the establishment in 2005 of the International Trifolium Network (ITN), a global consortium dedicated to building genetic and genomic capacity in this species and the translation of resources and information from the model legumes, particularly *M. truncatula* (Abberton, Spangenberg, Sledge, Young and Isobe, 2006).

GENETIC MANIPULATION IN FORAGE IMPROVEMENT

Several different genetic manipulation (or transformation) systems have been developed and are well established for all major forage grasses and legumes. Target traits for forage crop improvement can be categorised under three general headings concerned with (a) improving forage quality characteristics such as protein quality and stability, fermentable carbohydrate content and cell wall digestibility, (b) plant performance factors such as resistance to abiotic and biotic stresses, and (c) plant development processes.

Forage crops have also been transformed with a view to bio-farming and this is likely to be an area of increasing interest as we progress towards the environmental goal of lowering our carbon footprint by looking for novel sources of renewable energy.

Whereas conventional plant breeding is concerned mainly with transfer of large numbers of genes, the characteristics of which are known through phenotypic measurements, genetic manipulation is concerned with transfer of small numbers of genes with high precision. Successful genetic manipulation is therefore dependent upon detailed understanding of the physiological, morphological and biochemical basis of action of individually important genes as well as their identification and cloning. The pace of future development in this area is therefore dependent upon significant improvements, not just in the technology for transformation, but also in the detailed understanding of mechanisms that govern agronomically important trait characteristics.

Conclusions

Current agricultural targets include an increase in feed use efficiency by livestock to allow the maintenance or even increase in product yield while reducing nitrogen and energy inputs from feed. At the same time, with the development of new environmentally and nutritionally focused priorities such as sustainable agriculture, increased biodiversity, enhanced awareness of functional foods that offer human health benefits and pluralistic land use, the time is right to consider new priorities as breeding objectives. In so doing it is of considerable significance that the plant genome may be ultimately responsible for some key characteristics of rumen function that were previously thought to be influenced and controlled by microbial genes. Consequently, it is pertinent to ask, as we have done in this review, if the plant geneticist can take advantage of these new and emerging observations in the dissection and exploitation of novel traits in forage breeding programmes.

References

Abberton, M.T. and Marshall, A.H. (2005). Progress in breeding perennial clovers for temperate agriculture. Journal of Agricultural Science **143**, 117-135.

Abberton, M.T., Spangenberg, G., Sledge, M., Young, N. and Isobe, S. (2006) The International Trifolium Network. Proceedings of the International Conference on Legume Genetics and Genomics, Brisbane.

Andersson, B. and Aro, E.M. (1997). Proteolytic activities and proteases of plant chloroplasts. Physiologia Plantarum **100**, 780-793.

Armstead, I.P., Harper, J.A., Turner, L.B., Skøt, L., King, I.P., Humphreys, M.O., Morgan, W.G., Thomas, H.M. and Roderick, H.W. (2006). Introgression of crown rust (Puccinia coronata) resistance from meadow fescue (Festuca pratensis) into Italian ryegrass (Lolium multiflorum): genetic mapping and identification of associated molecular markers. Plant Pathology **55**, 62-67.

Barahona, R., Lascano, C.E., Narvaez, N., Owen, E., Morris, P. and Theodorou, M.K. (2003). In vitro degradability of mature and immature leaves of tropical forage legumes differing in condensed tannin and non-starch polysaccharide content and composition. Journal of the Science of Food and Agriculture

83, 1256-1266.

Barry, T.N. and McNabb, W.C. (1999). The implications of condensed tannins on the nutritive value of temperate forages fed to ruminants. British Journal of Nutrition **81**, 263-272.

Baumont, R. (1996). Palatability and feeding behaviour in ruminants. A review. Annales de Zootechie **45**, 385-400.

Beauchemin, K.A., Kreuzer, M., O'Mara, F. and McAllister, T.A. (2008). Nutritional management for enteric methane abatement: a review. Australian Journal of Experimental Agriculture **48**, 21-27.

Beauchemin, K.A., McGinn, S.M., Martinez, T.F. and McAllister, T.A. (2007). Use of condensed tannin extract from quebracho trees to reduce methane emissions from cattle. Journal of Animal Science **85**, 1990-1996.

Beha, E.M., Theodorou, M.K., Thomas, B.J. and Kingston-Smith, A.H. (2002). Grass cells ingested by ruminants undergo autolysis which differs from senescence: implications for grass breeding targets and livestock production. Plant Cell and Environment **25**, 1299-1312.

Beijer, W.H. (1952). Methane Fermentation in the Rumen of Cattle. Nature **170**, 576-577.

Blaxter, K.L. and Clapperton, J.L. (1965). Prediction of amount of methane produced by ruminants. British Journal of Nutrition **19**, 511-522.

Boadi, D., Benchaar, C., Chiquette, J. and Masse, D. (2004). Mitigation strategies to reduce enteric methane emissions from dairy cows: Update review. Canadian Journal of Animal Science **84**, 319-335.

Bowley, S.R. (1997) Breeding methods for forage legumes. In Biotechnology and the Improvement of Forage Legumes. pp. 25-42. Edited by McKersie B.D. and Brown D.C.W. Oxford University Press, Oxford.

Broderick, G.A., Walgenbach, R.P. and Maignan, S. (2001). Production of lactating dairy cows fed alfalfa or red clover silage at equal dry matter or crude protein contents in the diet. Journal of Dairy Science **84**, 1728-1737.

Brown, C.R. (1983). Banana polyphenol oxidase. School Science Review **64**, 690-695.

Brummer, E.C., Bouton, J.H. and Kochert, G. (1993). Development of an RFLP map in diploid alfalfa. *Theoretical and Applied Genetics* **86**, 329-332.

Cahill, D.J. and Schmidt, D.H. (2004) Use of marker assisted selection in a product development breeding program. *New directions for a diverse planet, Proceedings of the 4th International Crop Science Congress, Brisbane, Australia.* www.cropscience.org.au/icsc2004.

Cammell, S.B., Sutton, J.D., Beever, D.E., Humphries, D.J. and Phipps, R.H. (2000). The effect of crop maturity on the nutritional value of maize silage for lactating dairy cows 1. Energy and nitrogen utilization. *Animal Science* **71**, 381-390.

Carter, E.B., Theodorou, M.K. and Morris, P. (1997). Responses of Lotus corniculatus to environmental change.1. Effects of elevated CO2, temperature and drought on growth and plant development. *New Phytologist* **136**, 245-253.

Carter, E.B., Theodorou, M.K. and Morris, P. (1999). Responses of Lotus corniculatus to environmental change. 2. Effect of elevated CO2, temperature and drought on tissue digestion in relation to condensed tannin and carbohydrate accumulation. *Journal of the Science of Food and Agriculture* **79**, 1431-1440.

Carulla, J.E., Kreuzer, M., Machmuller, A. and Hess, H.D. (2005). Supplementation of *Acacia mearnsii* tannins decreases methanogenesis and urinary nitrogen in forage-fed sheep. *Australian Journal of Agricultural Research* **56**, 961-970.

Czerkawski, J.W., Blaxter, K.L. and Wainman, F.W. (1966). The effect of linseed oil and of linseed oil fatty acids incorporated in the diet on the metabolism of sheep. *British Journal of Nutrition* **20**, 485-494.

de Klein, C.A.M. and Eckard, R.J. (2008). Targeted technologies for nitrous oxide abatement from animal agriculture. *Australian Journal of Experimental Agriculture* **48**, 14-20.

del Pozo, O. and Lam, E. (1998). Caspases and programmed cell death in the hypersensitive response of plants to pathogens. *Current Biology* **8**, 1129-1132.

Dewhurst, R.J., Mitton, A.M., Offer, N.W. and Thomas, C. (1996). Effects of the composition of grass silages on milk production and nitrogen utilization by dairy cows. *Animal Science* **62**, 25-34.

Dixon, R.A. (2004) Molecular improvement of forages - from genomics to GMOs and welfare. *Molecular Breeding of Forage and Turf. Proceedings of the 3rd International Symposium, Dallas, Texas and Ardmore, Oklahoma.*

Dove, H., Wood, J.T., Simpson, R.J., Leury, B.J., Ciavarella, T.A., Gatford, K.L. and Siever-Kelly, C. (1999). Spray-topping annual grass pasture with glyphosate to delay loss of feeding value during summer. III. Quantitative basis of the alkane-based procedures for estimating diet selection and herbage intake by grazing sheep. *Australian Journal of Agricultural Research* **50**, 475-485.

Drew, M.C., He, C.J. and Morgan, P.W. (2000). Programmed cell death and aerenchyma formation in roots. *Trends in Plant Science* **5**, 123-127.

Duncan, R.R. and Carrow, R.N. (1999). Turfgrass molecular genetic improvement for abiotic/edaphic stress resistance. *Advances in Agronomy, Vol 67* **67**, 233-305.

Echt, C.S., Kidwell, K.K., Knapp, S.J., Osborn, T.C. and Mccoy, T.J. (1994). Linkage Mapping in Diploid Alfalfa (Medicago-Sativa). *Genome* **37**, 61-71.

Edwards, G.R., Parsons, A.J. and Rasmussen, S. (2007) High sugar ryegrasses for dairy systems. *Proceedings of the Dairy Science Symposium, University of Melbourne, 17-21 September 2007.*

Gatford, K.L., Simpson, R.J., Siever-Kelly, C., Leury, B.J., Dove, H. and Ciavarella, T.A. (1999). Spray-topping annual grass pasture with glyphosate to delay loss of feeding value during summer. I. Effects on pasture yield and nutritive value. *Australian Journal of Agricultural Research* **50**, 453-464.

Henry, R.J. (2001) *Plant Genotyping - The DNA Fingerprinting of Plants.* CABI Publishing: Wallingford.

Hess, H.D., Kreuzer, M., Diaz, T.E., Lascano, C.E., Carulla, J.E., Soliva, C.R. and Machmuller, A. (2003). Saponin rich tropical fruits affect fermentation and methanogenesis in faunated and defaunated rumen fluid. *Animal Feed Science and Technology* **109**, 79-94.

Hillman, K., Lloyd, D. and Williams, A.G. (1985). Use of a portable quadrupole mass-spectrometer for the measurement of dissolved-gas concentrations in ovine rumen liquor in situ. *Current Microbiology* **12**, 335-339.

Humphreys, M.W., Zwierzykowski, Z., Collin, H.A., Rogers, W.J., Zare, A.G. and Lesniewska, A. (2001) Androgenesis in grasses - methods and aspects for future breeding. *Proceedings of COST 824, Biotechnological Approaches for Utilization of Gametic Cells, Bled, Slovenia.*

Isobe, S., Klimenko, I., Ivashuta, S., Gau, M. and Kozlov, N.N. (2003). First RFLP linkage map of red clover (Trifolium pratense L.) based on cDNA probes and its transferability to other red clover germplasm. *Theoretical and Applied Genetics* **108**, 105-112.

Johnson, R.R. (1976). Influence of Carbohydrate Solubility on Non-Protein Nitrogen Utilization in Ruminant. *Journal of Animal Science* **43**, 184-191.

Jones, B.A., Muck, R.E. and Hatfield, R.D. (1995). Red clover extracts inhibit legume proteolysis. *Journal of the Science of Food and Agriculture* **67**, 329-333.

Jones, E.S., Hughes, L.J., Drayton, M.C., Abberton, M.T., Michaelson-Yeates, T.P.T., Bowen, C. and Forster, J.W. (2003). An SSR and AFLP molecular marker-based genetic map of white clover (Trifolium repens L.). *Plant Science* **165**, 531-539.

Jones, E.S., Mahoney, N.L., Hayward, M.D., Armstead, I.P., Jones, J.G., Humphreys, M.O., King, I.P., Kishida, T., Yamada, T., Balfourier, F., Charmet, G. and Forster, J.W. (2002). An enhanced molecular marker based genetic map of perennial ryegrass (Lolium perenne) reveals comparative relationships with other Poaceae genomes. *Genome* **45**, 282-295.

Kearsey, M.J. and Farquhar, A.G.L. (1998). QTL analysis in plants; where are we now? *Heredity* **80**, 137-142.

Kebreab, E., Clark, K., Wagner-Riddle, C. and France, J. (2006). Methane and nitrous oxide emissions from Canadian animal agriculture: A review.

Canadian Journal of Animal Science **86**, 135-158.

Kingston-Smith, A.H., Bollard, A.L., Humphreys, M.O. and Theodorou, M.K. (2002). An assessment of the ability of the stay-green phenotype in Lolium species to provide an improved protein supply for ruminants. *Annals of Botany* **89**, 731-740.

Kingston-Smith, A.H., Bollard, A.L., Thomas, B.J., Brooks, A.E. and Theodorou, M.K. (2003). Nutrient availability during the early stages of colonization of fresh forage by rumen micro-organisms. *New Phytologist* **158**, 119-130.

Kingston-Smith, A.H., Davies, T.E., Edwards, J.E. and Theodorou, M.K. (2008). From plants to animals; the role of plant cell death in ruminant herbivores. *Journal of Experimental Botany* **59**, 521-532.

Kingston-Smith, A.H., Merry, R.J., Leemans, D.K., Thomas, H. and Theodorou, M.K. (2005). Evidence in support of a role for plant-mediated proteolysis in the rumens of grazing animals. *British Journal of Nutrition* **93**, 73-79.

Kingston-Smith, A.H. and Theodorou, M.K. (2000). Post-ingestion metabolism of fresh forage. *New Phytologist* **148**, 37-55.

Kingston-Smith, A.H. and Thomas, H.M. (2003). Strategies of plant breeding for improved rumen function. *Annals of Applied Biology* **142**, 13-24.

Kiss, G.B., Csanadi, G., Kalman, K., Kalo, P. and Okresz, L. (1993). Construction of a Basic Genetic-Map for Alfalfa Using Rflp, Rapd, Isozyme and Morphological Markers. *Molecular & General Genetics* **238**, 129-137.

Kroll, J. and Rawel, H.M. (2001). Reactions of plant phenols with myoglobin: Influence of chemical structure of the phenolic compounds. *Journal of Food Science* **66**, 48-58.

Lee, M.R.F., Harris, L.J., Moorby, J.M., Humphreys, M.O., Theodorou, M.K., MacRae, J.C. and Scollan, N.D. (2002). Rumen metabolism and nitrogen flow to the small intestine in steers offered *Lolium perenne* containing different levels of water-soluble carbohydrate. *Animal Science* **74**, 587-596.

Lee, M.R.F., Jones, E.L., Moorby, J.M., Humphreys, M.O., Theodorou, M.K., MacRae, J.C. and Scollan, N.D. (2001). Production responses from lambs grazed on Lolium perenne selected for an elevated water-soluble carbohydrate concentration. *Animal Research* **50**, 441-449.

Lee, M.R.F., Olmos Colmenero, J.d.J., Winters, A.L., Scollan, N.D. and Minchin, F.R. (2006). Polyphenol oxidase activity in grass and its effect on plant-mediated lipolysis and proteolysis of Dactylis glomerata (cocksfoot) in a simulated rumen environment. *Journal of the Science of Food and Agriculture* **86**, 1503-1511.

Lee, M.R.F., Tweed, J.K.S., Minchin, F.R. and Winters, A.L. (2008). Red clover polyphenol oxidase: Activation, activity and efficacy under grazing. *Animal Feed Science and Technology* **In press**.

Lee, M.R.F., Winters, A.L., Scollan, N.D., Dewhurst, R.J., Theodorou, M.K. and

Minchin, F.R. (2004). Plant-mediated lipolysis and proteolysis in red clover with different polyphenol oxidase activities. *Journal of the Science of Food and Agriculture* **84**, 1639-1645.

Leury, B.J., Siever-Kelly, C., Gatford, K.L., Simpson, R.J. and Dove, H. (1999). Spray-topping annual grass pasture with glyphosate to delay loss of feeding value during summer. IV. Diet composition, herbage intake, and performance in grazing sheep. *Australian Journal of Agricultural Research* **50**, 487-495.

Lobley, G.E., Connell, A., Lomax, M.A., Brown, D.S., Milne, E., Calder, A.G. and Farningham, D.A.H. (1995). Hepatic detoxification of ammonia in the ovine liver: possible consequences for amino acid catabolism. *British Journal of Nutrition* **73**, 667-685.

Macheix, J.J., Sapis, J.C. and Fleurit, A. (1991). Phenolic compounds and polyphenol oxidase in relation to browning grapes and wines. *CRC Reviews of Food Science* **30**, 441-486.

Mackie, R.I. (2002). Mutualistic fermentative digestion in the gastrointestinal tract: Diversity and evolution. *Integrative and Comparative Biology* **42**, 319-326.

MacRae, J.C. (1976) From plant to animal protein. In *Reviews in Rural Science No 2*. Edited by Sutherland T.M., McWilliams J.R. and Leng R.A. University of New England Publishing Unit, Armidale, Australia.

MacRae, J.C., Campbell, D.R. and Eadie, J. (1975). Changes in Biochemical Composition of Herbage Upon Freezing and Thawing. *Journal of Agricultural Science* **84**, 125-131.

Matile, P. (1997) The vacuole and cell senescence. In *The Plant Vacuole; Advances in Botanical Research Volume 25*. pp. 87-112. Edited by Leigh R.A. and Sanders D. Academic Press, London.

Matile, P., Hortensteiner, S. and Thomas, H. (1999). Chlorophyll degradation. *Annual Review of Plant Physiology and Plant Molecular Biology* **50**, 67-95.

McCouch, S.R. and Doerge, R.W. (1995). QTL Mapping in Rice. *Trends in Genetics* **11**, 482-487.

Merry, R.J., Lee, M.R.F., Davies, D.R., Dewhurst, R.J., Moorby, J.M., Scollan, N.D. and Theodorou, M.K. (2006). Effects of high-sugar ryegrass silage and mixtures with red clover silage on ruminant digestion. 1. In vitro and in vivo studies of nitrogen utilization. *Journal of Animal Science* **84**, 3049-3060.

Miller, L.A., Moorby, J.M., Davies, D.R., Humphreys, M.O., Scollan, N.D., MacRae, J.C. and Theodorou, M.K. (2001). Increased concentration of water-soluble carbohydrate in perennial ryegrass (Lolium perenne L.): Milk production from late-lactation dairy cows. *Grass and Forage Science* **56**, 383-394.

Miller, L.A., Theodorou, M.K., MacRae, J.C., Evans, R.T., Humphreys, M.O., Scollan, N.D. and Moorby, J.M. (2000) Efficiency of nitrogen use by dairy cows offered perennial ryegrass with high water soluble carbohydrate concentrations. *British Grassland Society Sixth Research Conference, Aberdeen, UK.*

Min, B.R., Barry, T.N., Attwood, G.T. and McNabb, W.C. (2003). The effect of condensed tannins on the nutrition and health of ruminants fed fresh temperate forages: a review. *Animal Feed Science and Technology* **106**, 3-19.

Mittler, R., Lam, E., Shulaev, V. and Cohen, M. (1999). Signals controlling the expression of cytosolic ascorbate peroxidase during pathogen-induced programmed cell death in tobacco. *Plant Molecular Biology* **39**, 1025-1035.

Mohan, M., Nair, S., Bhagwat, A., Krishna, T.G., Yano, M., Bhatia, C.R. and Sasaki, T. (1997). Genome mapping, molecular markers and marker-assisted selection in crop plants. *Molecular Breeding* **3**, 87-103.

Monteny, G.J., Bannink, A. and Chadwick, D. (2006). Greenhouse gas abatement strategies for animal husbandry. *Agriculture Ecosystems & Environment* **112**, 163-170.

Moorby, J.M., Evans, R.T., Scollan, N.D., MacRae, J.C. and Theodorou, M.K. (2006). Increased concentration of water-soluble carbohydrate in perennial ryegrass (*Lolium perenne* L.). Evaluation in dairy cows in early lactation. *Grass and Forage Science* **61**, 52-59.

Ramírez-Restrepo, C.A. and Barry, T.N. (2005). Alternative temperate forages containing secondary compounds for improving sustainable productivity in grazing ruminants. *Animal Feed Science and Technology* **120**, 179-201.

Ryerson, D.E. and Heath, M.C. (1996). Cleavage of nuclear DNA into oligonucleosomal fragments during cell death induced by fungal infection or by abiotic treatments. *Plant Cell* **8**, 393-402.

Serraj, R., Hash, C.T., Rizvi, S.M.H., Sharma, A., Yadav, R.S. and Bidinger, F.R. (2005). Recent advances in marker-assisted selection for drought tolerance in pearl millet. *Plant Production Science* **8**, 334-337.

Siddons, R.C., Paradine, J., Gale, D.L. and Evans, R.T. (1985). Estimation of the Degradability of Dietary-Protein in the Sheep Rumen by Invivo and Invitro Procedures. *British Journal of Nutrition* **54**, 545-561.

Siever-Kelly, C., Leury, B.J., Gatford, K.L., Simpson, R.J. and Dove, H. (1999). Spray-topping annual grass pasture with glyphosate to delay loss of feeding value during summer. II. Herbage intake, digestibility, and diet selection in penned sheep. *Australian Journal of Agricultural Research* **50**, 465-474.

Smith, P., Martino, D., Cai, Z., Gwary, D., Janzen, H., Kumar, P., McCarl, B., Ogle, S., O'Mara, F., Rice, C., Scholes, B. and Sirotenko, O. (2007) Agriculture.

In *Climate Change 2007: Mitigation. Contribution of Working Group III to the Fourth Assessment Report of the Intergovernmental Panel on Climate Change* pp. 497-540. Edited by Metz B., Davidson O.R., Bosch P.R., Dave R. and Meyer L.A. Cambridge University Press, Cambridge, United Kingdom and New York, NY, USA.

Spangenberg, G., Kalla, R., Lidgett, A., Sawbridge, T., Ong, E.K. and John, U. (2001) Breeding forage plants in the genome era. *Proceedings of the 2nd international Symposium, Molecular Breeding of Forage Crops, Lorne and Hamilton, Victoria, Australia.*

Tas, B.M., Taweel, H.Z., Smit, H.J., Elgersma, A., Dijkstra, J. and Tamminga, S. (2006a). Effects of perennial ryegrass cultivars on milk yield and nitrogen utilization in grazing dairy cows. *Journal of Dairy Science* **89**, 3494-3500.

Tas, B.M., Taweel, H.Z., Smit, H.J., Elgersma, A., Dijkstra, J. and Tamminga, S. (2006b). Utilisation of N in perennial ryegrass cultivars by stall-fed lactating dairy cows. *Livestock Science* **100**, 159-168.

Taweel, H.Z., Tas, B.M., Smit, H.J., Elgersma, A., Dijkstra, J. and Tamminga, S. (2005). Effects of feeding perennial ryegrass with an elevated concentration of water-soluble carbohydrates on intake, rumen function and performance of dairy cows. *Animal Feed Science and Technology* **121**, 243-256.

Taylor, N.L. (2008). A century of clover breeding developments in the United States. *Crop Science* **48**, 1-13.

Theodorou, M.K., Kingston-Smith, A.H., Winters, A.L., Lee, M.R.F., Minchin, F.R., Morris, P. and MacRae, J. (2006). Polyphenols and their influence on gut function and health in ruminants: a review. *Environmental Chemistry Letters* **4**, 121-126.

Theodorou, M.K., Merry, R.J. and Thomas, H. (1996). Is proteolysis in the rumen of grazing animals mediated by plant enzymes? *British Journal of Nutrition* **75**, 507-508.

Thomas, H. (1987). Sid - a Mendelian Locus Controlling Thylakoid Membrane Disassembly in Senescing Leaves of Festuca-Pratensis. *Theoretical and Applied Genetics* **73**, 551-555.

Thomas, H., Evans, C., Thomas, H.M., Humphreys, M.W., Morgan, G., Hauck, B. and Donnison, I. (1997). Introgression, tagging and expression of a leaf senescence gene in Festulolium. *New Phytologist* **137**, 29-34.

Thomas, H., Morgan, W.G., Thomas, A.M. and Ougham, H.J. (1999). Expression of the stay-green character introgressed into Lolium temulentum Ceres from a senescence mutant of Festuca pratensis. *Theoretical and Applied Genetics* **99**, 92-99.

Thomas, H., Ougham, H.J. and Davies, T.G.E. (1992). Leaf Senescence in a Nonyellowing Mutant of Festuca-Pratensis - Transcripts and Translation

Products. *Journal of Plant Physiology* **139**, 403-412.

Thomas, H. and Smart, C.M. (1993). Crops That Stay Green. *Annals of Applied Biology* **123**, 193-219.

Thomas, H.M., Humphreys, M.W. and King, I.P. (2001) Molecular markers and marker-assisted selection in forage grasses. *Plant Breeding: Sustaining the Future. Abstracts 16th Eucarpia Congress, Edinburgh.* Abstract O1.3.

Thorogood, D. (1996). Varietal colour of Lolium perenne L turfgrass and its interaction with environmental conditions. *Plant Varieties and Seeds* **9**, 15-20.

Thorogood, D. and Laroche, S. (2001) QTL analysis of chlorophyll retention during leaf senescence in perennial ryegrass. *Plant Breeding: Sustaining the Future. Abstracts of 16th Eucarpia Congress, Edinburgh, UK.*

Turner, L.B., Cairns, A.J., Armstead, I.P., Ashton, J., Skot, K., Whittaker, D. and Humphreys, M.O. (2006). Dissecting the regulation of fructan metabolism in perennial ryegrass (Lolium perenne) with quantitative trait locus mapping. *New Phytologist* **169**, 45-57.

Turner, L.B., Cairns, A.J., Armstead, I.P., Thomas, H., Humphreys, M.W. and Humphreys, M.O. (2008). Does fructan have a functional role in physiological traits? Investigation by quantitative trait locus mapping. *New Phytologist* **179**, 765-775.

van Loo, E.N., Dolstra, O., Humphreys, M.O., Wolters, L., Luessink, W., de Riek, W. and Bark, N. (2003). Lower nitrogen losses through marker assisted selection for nitrogen use efficiency and feeding value (NIMGRASS). *Vorträge Pflanzenzüchtung* **59**, 270-279.

Van Nevel, C.J. and Demeyer, D.I. (1996). Control of rumen methanogenesis. *Environmental Monitoring And Assessment* **42**, 73-97.

Webb, K.J. and Abberton, M.T. (1999) Molecular genetics of white clover. *Crop Development for Cool and Wet Climate of Europe, COST 814 Workshop, University of Navarra, Pamplona, Spain.* 53-63.

Webb, K.J., Abberton, M.T. and Young, S.R. (2004) Molecular genetics of white clover. In *Applied Genetics of Leguminosae Biotechnology.* pp. 239-253. Edited by Jaiwal J.K. and Singh R.P. Kluwer Academic Publishers, Dordrecht.

Williams, W.M., Easton, H.S. and Jones, C.S. (2007). Future options and targets for pasture plant breeding in New Zealand. *New Zealand Journal of Agricultural Research* **50**, 223-248.

Wilson, J.R. and Mertens, D.R. (1995). Cell Wall Accessibility and Cell Structure Limitations to Microbial Digestion of Forage. *Crop Science* **35**, 251-259.

Winters, A.L. and Minchin, F.R. (2002) The effect of PPO on the protein content of ensiled red clover. *Proceedings of the XIIIth International Silage Conference.* 84-85.

Winters, A.L., Minchin, F.R., Merry, R.J. and Morris, P. (2003) Comparison of polyphenol oxidase activity in red clover and perennial ryegrass. In *Crop Quality: Its role in sustainable livestock production*. Edited by Abberton M.T., Andrews M., Skøt L. and Theodorou M.K. The Association of Applied Biologists, Warwick.

Zhu, W.Y., Kingston-Smith, A.H., Troncoso, D., Merry, R.J., Davies, D.R., Pichard, G., Thomas, H. and Theodorou, M.K. (1999). Evidence of a role for plant proteases in the degradation of herbage proteins in the rumen of grazing cattle. *Journal of Dairy Science* **82**, 2651-2658.

4

IMPROVING FEED EFFICIENCY IN CATTLE WITH RESIDUAL FEED INTAKE

DONAGH P. BERRY
Teagasc, Moorepark Dairy Production Research Centre, Fermoy, Co. Cork, Ireland

Introduction

The profitability of any farming enterprise, including dairy and beef production, is a function of revenues and costs. Revenues, which in dairy and beef herds are mostly reflected in milk and livestock sales, are relatively easy to compute and monitor. Some costs on the other hand, such as feed costs, are more difficult to compute and monitor. Until recently, breeding programs in dairy and beef cattle, with some exceptions, have focused on output, attributable mainly to the routine availability of data for genetic evaluations. Beef cattle breeding programs have sought faster-growing, leaner animals while selection in dairy cattle in most countries until recently has focused on increased milk production. Both selection practices have led to increased mature size, which has implications for feed inputs and thus production efficiency and profitability.

As trade barriers and tariffs, especially those applied to produce entering the EU, continue to be threatened under WTO negotiations, the food supply within the EU is likely to increase. Although some commentators suggest that, at least in Western Europe, consumers will be willing to pay more for "safe" food, the general experience to date does not always support this. This influx of food produce into the EU is likely to curtail any increases in real term farm gate prices and squeeze farm profit margins. Producers, however, have little influence on the market price of their products, other than through improved quality, which emphasises the importance of controlling input costs.

Articles relating to feed efficiency are becoming increasingly common in the scientific literature. A review of the literature was undertaken using PubMed and Cab abstracts. The search criteria were that all publications had to be in scientific journals, and the word "cattle" had to be mentioned in either the title or the abstract.

Only papers that cited the phrases "residual feed intake", "net feed efficiency", "feed efficiency" or "feed conversion" were retained. Where possible a distinction was made, based on the title, abstract and/or keywords, between solely dairy, solely beef cattle, and "other". The "other" group included studies that did not specify type of cattle and studies that related to both dairy and beef animals. A further distinction was made if the study related in some way to genetics (e.g., estimates of genetic variation using mixed models or quantification of breed effects). Figure 1 summarises the number of scientific publications reporting traits related to feed efficiency over the past four decades. Clearly the number of such publications has increased with time (Figure 1a) although this is in line with the total number of publications across the animal science category. However, the proportion of publications on feed efficiency with an element of animal breeding or genetics has increased mainly in the past decade. Most of the publications on feed efficiency are in beef cattle (Figure 1b) although interest in dairy cattle, mainly in the area of genetics, has grown in recent years. Furthermore, there is a clear trend over the past decade to define feed efficiency as residual feed intake (Figure 1c).

Importance of feed efficiency in dairy and beef cattle production systems

In 2025, the world population is expected to be 1.6 billion larger than it was in 2002 (United Nations, 2004); in other words a 25% increase in population size. Assuming per capita consumption of meat and milk products remains constant this is likely to lead to a 25% increase in demand, although there may be some displacing of beef products with white meat or other products. However, Elam (2004) showed that as peoples' incomes increase, they tend to eat more meat. Furthermore, the proliferation of refrigeration and diversification of dairy products may also result in an increase in per capita consumption of dairy produce. This increased demand for dairy and beef produce will have to be met on roughly the same land area for crops and grass as well as competing against the ever increasing demand from non-agricultural use of crops and agricultural land.

Nearly one-third of the land area of the US currently planted to principal crops is sown with maize, sorghum, barley or oats. There is a ever growing non-agricultural demand for in particular maize, for the production of for example ethanols. In the US this is facilitated mainly by the US Energy Policy Act of 2005 as well as spiralling crude oil prices. The use of maize in ethanol production has tripled in the US in the 21st century and this growth is likely to continue. During the 2005/2006 crop season, about 14% of maize grown in the US was refined into ethanol which is expected to double by 2016 (Westcott, 2007). In early 2007, ethanol refineries in the US could produce 5.6 billion gallons of ethanol and if all the factories that

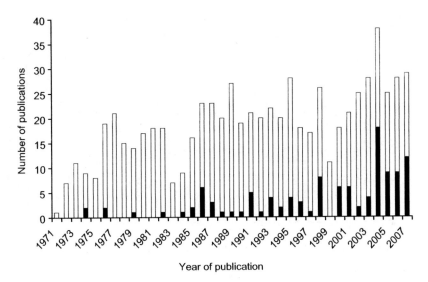

Figure 1a. Number of publications related to feed efficiency from 1970 to 2007 related to genetics (black) and non-genetics (white).

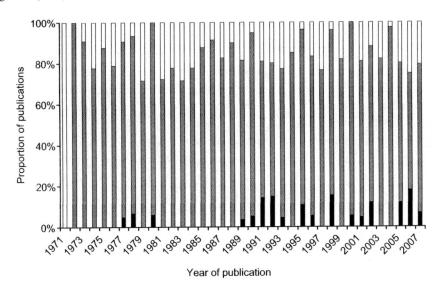

Figure 1b. Proportion of feed-efficiency related publications related to dairy animals (black), beef animals (grey) and unspecified or both dairy and beef animals (white) from 1970 to 2007.

were under construction at that time started to refine ethanol, the total ethanol capacity of the US could be 11 billion gallons by 2011 (Hoffman et al., 2007). As well as reducing the supply of maize to the agricultural markets, farmers may plant greater areas of maize, thereby displacing other crops such as grass, cereals, soya and other feed crops.

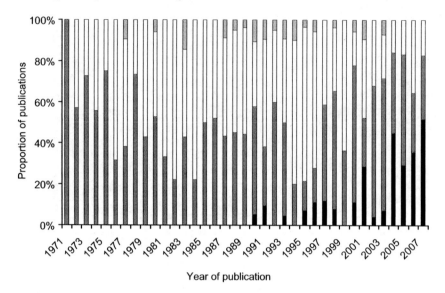

Figure 1c. Proportion of feed-efficiency related publications using the phrase residual feed intake (black), feed efficiency (grey), feed conversion (white) or a mixture (light grey) from 1970 to 2007.

To meet the expected future demands of the world's population from the same land area, several things will have to improve, including not only crop yield per hectare, but also improved feed efficiency in cattle (as well as other species). Improved utilisation of feed is also important for the individual farmer for several reasons: 1) approximately 65 to 75% of total dietary energy intake of individual beef breeding cows is used solely for body maintenance (Ferrell and Jenkins, 1985; Montano-Bermudez et al., 1990) and the beef cow breeding herd uses 65 to 85% of the energy required in a beef production system (Montano-Bermudez et al. 1990). Similarly, feed costs account for approximately 80% of total variable costs associated with pastoral milk production in dairy cows (Shalloo et al., 2004); 2) reduced security for the continuous availability of feedstuffs for animals especially at a reasonable price; 3) a 5% improvement in feed efficiency in growing beef cattle has a four-times greater economic impact than a 5% improvement in average daily gain (Gibb and McAllister, 1999); 4) increasing feed efficiency may lead to a reduction in nutrient excretion (Herd et al., 2002) and methane emissions (Hegarty et al., 2007; Nkrumah et al., 2006) thereby aiding environmental sustainability. Figure 2 illustrates the trend in nominal prices for barley and soya over the past two decades in the UK. Although cyclical trends in barley and soya prices are evident over the past 20 years, nominal prices increased dramatically in the past year and are unlikely to ease off in the foreseeable future.

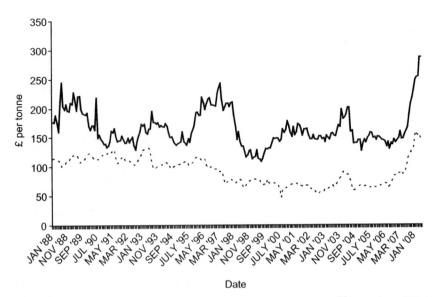

Figure 2. Trend in nominal prices for barley (broken line) and soya (continuous line) in the UK from 1988 to 2008 (*Source: DEFRA, 2008*)

Improved feed efficiency is also important in production systems relying heavily on grazed grass as the basal diet because improved feed efficiency allows either more animals to be stocked per unit area (assuming no other constraint such as environmental load constraints in the nitrates directive), or reduced inputs into the farming system (such as fertilizer or supplementary feed), or exploitation of the opportunity cost of land. Furthermore, economic efficiency in pastoral production systems may be improved by increasing dry matter intake, because intake of pasture is generally a factor limiting productivity; by increasing dry matter intake, the potential to displace expensive concentrates with less expensive forages is increased.

Measures of feed efficiency

A plethora of definitions of efficiency is used worldwide. Some definitions express efficiency on a per animal basis, either as ratios or residuals from regression models; others express efficiency per unit area or production system. Furthermore, the definitions used are not always consistent across studies or across time. Nevertheless, irrespective of the definition used, almost all efficiency measures relate inputs to outputs. Whatever the measure of feed efficiency, it should be easily measured with a high degree of accuracy, preferably be under genetic control with no antagonistic correlations with other economically important traits, be repeatable across time, applicable across different production systems, and preferably relatively easy to compute and explain to the end user.

Feed conversion ratio (FCR) is commonly used in beef cattle production and is generally defined as dry matter intake divided by average daily gain, although the converse is sometimes used. Animals with a lower FCR (using the definition above) are more efficient.

Feed conversion efficiency (FCE; Brody, 1945), also called gross feed efficiency, is more typically used in dairy production systems and is opposite in definition to FCR as defined in beef cattle. FCE is usually defined as kilograms milk output (usually milk solids output or milk yield corrected to a standard composition) divided by kilograms intake (usually dry matter intake). A higher value indicates greater efficiency.

Partial efficiency of growth (Kellner, 1909) is the efficiency of growth (i.e., the ratio of weight gain to feed) after accounting for energy requirements for maintenance. This may be calculated as average daily live-weight gain divided by average feed intake less the feed intake required for maintenance. Maintenance requirements can be estimated using feed tables and average body weight during the measurement period. However, this assumes no difference among animals of the same live-weight in maintenance efficiency, which is not necessarily true (see Archer et al., 1999); maintenance efficiency may be defined as the ratio of body weight to feed intake at zero body weight change (Archer et al., 1999).

Net feed efficiency (NFE; Exton et al., 2000), which is now more commonly referred to as residual feed intake (RFI), is increasing in popularity (Figure 1c), and RFI will be used throughout this chapter as an indicator of efficiency. Koch et al. (1963) appear to have been the first to propose the use of RFI as a measure of feed efficiency in cattle. Residual feed intake is defined as the difference between actual and predicted feed intake; in other words it is the feed intake that cannot be accounted for by production and maintenance. This unexplained feed intake or "residual" can be due to random noise, such as measurement error, due to bias in the regression coefficients for the respective regressors, or due to true differences in efficiency among animals. An example of the calculation of RFI is given in Figure 3. Because RFI is the residual from a multiple regression model, assuming linearity, the variance for RFI will be lower than the variance for feed intake, the magnitude of the difference depending on the how much variation in feed intake is unexplained by the model. The units of RFI are the units of the left hand side of the equation, such as kg dry matter or energy intake. Animals with positive RFI are less efficient than average; animals with negative RFI are more efficient than average.

Residual feed intake is therefore calculated by subtracting from actual feed (energy) intake, expected feed (energy) requirements, based on "energy sinks" such as average daily gain and metabolic live-weight as well as any energy that is "exported". However, differences in RFI among animals may also be due to differences in composition of weight gain because there is a greater energy requirement for putting on fat, compared to protein and water. However, protein requires more energy to maintain. For this reason factors such as body fat depth (measured by ultrasound scan) may also been used as a regressor in models to predict RFI. An intercept is included in the model if it is significantly different from zero. Fixed effects such as contemporary group may be included in the model as main effects as well as possibly interacting with energy sinks.

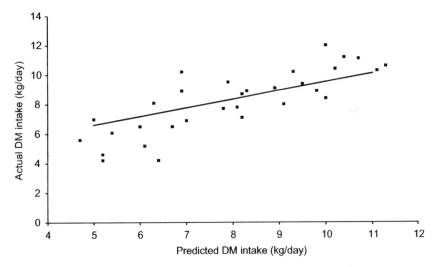

Figure 3. Example of actual (square dots) and predicted (continuous line) dry matter intake. Dots above the predicted DM intake line have positive RFI values (less efficient); animals below the predicted DM intake line have negative RFI values (more efficient).

Expected energy intake in the model may be calculated from energy tables (e.g. NRC, 2001) or other sources as undertaken by Arthur et al. (2001a). More commonly, it is calculated within the sample population under investigation and assumed to represent the residuals from a least squares regression model. This model would regress energy intake against energy sinks such as average daily live-weight gain and metabolic live-weight as well as any energy forms that are exported such as milk yield in lactating cows. Metabolic live weight is usually represented as live weight half way through the experiment raised to the power of 0.75, although a value of 0.73 has also been used (Arthur et al., 1996; Archer et al., 2002). The advantage of using energy tables in the calculation of expected energy requirements is that, assuming the same tables are used, results across populations are directly comparable, whereas residuals from a regression model are specific to the population under investigation and hence results from sample populations are not directly comparable.

Other measures of efficiency include the Kleiber ratio (Kleiber, 1961) which is the average daily live-weight gain per unit metabolic live-weight, and relative growth rate (Fitzhugh and Taylor, 1971), which is defined as growth relative to instantaneous body size. Relative growth rate may be calculated as the logarithm of live weight at the end of the test period less the logarithm of live weight at the end of the test period divided by the days in test, all multiplied by 100.

Differences among measures of feed efficiency

There are several advantages and disadvantages of different feed efficiency measures. Ratio measures, such as feed conversion efficiency and feed conversion rate, are not optimal because 1) they can lead to an increase in the error variance as a proportion of the total variance in the statistical analysis, 2) the measure will be strongly correlated with its component traits, and 3) most do not directly distinguish between the energy used for separate functions. With the exception of RFI, most of the other feed efficiency related measures are related to body size and/or growth rate. This complicates predicted responses to genetic selection due to antagonism between the desirable response in the numerator and the demoninator and the unknown relative selection pressure on each. A disproportionate amount of selection pressure will be exerted on the trait in the ratio with the higher genetic variance (Sutherland, 1965). Inclusion of ratio traits in breeding goals is also problematic when one of the component traits is itself a breeding goal. Furthermore, relationships between the feed efficiency variable and other economically important traits may imply (unless undertaken using a selection index) correlated responses in other traits which may not always be favourable. Nonetheless, most of these ratio measures of feed efficiency, as well as being comparable across populations, are easy to calculate and to explain to the end user.

Net feed efficiency or RFI, on the other hand, is by definition phenotypically (or genetically if the trait is defined as such) independent of growth rate and live weight, as well as any other trait that is included in the regression model. This is advantageous because it allows comparison of animals differing in their performance for the regressors. However, if RFI is calculated from phenotypic regression of intake on animal production (e.g., weight and growth in beef cattle; weight, milk production and body tissue loss in dairy cattle), although this implies phenotypic independence between RFI and the regressors, it does not necessarily imply genetic independence (Kennedy et al., 1993) unless the heritability estimates of the feed intake and the production traits are identical and the residual covariance between the traits is equal to the genetic covariance. Kennedy et al. (1993) showed that the genetic correlation between phenotypic RFI and both feed intake and the regressor traits is dependent on the heritability (heritability is explained later) of feed intake and the regressor traits as well as the residual and genetic correlation between them. In general, as the genetic correlation between the regressor traits and feed intake becomes more positive, the genetic correlation between RFI and the regressor traits also becomes more positive (i.e., unfavourable) unless the residual correlation between feed intake and the regressor traits is also strongly positive. Negative (i.e., favourable) genetic correlations between RFI and the regressor traits are evident when the genetic correlation between feed intake and the regressor traits is weak and the residual correlation is strongly positive. Although most estimates of genetic correlations, albeit predominantly in beef cattle, between RFI derived from phenotypic regression and production traits are not different from zero, genetic regression is also possible (Crews, 2005) to ensure zero genetic covariances between RFI and the regressors. However, selection on RFI derived from genetic regression is equivalent to using a multi-trait (restricted) selection index containing the regressor traits (Kennedy et al., 1993) but is dependent on knowing the true genetic covariances between feed intake and the regressor traits. Inclusion of RFI in a breeding goal will also require alterations to economic weights on some traits to avoid double counting. This will increase the requirement for greater explanation of the breeding goal and may confuse the end user. Other disadvantages are that, if estimated using least squares regressions then it is not easily possible to compare across populations unless the original data from all populations are available. Furthermore, RFI cannot be estimated for individual animals and needs several animals to provide accurate comparison.

The main factor limiting the use of most measures of feed efficiency is availability of accurate data on feed intake. This is a disadvantage of all measures of feed efficiency except the Kleiber ratio and relative growth rate, which do not require feed intake data, despite both been strongly genetically correlated with feed conversion ratio (Arthur et al., 2001a).

Measurement of feed efficiency related variables

Measurement of feed efficiency related variables requires data on feed intake (and possibly energy content of the diet depending on the variable being calculated) and measures of energy sinks such as live weight, live-weight gain, milk production and change in body composition. Measurement of most of these traits is costly although economic analyses in beef cattle (Exton et al., 2000) have shown the benefit to the producer and industry of performance testing for feed efficiency. In estimating regression coefficients using traditional least squares methodology, as is generally done for the quantification of RFI, one assumes no measurement error in the independent variables which will not be true for traits such as average daily gain; errors will be lower for traits based on averages such as mean live

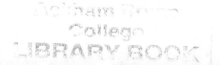

weight. Measurement error will bias the regression coefficients (Robinson, 2005) and therefore it is vital that all regressors are measured as accurately as possible. Because of this, several studies have attempted to quantify the optimal length of the test period to obtain accurate predictions of feed efficiency.

Accurate measurement of average daily gain appears to be the main factor influencing optimal length of the test period. Archer et al. (1997) reported that if feed intake is measured daily then 35 days is sufficient for accurate quantification of individual animal feed intake, but 70 days, with animals weighed fortnightly, is required to measure growth rate (and thus feed efficiency related traits). Work in South Africa (Archer and Bergh, 2000) indicated that a test period of 42 to 56 days was adequate to accurately measure growth rate; feed intake required a testing period of 56 to 70 days and RFI required 70 to 84 days. A testing period of 112 days is currently used in South Africa (Scholtz et al., 1998). Brown et al. (1991) evaluated the impact of reducing the length of the testing period from 140 days to either 112 days or 84 days on 1,830 individually-fed bulls representing 13 different breeds. The rank correlations between sires ranked for average daily gain, feed intake and feed conversion using the three periods were all greater than 0.90, suggesting that they ranked similarly irrespective of the length of the test period. Brown et al. (1991) concluded that there was no advantage of a test period longer than 112 days. Using automatic scales weighing the animal each time it ate, Kearney et al. (2004) suggested that with the use of a random coefficient regression model including a cubic spline for time to estimate average daily gain, a 56-day testing period was adequate to achieve sufficient precision on growth rate.

It appears that the optimal length of test depends on the stage of life in which the animal is measured. Hebart et al. (2004) reported that 70 days was required to get an accurate estimate of feed intake for growing cattle (i.e., post-weaning), but only 50 days was required for finishing cattle, although the effect may have been confounded with breed of animal and the slight difference in feeding systems. Currently test periods of 112 to 168 days are used in North America (Beef Improvement Federation, 1996). In Ireland, a centralised beef performance station is operated by the Irish Cattle Breeding Federation and they test approximately 150 to 200 beef bulls annually. The length of the test period is over 120 days. These data are included in national genetic evaluations.

Systematic environmental effects usually accounted for when analysing data from centralised test stations include: contemporary group (defined as the animals on test at a given time, or the animals in a pen within the test station, or the animals on test at a given time originating from the same herd); age of the animal at the start of test; breed of the animal; and age of the dam when the animal was born. To estimate genetic variation, animal (or sire) may be included as a random effect, with relationships among animals/sires described using a numerator relationship matrix. A maternal genetic component may also be fitted. Other fixed effects may include length of acclimatisation period (should be at least 21 days), live-weight gain prior to entering the central test station (although this may remove some of the genetic variation in daily gain on test) and, if using repeated measures, some account for the test-day as well as a permanent environmental effect fitted as a random effect. Depending on the number of animals originating from each herd and the definition of contemporary group, herd of origin may be included in the model as a fixed or random effect. However, few studies have investigated the effect of herd of origin on feed efficiency or related traits (Liu et al. 1995; Herd and Bishop, 2000; Berry et al., 2007a)

Biological basis for differences in feed efficiency

Following one generation of selection for RFI, Richardson and Herd (2004) suggested that, based on blood metabolic profiles, differences among animals in RFI could be attributable to differences in body composition (5%), activity (10%), ability to digest a diet (10%), heat increment from fermentation (9%), feeding behaviour (2%), protein turnover, stress and metabolism (37%); they were unable to explain the remaining 27% of variation in RFI.

Feed energy consumed may be partitioned into energy required for maintenance and energy required for production. Maintenance includes the energy required for basal metabolism, immune function, activity and maintenance of body temperature, which in turn includes the energy requirement for protein and fat synthesis and turnover. Differences in maintenance efficiency undoubtedly play a large role in differences in RFI; Herd and Bishop (2000) reported a strong genetic correlation (0.93) between maintenance energy requirement per kilogram metabolic live weight and RFI in young Hereford bulls. Ball and Thompson (1995) reported lower maintenance requirements for fatter sheep compared to leaner sheep at the same live weight. This is because, although protein synthesis requires less energy than fat synthesis, protein is continually degraded and resynthesised resulting in lower maintenance efficiency than fat. DiCostanzo et al. (1990) estimated in beef cows that 804 kJ of energy is required to maintain 1 kg of protein and 86.7 kJ to maintain 1 kg of fat. This is substantiated by data from the Trangie experiment from NSW, Australia (Richardson et al., 2004), where a positive correlation was found between plasma urea concentration at weaning and RFI in the steer progeny of animals selected for low RFI (i.e., more efficient animals had lower plasma urea content). Urea is a by-product of protein degradation (Cameron, 1992) suggesting lower protein degradation in the more efficient animals, although other factors can also contribute to differences in plasma urea content. Additionally, Richardson et al. (2004) reported higher blood viscosity in less efficient animals, which may be due to a combination of factors, including greater concentrations of plasma proteins as would be expected with greater protein degradation.

Differences in body composition do not account for all differences in maintenance requirements among animals; Taylor et al. (1986) reported differences in maintenance requirements between dairy and beef animals of similar body composition. Ferrell and Jenkins (1985) reported that energy expenditure by the main visceral organs make up a major proportion of the energy required for basal metabolism, suggesting that the size and activity of these organs is also likely to contribute to differences in energy for maintenance. This is substantiated by the greater dry matter intake in high-RFI animals relative to their contemporaries growing at the same rate of gain and same live weight (i.e., the mathematical definition of RFI) thereby requiring more energy for digestion and metabolism, and also by the lower weights of liver, small and large intestine and stomach in more efficient steers (Basarab et al. 2003). Basarab et al. (2003) reported that less efficient animals consumed 11.3% more ME intake and produced 10.3% more heat than their more efficient counterparts. Although lower heat production implies greater efficiency, if heat production is linked to important physiological processes then selection for reduced heat production may not be desirable. Furthermore, daily methane emissions were lower in low-RFI animals (Hegarty et al., 2007) and were consistent with expectations based on differences in dry matter intake among animals.

Another factor that may help to explain differences in energy required for maintenance among animals is level of activity (Basarab et al. 2003). The energy required for a 500 kg cow is 5 MJ/day for standing versus lying, 1.12 MJ/day for chewing, 0.13 MJ each time she lies down and stands up, and 1.25 MJ for walking 1 km on flat terrain (SCA, 1990). Based on these figures, Waghorn and Dewhurst (2007) suggested that small changes in activity may explain 1% of the variation in gross feed efficiency, although reduction in eating and/or chewing may have implications for feed intake and digestion. Richardson et al. (2000) suggested that approximately 10% of observed variation in RFI was due to differences in activity as measured using a pedometer. However, the contribution of differences in activity to differences in RFI seem to be greater in other species such as chickens (Luiting et al. (1991) where it has been suggested that 79% of the genetic difference in RFI between lines could be related to differences in activity.

Richardson and Herd (2004) reported that differences among animals in their ability to digest a given diet explained 10% of the differences among animals in RFI. Berry et al. (2007b) reported significant genetic variation among dairy cows in their ability to digest a predominantly grazed grass diet. Richardson et al. (1996) reported differences among animals varying in RFI in their ability to digest their feed. However, the associations between RFI and diet digestibility were inconclusive (Richardson et al., 2004). Nonetheless, an association would be expected, because approximately 16 to 40% of energy ingested is lost in faeces and 4 to 8% is lost as methane.

Approximately 65% of digestion occurs in the rumen, so the microbial population of the rumen affects the quantity and type of nutrients available to the individual. Hegarty (2004) concluded that because it is difficult to identify distinct rumen microbial populations, and to count and culture individual species within animals, selection for numbers or type of rumen microbes will not be fruitful. Hegarty (2004) went on to suggest that differences in diet selection, eating rate and digesta kinetics may be more appropriate traits to measure and include in any breeding goal for improved feed efficiency.

Where RFI is calculated using daily gain as the regressor, differences among animals may be attributable to differences in composition of the live-weight gain, just as differences in maintenance efficiency can be attributed to differences in body composition. Water has a lower energy content than protein which, in turn, has a lower energy content than fat (Ferrell and Jenkins, 1998). Basarab et al. (2003) reported positive correlations between RFI and change in ultrasound backfat thickness (r=0.22) and ultrasound marbling (r=0.22), and concluded that calculation of RFI should take account of changes in ultrasound backfat thickness and marbling score. Similarly, in lactating dairy cattle, differences among animals in RFI may be due to differences in composition of the milk. Therefore, it is important that milk solids or solids corrected milk are used in calculations.

Controlled experiments on divergent selection for feed efficiency

In order to elucidate biological differences among animals differing in a trait of interest, selection experiments that divergently select for the trait of interest are usually undertaken, or a sample of diverse animals are identified from a population and managed in a controlled environment.

The Trangie project was undertaken at the Agricultural Research Center at Trangie in New South Wales, Australia from 1993 to 2000. Briefly, Angus, Hereford, and Shorthorn bulls and heifers underwent a post-weaning performance test. After the test the heifers entered the cow herd and were given at least two opportunities to calve. The "low efficiency" cows (based on their post-weaning test), were put in calf to "low efficiency" bulls (also identified from their post-weaning test); the "high efficiency" cows were mated to "high efficiency" bulls. After the birth of their second calf, cows were not re-mated and were once again tested for differences in feed efficiency approximately 10 weeks after weaning their second calf.

The Beef CRC I project was undertaken by the Cooperative Research Center for Cattle and Beef Quality from 1993 to 2000 (Bindon, 2001). Angus, Hereford, Shorthorn, Murray Grey, Brahman, Santa Gertrudis and Belmont Red steers (n=1,309) and heifers (n=172) were used in the study and they were fed on a grain-based diet. Animals were on test for up to 79 days; more details are given by

Robinson et al. (1999). The second phase of the Beef CRC I project (called Beef CRC II project) started in 1999 and was part of a larger integrated project looking at factors such as meat quality.

One objective of these studies was to gather sufficient, high quality data for estimation of genetic parameters as well as validating those genetic parameters through generations of divergent selection. The Trangie study proved that the genetic parameters estimated were realised following five years of selection (approximately two generations). Selection for low RFI (i.e., more efficient animals) resulted in progeny that ate less, were slightly leaner, but otherwise had similar performance to their high RFI contemporaries up to 1 year of age (Arthur et al., 2004). When steers were slaughtered following one generation of selection on RFI, there was no difference among the high or low RFI steers in carcass weight, killing out percentage, or eye muscle area, although the more efficient steers had slightly less subcutaneous fat over the rib than the less efficient animals (McDonagh et al., 2001). There was no difference among animals in the content of intramuscular fat, marbling score, meat colour or fat colour in samples taken from the *M. longissimus dorsi*, although the level of calpastatin was 13% higher in the high-efficiency animals compared to their low efficiency counterparts (McDonagh et al., 2001).

These studies were also used to quantify the associations between traits measured in weanlings and those in mature cows. Archer et al. (2002) calculated RFI in second parity beef cows using the same prediction equations are used for weanlings. The cows were put on test for 70 days after a 14 to 21 days acclimatisation period; the test started 10 weeks after weaning their second calf (approximately 350 days post-calving). The results showed that RFI measured at weaning was strongly genetically correlated with RFI measured in these cows (r=0.98), although selection for RFI may be expected to increase cow body size since a negative genetic correlation (-0.22) was estimated.

Relatively small experimental studies facilitate testing of potential bio-markers for identifying animals differing in feed efficiency. One of the strongest conclusions from the Beef CRC II project was the potential of IGF-1 as a physiological biomarker for feed efficiency in cattle (Richardson et al. 2002). Similar results have been reported by others (Moore et al., 2003). Selection for low IGF-1 may therefore improve RFI; however, this may have implications for reproductive performance, especially in dairy cows, since high IGF-1 is associated with positive energy balance (a similar trait to RFI) and subsequently luteal activity (Spicer et al., 1990). Furthermore, the potential importance of physiological biomarkers for the identification of genetically different animals at a young age is likely to be reduced in the near future with relatively cheap, high throughput genotyping platforms available. However, these genotyping approaches do not currently distinguish between genes that are differentially expressed, for example due to DNA methylation. Transcriptomics, metabolomics and proteomics offer the potential to quantify differential expression of some genes, but the most appropriate tissues to biopsy, and when to biopsy, are still largely unknown.

Two experiments in Limousin and Simmental beef cattle selected divergently for RFI are underway at two separate locations in Ireland, with one breed located in each research station. In one experiment run by Teagasc, approximately 90 purebred Simmental or Simmental x Holstein-Friesian weanling heifers were purchased from commercial herds in 2005. RFI was determined when heifers were fed indoors as weanlings, and at 15 months of age the heifers were separated into high and low RFI and mated to respective high and low RFI Simmental sires; estimates of genetic merit for RFI of the sires was based on the national performance test. A herd of approximately 80 cows is now in place, and measurements of feed intake, feeding behaviour, gastrointensinal tract digestion, rumen fermentation, blood metabolic, hormonal, haematological and immunological profiles, reproductive performance, and carcass traits will be made, as well as detailed structural and functional genomic measures. In the second experiment, led by University College Dublin, approximately 100 female Limousin calves were purchased at 2 to 4 weeks of age from Holstein-Friesian dams and brought to the research station. Total daily feed intakes of milk and concentrate were measured to 10 weeks of age. Lumbar muscle and fat accretion were measured ultrasonically on 3 occasions. Animals grazed following weaning and were rehoused at 8 months of age and fed on a maize silage and concentrate diet (30:70 on a dry matter basis). Animals were categorised into quartiles of RFI and the extreme quartiles were retained for further studies, such as differences in methane emissions. Transcriptomic analysis of tissue was also undertaken. RFI was calculated also at grass and at rehousing to quantify the repeatability of RFI across an animal's life.

DairyNZ, formerly Dexcel, in New Zealand have also initiated a large study to identify dairy cows differing in feed conversion efficiency. The first group (n=171) of Holstein-Friesian dairy calves was sourced in spring 2007; this is expected to be followed by a further 550 purchased in spring 2008 and 550 more in spring 2009. The first group of calves were transported to a commercial rearing facility until weaning, after which they were moved to a DairyNZ farm and eventually to a commercial farm. They will remain there until a specially commissioned feeding facility is ready. This facility will have automated feed weighing and recording for individual animals. The animals will be fed cubed lucerne to get over the difficulty of measuring intake while grazing as well as the difficulty of feeding a bulky feed such as grass in a confinement system. Lucerne is similar to pasture and has adequate fibre length compared with pelleted feeds. Following the initial feeding trial the 10% highest and lowest calves ranked on feed conversion efficiency will be retained and intakes will be measured on these calves when they are in their second lactation. The main objective of the trial is to identify genetic markers for feed conversion efficiency. A similar trial is being run by Dairy CRC in Australia.

Non-genetic factors affecting feed efficiency related traits

Other than the factors included in the calculation of feed efficiency related variables, such as live-weight and growth rate or milk production, many non-genetic factors are associated with feed efficiency, although the effects of some can be minimised through use of RFI as a measure of feed efficiency.

Feed conversion efficiency will, on average, be better in early lactation cows since these cows will generally be mobilising body tissue reserves towards milk production. However, the equation used to derive RFI should account for changes in body condition and/or live weight. As previously discussed, in growing cattle change in body fat should also be accounted for, although arguments can be made to the contrary. Assuming no genetic change over time, younger lactating animals will tend to have poorer feed conversion efficiency than older animals because two-year old animals are approximately 80 to 90% of their mature weight (Berry et al., 2005) and are therefore partitioning ingested energy towards growth. This could be (partly) accounted for by including live-weight change and body condition score change in the equation for prediction of RFI. Similarly, pregnant animals will partition energy towards the growing foetus, which will not be the case for non-pregnant animals. However, this effect is likely to be restricted to the last trimester of pregnancy. Stressors such as climate (e.g., heat stress), pathogen load, or metabolic disease will also affect feed efficiency. A common metabolic disease in cattle fed a high concentrate diet is acidosis, caused by lowering of rumen pH. Subacute acidosis is more common that acute acidosis and the main effect is a reduction in feed intake followed by a decline in performance. Reducing the rate and amount of starch being digested in the rumen decreases the risk of rumen acidosis, although this may subsequently lead to hindgut acidosis. Inclusion of roughage in the diet will help minimise the risk of acidosis by diluting the starch content of the diet, reducing total intake of starch, increasing rumination and salivary flow to buffer the rumen contents, and increasing rate of passage of digesta through the rumen.

Feed efficiency may be altered through other nutritional means and feeding practices. The potential to alter feed efficiency nutritionally is probably greater in ruminants than monogastrics because feed is fermented by rumen microflora. The rumen affects feed conversion through the process of fermentation as well as the products available to the host tissues (Waghorn and Dewhurst, 2007)

Feed additives such as ionophores and antibiotics have been shown to improve feed efficiency (Sprott et al., 1988), although both are prohibited as feed additives in EU cattle. Ionophores improve feed efficiency by increasing the amount of propionate produced in the rumen and decreasing the amount of energy lost as methane. Ionophores also decrease the breakdown of feed protein and may decrease synthesis of microbial protein, which are important for cattle fed high roughage diets. Ionophores may also reduce the incidence of subacute acidosis. In the US, antibiotics are mainly included in feed to reduce the incidence of liver abscesses. Other feed additives include those that inhibit ovulation and suppress oestrus; results from these additives are variable.

"Limit feeding" (i.e., restricting feed intake without compromising performance) has been proposed as a means of increasing feed efficiency. Results from some US studies (Galyean, 1996; Hicks et al. 1990) indicate beneficial effects of moderate feed restriction. However, the economic benefits of feed restriction are questionable (Mathison and Engstrom, 1995) and appear to depend on diet (Mathison and Engstrom, 1995; Delphino et al., 1988) and climate (McKinnon et al., 2001). Possible reasons why restricted feeding might improve feed efficiency are: 1) organic matter digestibility of a constant diet decreases per unit increase in intake above maintenance; 2) efficiency of utilisation of metabolisable energy intake decreases as metabolisable energy intake increases; 3) maintenance requirements might be lower if weight and activity of the gastrointestinal organs and liver are reduced; and 4) heat increment of feeding might be reduced by lower intake.

Genetics of feed efficiency related traits

Several studies have investigated the presence of genetic variation in feed efficiency related measures in both dairy and beef cattle. The presence of genetic variation may be detected using several approaches, such as comparison of breeds or strains within breeds managed under a controlled environment, or estimating genetic variance components using statistical analysis of large datasets.

Narrow sense heritability is a statistic which describes the proportion of phenotypic differences among individual attributable to differences in additive genes. Heritability estimates vary from zero to one; the greater the heritability estimate the greater the expected influence of additive genes on the trait under investigation. Heritabilities are estimated by using mixed model analysis of usually large datasets (i.e., thousands of animals) where the observations are adjusted for systematic environmental effects (e.g., herd, year, age of animal) and the remaining variation is partitioned into variance components such as the variation attributable to genetics and the unexplained variation (i.e., the residual variation). Genetic variation is estimated by exploiting the known relationships among animals through the use of an average relationship matrix. Several heritability estimates have been published for dairy and beef cattle for feed efficiency related traits and are reviewed in greater detail elsewhere (Koots et al., 1994b). Heritability estimates for FCR or FCE vary from 0.16 to 0.35 (SE vary from 0.09 to 0.27; some SE not provided) in beef cattle (Gengler et al., 1995; Brelin and Brannang, 1982; Fan et al., 1995; Bishop et al., 1991; Arthur et al., 1997) and from 0.21 to 0.48 in dairy cattle (Venge, 1956; Mason et al., 1957). However, in the latter studies on lactating dairy cows, cows were fed according to yield which may bias the results because this will induce a strong correlation between feed intake and milk yield.

Heritability estimates for RFI in growing cattle vary from 0.14 to 0.44 (SE vary from 0.07 to 0.23) in beef cattle (Brelin and Brannang, 1982; Fan et al., 1995; Koch et al., 1963; Arthur et al., 1997) and 0.22 (SE vary from 0.11) in dairy cattle (Korver et al., 1991). However, heritability estimates for RFI in these studies are calculated from phenotypic regression and some genetic variation may be due to genetic correlations with the regressor traits (Kennedy et al., 1993). Nonetheless, the genetic correlations reported by both Brelin and Brannang (1982) and Korver et al. (1991) between phenotypic RFI and production were close to zero, suggesting that the heritability estimates reported, for these two studies at least, may be an accurate estimate of the true genetic variation in RFI. In contrast, Veerkamp et al. (1995) observed a reduction in the heritability for RFI from 0.32 to 0.05 when estimated using genetic regression compared to phenotypic regression, although they concluded that the estimate of 0.05 was likely to be biased downwards. Furthermore, Kennedy et al. (1993) demonstrated that if feed intake and the regressor traits are normally distributed, then the heritability of RFI can be calculated from heritability of feed intake and the regressor traits, as well as the genetic and residual correlations between feed intake and regressor traits. As heritability for feed intake or the regressor traits increases, heritability for RFI also increases. As the genetic correlation between feed intake and the regressor traits increases, heritability for RFI decreases due mainly to a reduction in the genetic variance of RFI, the absolute effect being greater as the heritabilities of feed intake and the regressor traits increase. As the residual correlation between feed intake and the regressor traits increases, heritability for RFI increases due mainly to a reduction in the phenotypic variance for RFI.

Heritability estimates of RFI in lactating dairy cattle vary from 0.12 to 0.38 (van Arendonk et al., 1991; Kennedy et al., 1993; Veerkamp et al., 1995) although estimates vary with stage of lactation (van Elzakker and van Arendonk, 1993). In contrast, some studies have reported no genetic variation in RFI in lactating dairy cows (Ngwerume and Mao, 1992; Svendsen et al., 1993). Veerkamp and Emmans (1995) discuss the genetics of RFI in lactating dairy cattle in more detail. Little is known on the genetic variation in RFI in lactating beef cows.

Genetic correlations between traits describe the strength of the linear relationship between the true genetic merit of animals for the traits in question. Genetic correlations can arise through pleiotrophy (i.e., a gene affects more than one trait) or through linkage (i.e., two genes affecting different traits reside close to each other on a chromosome and are usually inherited together).

Estimates of genetic correlations between feed efficiency related traits appear in general to be strong (Herd and Bishop, 2000; Arthur et al., 2001a). Arthur et al. (2001a) reported strong genetic correlations between relative growth rate, partial efficiency of growth, feed conversion ratio and RFI; the absolute genetic correlations varied from 0.56 to 0.94. The genetic correlation between Kleiber ratio and both relative growth rate and feed conversion ratio was 0.99 and -0.81, respectively (Arthur et al., 2001a). The genetic correlation between RFI and Kleiber ratio was -0.40 (Arthur et al., 2001a). Therefore, despite the differences in definitions of the various measures of feed efficiency, the genes affecting most traits are probably the same or reside closely together on the genome. Genetic correlations between RFI and feed intake (0.50 to 0.79; Herd and Bishop, 2000; Arthur et al., 2001a) were moderate to strong while the genetic correlation with metabolic live weight was lower but not different from zero (r=0.22; SE=0.29; Herd and Bishop, 2000). Arthur et al. (2001a) reported a genetic correlation of -0.02 between RFI calculated using standard feed tables and live weight, and the genetic correlation between RFI calculated using least squares phenotypic regression and live-weight was 0.32, which was not significantly different from the correlation between feed conversion ratio and live weight.

Several studies have reported strong genetic correlations between feed conversion efficiency and growth rate in beef cattle or milk production in dairy cattle; Koots et al. (1994a) in a meta-analysis of published papers on the genetics of feed efficiency in beef cattle, reported genetic correlations between FCR and live weight and growth rate ranging from -0.71 to -0.50. This has led to some suggesting that selection for increased growth rate or milk production will result in a favourable correlated response in feed efficiency because with higher output the influence of maintenance is diluted. Furthermore, if heritability for feed efficiency is lower than that for a performance trait, and the genetic correlation between the two traits is strong, then selection on the performance trait may be more efficient that direct selection on feed efficiency. Although this may appear to be a good strategy, and one could argue that it is for farmers solely producing animals for slaughter, these correlated responses have implications for mature cow weight which is strongly positively genetically correlated with growth rate of younger animals (Herd and Bishop, 2000). Therefore, continued selection for improved (i.e., lower) FCR without cognisance of other traits will lead to a heavier national beef cow herd with the consequence of greater maintenance requirements. When considering a cow-calf production system, Thompson and Barlow (1986) estimated that the dam consumed 89% of the total feed costs; they concluded that one of the most efficient ways to improve overall efficiency of the production system would be to decrease the maintenance requirements (i.e., live weight) of the breeding cows. The implications of selection for feed efficiency in a dairy herd are less well known and understood.

There has not been as much research in the detection of genes or quantitative trait loci (QTL; regions of the genome associated with a trait) for feed efficiency as for other production traits, due mainly to the lack of high quality phenotypic data on a large number of animals with DNA available for genotyping. However, Barendse et al. (2007) in a whole genome association study using 8786 polymorphic single nucleotide polymorphisms (SNP; pronounced "snip" is a segment of the DNA sequence which shows variation among animals) reported associations between many SNPs and RFI in cattle; 20 of the SNPs they identified explained 76% of the genetic variation in RFI. Sherman et al. (2008) identified several SNPs associated with RFI in beef steers with the allelic substitution effect of the largest SNP on BTA2 being -0.25 kg DM/day for RFI. Considerably more work is needed to fine map and identify causative mutations affecting RFI, but results to date are promising. More in-depth knowledge of the physiological pathways underpinning differences in feed efficiency among animals will help to identify and target research in functional or positional candidate genes. The use of genes that have a known effect on feed efficiency is useful in breeding programs, given that measurement of feed efficiency is resource intensive.

There appears to be no limitation to the response to selection on RFI. Response to genetic selection for any trait may be limited by a lack of genetic variation; however, there is no evidence to suggest that genetic variation in traits currently under selection in dairy and beef cattle is reducing, due mainly to the contribution of large numbers of genes to each trait, genetic mutations and the recent broadening of breeding goals in most countries. Furthermore, cattle have evolved on a predominantly high fibre diet with little or no selection pressure on efficiency of utilisation of high concentrate diets (e.g., efficiency of starch digestion) and thus there is likely to be considerable variation in such characteristics among animals. The threat of negligible genetic variation is further minimised by the proliferation of crossbreeding. Nevertheless, selection on individual genes (e.g., marker or gene assisted selection) can lead to fixation of genes over time. Antagonistic genetic correlations between RFI and other traits, especially those associated with fitness and viability may also hamper genetic gain in RFI. Although there is currently no strong evidence to suggest any strong antagonistic genetic correlations, antagonistic genetic correlations can develop over time if selection pressure is placed on both traits, although this will not happen for many generations and is not an immediate cause for concern. Long generation intervals in dairy and beef cattle (McParland et al., 2007) will slow down any exhaustion of genetic variation or development of antagonistic correlations with fitness traits, although advances in reproductive technologies and genomic techniques and exploitation will undoubtedly lead to a considerable reduction in generation interval in the near future.

Future research

Most research in feed efficiency has focused firstly on beef cattle production systems (Figure 1b) and secondly on younger animals in beef cattle production systems. Because of the low reproductive rate of cattle, we need to know the impact of breeding programs incorporating some measure of efficiency, on the efficiency of the entire production system. To do this, phenotypic and genetic (co)variances between different efficiency measures at different ages are required, as well as (co) variances with other traits affecting overall system efficiency. Few studies have attempted to estimate the genetic correlation between RFI in young and mature animals, although Archer et al. (2002) suggested the correlation in beef cattle was almost unity (0.98). Similarly, Nieuwhof et al. (1992) estimated a moderate positive (0.58) genetic correlation between RFI in growing heifers and lactating heifers (RFI in lactating heifers was calculated using a multiple regression model including metabolic live weight, live-weight change and fat and protein corrected milk yield) in the first 105 days of lactation, suggesting that selection for RFI in growing heifers will result in more efficient lactating heifers, at least in early to mid lactation. However, studies on this topic are limited and do not quantify effects on other performance traits such as fertility and health. Nevertheless, research is underway, for example in Australasia, which may help answer this question. Less still is known about the genetic correlation between RFI in growing bulls and RFI in lactating heifers; Nieuwhof et al. (1992) did not estimate this genetic correlation, but reported a moderate genetic correlation (0.40) between gross feed efficiency in growing dairy bulls and lactating heifers.

In order to investigate the potential of RFI in dairy cattle, more research is needed on how to measure and calculate feed efficiency in dairy cows. This is becoming increasingly important with the proliferation of alternative dairy breeds, such as the Jersey, which have been shown to be more efficient converters of feed to milk than the Holstein (Grainger and Goddard, 2007). Unlike growing beef cattle, dairy cows undergo lactation cycles characterised by rapid catabolism of body reserves immediately post calving, following anabolism of body reserves during the non-lactating period. Any measure of feed efficiency in dairy cattle must take account of the contribution of mobilisation of body reserves to the energy supply of the animal. Failure to account for this is mathematically equivalent to energy balance, a term commonly used in dairy cattle. Therefore, feed efficiency should be undertaken across at least the whole inter-calving interval, but preferably across an animal's lifetime. To illustrate this, dairy cows of higher genetic potential for milk production lose more body condition in early lactation (McCarthy et al., 2007) and may therefore be viewed as being efficient in early lactation. However, these animals must reach their target body condition score by the start of their subsequent lactation and during this period of anabolism of body reserves they will be viewed as being inefficient. The importance of taking cognisance of this cyclic phenomenon in dairy cows is greater in grass-based seasonal calving herds where early lactation coincides with the feeding of the relatively cheap grazed grass and the non-lactating period coincides with the feeding of more expensive feed. Not only is the energy requirement of gaining body condition more than the energy obtained from mobilising body condition (Jarrige, 1989), but also the cost of the energy source differs. Furthermore, dairy (Roche et al., 2007) and beef (Drennan and Berry, 2007) cows that lose more body condition post-calving (i.e., more efficient during that period of time) are predisposed to inferior fertility. Also, excessive body condition score loss in early lactation has been associated with reduced health, although the effect is not always consistent across parities (Berry et al., 2007c). Some studies that attempted to measure RFI in dairy cattle have included change in live weight in the prediction equations; however, changes in live weight (especially in early lactation) are due to differences in gut fill as well as differences in composition of mobilised tissue (i.e., proportion of fat relative to protein), which varies with body condition score of the animal. Furthermore, accounting for live-weight change over a given time period, especially over a long period, does not reflect changes that occurred during that period (i.e., an animal may have lost considerable weight initially but regained some or all of that weight before the next measurement). More appropriate modelling of such phenomena requires immediate attention.

Breeding programs for dairy production, with the exception of a few countries, have selected aggressively for milk production, with some breeders also placing emphasis on angularity (i.e., low body condition score) as a desirable trait. Selection for increased production is expected to improve feed efficiency due to the dilution effect on maintenance. However, this breeding strategy has played a major role in the observed deterioration of fertility within the Holstein-Friesian breed due to the antagonistic genetic correlations between milk production and fertility. Richardson et al. (2001) reported lower carcass fat content in Angus steer progeny of low RFI (i.e., efficient), and Arthur et al. (2001b) reported positive correlations between RFI and ultrasound backfat thickness ($r=0.14$) and rump P8 fat depth ($r=0.11$). This suggests that selection for RFI in young growing animals may genetically lower body fat (and therefore possibly body condition score) which has been shown to be genetically (Berry et al., 2003) and phenotypically (Roche et al., 2007; Drennan and Berry, 2007) correlated with inferior fertility. However, Arthur et al. (1999) reported no change in subcutaneous fat depth in cows following divergent selection on post-weaning RFI. Nonetheless, this must be thoroughly investigated prior to any concrete recommendations on selection for RFI. One option to potentially alleviate this correlation may be to include (change in) body condition score in the prediction of RFI, although this does not guarantee genetic independence and will require waiting until the animal is lactating unless a good predictor trait measured early in life can be identified. Another option is to include body condition score, or even better fertility and health, in a balanced breeding goal with RFI with the appropriate weightings.

The main limitation to inclusion of feed efficiency (or feed intake) related traits in breeding goals for dairy and beef cattle is availability of sufficient high quality phenotypic data on feed intake to estimate breeding values. The problem is greater in dairy cattle, because beef breeding programs generally include a performance test. Lack of data is also a problem in production systems where the majority of the diet is grazed grass. Measuring feed efficiency in confinement systems is easier because actual feed intake and diet composition can be measured more easily; hence, most published studies on feed intake or efficiency related parameters are based on animals fed indoors. Harvesting fresh pasture for feeding to animals indoors may provide a more accurate measure of feed intake, but this removes any potential effect of grazing behaviour which is known to exist among dairy cattle (Linnane et al., 2004) and to a lesser extent any potential difference among animals in diet selection, which has been shown to exist in sheep and goats (Penning et al., 1997) and dairy cattle (Weller and Phipps, 1986). Use of indigestible markers, such as chromic oxide or n-alkanes, to measure feed intake in grazing animals requires uniform pastures, known dose quantities (which is particularly important if using a controlled release device), freedom from contamination as well as the sample of the pasture to be representative of what the cows actually ate. Also, inter-cow variation in digestibility of the marker can affect the results. Estimation of genetic parameters and identification of QTL require access to large quantities of accurate phenotypes. Unfortunately considerable resources are being expended on genetic (both quantitative and molecular) analyses of data on some measure of feed efficiency, but there is little research on more accurate modelling of feed efficiency to provide superior quality phenotypes. This is particularly true for lactating dairy cows not fed in confinement. This should be one of the highest research priorities in the area of feed efficiency, and also for other traits. High quality phenotypes are key to maximising genetic gain in feed efficiency.

Fortunately, it is possible to genetically select for a goal trait (e.g., feed efficiency) without the necessity to measure the goal trait itself. A multi-trait selection index could be developed where the marginal cost of measuring the traits genetically correlated with the goal trait is low. Examples of such a trait include linear type traits, which have been shown to be associated with live weight. However, some of these traits may not be strongly correlated with RFI because RFI is phenotypically independent of live weight. Irrespective of the predictor trait(s) used, the accuracy of breeding values estimated for the goal trait will never be greater than the genetic correlation with the predictor trait. Nonetheless, potential predictor traits that can be preferably measured early in life at a relatively low marginal cost on a large number of animals should be investigated.

Detection of QTLs or genes associated with feed efficiency will also facilitate genetic selection on feed efficiency without the requirement for continuous measurement of feed efficiency. However, many genes are likely to affect feed efficiency, each with a small additive effect, so they will be difficult to identify accurately. Selection of plausible functional candidate genes potentially related to feed efficiency is an obvious start, and research on this is underway across the world. However, detection and validation of genes or causative mutations for feed efficiency is extremely resource intensive, both in the generation of high quality phenotypes on a large number of animals and in the analysis of the accruing data; costs associated with genotyping of animals are decreasing and are not major. If identified, the alleles may not be segregating in the population of interest or may have a very small effect; if the effect is large and the favourable allele is not fixed in the population then questions must be asked as to why it is not fixed. Research to develop a greater understanding of the biological pathways underpinning differences in RFI will be crucial in identifying potential functional or positional candidate genes.

The availability of high throughput, large scale genotyping platforms offers the potential to undertake genome wide selection (Meuwissen et al., 2001) for feed efficiency if sufficient phenotypes are available on genotyped animals to "train" the SNPs. However, the breakdown of linkage disequilibrium between informative SNPs and the causative mutation over generations may still require phenotyping of animals to maintain high accuracies with genomic selection. Furthermore, linkage phases may not apply or actually may be reversed across breeds; therefore, given the current number of SNPs on the bovine chip (54,001) genomic selection is really only applicable within breeds. This may be less of an issue as the number of SNPs on these chips increases (de Roos et al., 2008), or the whole genome sequencing of a large number of animals become feasible. Optimal use of these new technologies should be fully researched alongside optimal design of breeding programs.

An often neglected research topic is the area of social science and extension techniques, to educate the end user of the benefits of feed efficiency and the tools at their disposal. In order to maximise the full exploitation of research in feed efficiency by the end user, it is vital that extension techniques are tailored towards full understanding of the technology by the end user and the reasons for any lack of uptake are identified and addressed. What should be disseminated to herdowners are the benefits of genetic selection for such traits. Unlike most non-genetic methods of improving feed efficiency, genetic improvement is permanent and cumulative, and does not necessarily incur any future costs after the selection of the superior germplasm. Hence, any "good genes" introduced to a herd via superior germplasm will remain in the herd for some time and their effect can be augmented by additional selection for RFI. The opposite is true for genetic selection against superior RFI or the introduction of "bad genes" into the herd.

Other areas of future research include more studies on the association between feed intake and feed efficiency related variables measured in performance stations and subsequent progeny (male and female) performance in commercial environments; in other words, the potential existence of genotype by environment interactions. Epigenetics refers to changes in gene expression without a change in the underlying DNA sequence and is a growing scientific field that could contribute to differences among animals in feed efficiency.

Conclusions

Reduced profit margins in most dairy and beef herds necessitate more emphasis being placed on costs of production, as well as trying to improve the quality of the product produced. Feed costs constitute the majority of the variable costs of production on most farms. Several measures of feed efficiency exist, but in recent years the measure of choice is residual fed intake (RFI), which is defined as the difference between actual and expected feed intake for the given level of performance. Genetic analyses indicate that selection for improved (i.e., more negative) RFI is feasible although a separate trait, RFI, does not necessarily have to be computed if incorporated within a breeding goal. Advances in molecular genetics and technology platforms will soon facilitate more accurate differentiation among animals for some measure of RFI without having phenotypic information on these animals (or relatives). The value of RFI in a breeding program will depend on a number of factors including how accurately it is measured, as well as its economic value and correlations with other performance traits. There is a considerable amount of research still to be undertaken in this area, particularly in lactating dairy cows.

References

Archer, J.A., Arthur, P.F., Herd, R.M., Parnell, and Pitchford, W.S. (1997). Optimum postweaning test for measurement of growth rate, feed intake and feed efficiency in British breed cattle. *Journal of Animal Science.* **75,** 2024-2032.

Archer, J.A., Reverter, A., Herd, R.M., Johnston, D.J., and Arthur, P.F. (2002). Genetic variation in feed intake and efficiency of mature beef cows and relationships with postweaning measurements. In: Proceedings of the 7th World Congress on Genetics Applied to Livestock Production. **31,** 221-224. Edited by Organising committee. 7th WCGALP August 19-23, Montpellier, France.

Archer, J.A., and Bergh, L. (2000). Duration of performance tests for growth rate, feed intake and feed efficiency in four biological types of beef cattle. *Livestock Production Science.* 65: 47-55.

Archer, J.A., Richardson, E.C., Herd, R.M. and Arthur, P.F. (1999). Potential for selection to improve efficiency of feed use in beef cattle: a review. *Australian Journal of Agricultural Research*. **50**, 147-161.

Arthur, P.F., Renand, G, and Krauss, D. (2001a) Genetic and phenotypic relationships among different measures of growth and feed efficiency in young Charolais bulls. *Livestock Production Science*. **68**, 131-139.

Arthur, P.F., Archer, J.A., Johnson, D.J., Herd, R.M., Richardson, E.C. and Parnell, P.F. (2001b). Genetic and phenotypic variance and covariance components for feed intake, feed efficiency and other postweaning traits in Angus cattle. *Journal of Animal Science*. **79**, 2805-2811.

Arthur, P.F., Herd, R.M., Wright, J., Xu, G., Dibley, K. and Richardson, E.C. (1996). Net feed conversion efficiency and it relationship with other traits in beef cattle. *Proceedings of the Australian Society of Animal Production*. **21**, 107-110

Arthur, P.F., Archer, J.A., Herd, R.M., and Richardson, E.C. (1999). Relationship between postweaning growth, net feed intake and cow performance. Pages 484-487 In: Proceedings of the 13th Conference on the Association for the Advancements of Animal Breeding and Genetics 5-7 July 1999, Mandurah, Australia.

Arthur, P.F., Archer, J.A., Herd, R.M., Richardson, E.C., Exton, S.C., Wright, J.H., Dibley, K.C.P. and Burton, D.A. (1997). Genetic and phenotypic variation in feed intake, feed efficiency and growth in beef cattle. *Proceedings of the 12th Conference of the Association for the Advancement of Animal Breeding and Genetics*. **12**, 234-237. 6th – 10th April 1997. Dubbo, New South Wales

Barendse, W., Reverter, A., Bunch, R.J., Harrison, B.E., Barris, W., Thomas, M.B. (2007). A validated whole-genome association study of efficient food conversion in cattle. *Genetics*. **176**, 1893-1905.

Ball, A.J. and Thompson, J.M. (1995). the effect of selection for differences in ultrasonic backfat depth on the feed utilisation for maintenance and biological efficiency in sheep. *Proceedings of the Australian Association of Animal Breeding and Genetics*. **11**, 403-417. 3-5 July 1995. Melbourne, Australia

Basarab, J.A., Price, M.A., Aalhus, J.L., Okine, E.K., Snelling, W.M. and Lyle, K.L. (2003). Residual feed intake and body composition in young growing cattle. *Canadian Journal of Animal Science*. **83,** 189-204.

Beef Improvement Federation. 1996. "Guidelines for Uniform Beef Improvement Programs" 7th Edition. Eds C. Bailey. Beef Improvement Federation, Raleigh NC, USA.

Berry, D.P., Evans, R.D. and Amer, P.R. (2007a). Length of beef performance test period at Tully, Ireland. Technical report to the Irish Cattle Breeding Federation. July 2007. (http:www.icbf.com) Accessed August 2008

Berry, D.P., Buckley, F., Dillon, P.G., Evans, R.D., Rath, M. and Veerkamp, R.F. (2003). Genetic parameters for body condition score, body weight, milk yield, and fertility estimated using random regression models. *Journal of Dairy Science*. **86**, 3704-3717.

Berry, D.P., Horan, B., and Dillon, P.G. (2005). Comparison of growth curves of three strains of female dairy cattle. *Animal Science* **80,** 151-160

Berry, D.P., Horan, B., O'Donovan, M., Buckley, F., Kennedy, E., McEvoy, M. and Dillon, P. (2007b) Genetics of grass dry matter intake, energy balance and digestibility in grazing Irish dairy cows. *Journal of Dairy Science* **90,** 4835-4845

Berry, D.P., Lee J.M., Macdonald, K.A., Stafford, K., Matthews, L., and Roche, J.R. (2007c). Associations among body condition score, body weight, somatic cell count, and clinical mastitis in seasonally calving dairy cattle. *Journal of Dairy Science* **90,** 637-648

Bindon, B.M. (2001). Genesis of the Cooperative Research Center for Cattle and Beef Industry: integration of resources for beef quality research (1993-2000). *Australian Journal of Experimental Agriculture* **41**, 843-853.

Bishop, M.D., Davis, M.E., Harvey, W.R., Wilson, G.R. and VanStavern, B.D. (1991). Divergent selection for postweaning feed conversion in Angus beef cattle: II. Genetic and phenotypic correlations and realised heritability estimates. *Journal of Animal Science* **69**, 4360-4367.

Brelin, B., and Brannang, E. (1982). Phenotypic and genetic variation in feed efficiency of growing cattle and their relationship with growth rate, carcass traits and metabolic efficiency. *Swedish Journal of Agricultural Research* **12**, 29-34.

Brody, S., (1945). *Bioenergetics and Growth*. Rheinhold, New York.

Brown, A.H., Chewning, J.J., Johnson, Z.B., Loe, W.C., and Brown, C.J. (1991). Effects of 84-, 112-, and 140-day postweaning feelot performance tests for beef bulls. *Journal of Animal Science* **69**, 451-461.

Cameron, N.D. (1992). Correlated physiological responses to selection for carcass lean content in sheep. *Livestock Production Science*. **30,** 53-68.

Crews, D.H. Jr. (2005). Genetics of efficient feed utilization and national cattle evaluation: a review. *Genetics and Molecular Research* **4**, 152-165

de Roos, A. P. W., Hayes, B. J., Spelman, R. J. and Goddard, M. E. (2008). Linkage disequilibrium and persistence of phase in Holstein-Friesian, Jersey and Angus cattle. *Genetics*. **179**, 1503-1512

Delphino, J., Mathison, G.W., and Smith, M.W. (1988). Effect of lasolocid on feedlot performance and energy partitioning in cattle. *Canadian Journal of Animal Science*. **66,** 136

Department for Environment, Food and Rural Affairs (DEFRA). (2008) https://statistics.defra.gov.uk/esg/publications/amr/feedingstuffs.xls Accessed 20th July 2008

DiCostanzo, A., Meiske, J.C., Plegge, S.D., Peters, T.M. and Goodrich, R.D. (1990). Within-herd variation in energy utilisation of maintenance and gain in beef cows. *Journal of Animal Science* **68**, 2156-2165.

Drennan, M.J. and Berry, D.P. (2006). Factors affecting body condition score, live weight and reproductive performance in spring-cavling suckler cows. *Irish Journal of Agricultural and Food Research* **45,** 25-38

Elam, T.E. (2004). Meetign growing meat demand for the future while protectig environment will be a challenge. *Feedstuffs* **4**, 23-28

Exton, S.C., Herd, R.M., Davies, L., Archer, J.A., and Arthur, P.F. (2000). Commercial benefits to the beef industry for genetic improvement in net fed efficiency. *Asian-Australian Journal of Animal Science.* **13**, 338-341

Fan, L.Q., Bailey, D.R.C., and Shannon, N.H. (1995). Genetic parameter estimation of post-weaning gain, feed intake and feed efficiency for Hereford and Angus bulls fed two concentrate diets. *Journal of Animal Science* **73**, 365-372.

Ferrell, C.L., and Jenkins, T.G. (1985). Cow type and the nutritional environment: nutritional aspects. *Journal of Animal Science* **61**, 725-741.

Fitzhugh, H.A. and Taylor, C.S. (1971). Genetic analysis of degree of maturity. *Journal of Animal Science.* **33**, 717-725.

Galyean, M.L. (1996). Protein levels in beef cattle finishing diets: industry applications, University research and system results. *Journal of Animal Science* **74**, 2860-2870.

Gengler, N., Seutin, C., Boonen, F., and van Vleck, L.D. (1995). Estimation of genetic parameters for growth, feed consumption, and conformation traits for double muscled Belgian Blue bulls performance tested in Belgium. *Journal of Animal Science* **73**, 3269-3273.

Gibb, D.J., and McAllister, T.A. (1999). The impact of feed intake and feeding behaviour of cattle on feedlot and feedbunk management. Pages 101-116. Eds. D. Korver and J. Morrison. Proceedings of the 20th Western Nutrition Conference. 17th – 18th September, 1999. Calgary, Alberta, Canada.

Grainger, C. and Goddard, M.E. (2007). A review of the effects of dairy breed on feed conversion efficiency. pp 84-92 In: Meeting the challenges for Pasture-Based Dairying. Proceedings of the Australasian Dairy Science Symposium, September 2007. Melbourne, Australia. Eds.Chapman, D.F., D.A. Clark, K.L. Macmillan and D.P. Nation. National Dairy Alliance. Melbourne, Australia.

Hebart, M.L., Pitchford, W.S., Arthur, P.F., Archer, J.A., Herd, R.M., and Bottema, C.D.K. (2004). Effect of missing data on the estimate of average daily feed intake in beef cattle. *Australian Journal of Experimental Agriculture* **44**, 415-421.

Hegarty, R.S. (2004). Genotype differences and their impact on digestive tract function of ruminants: a review. *Australian Journal of Experimental*

Agriculture. **44**, 459-467.

Hegarty, R.S., Goopy, J.P., Herd, R.M. and McCorkell, B. (2007). Cattle selected for lower residual feed intake have reduced daily methane production. *Journal of Animal Science*. **85**, 1479-1486.

Herd, R.M. and Bishop, S.C. (2000). Genetic variation in residual feed intake and its association with other production traits in British Hereford cattle. *Livestock Production Science*. **63**, 111-119.

Herd, R.M., Arthur, P.F. and Hegarty, R.S. (2002). Potential to reduce greenhouse gas emissions from beef production by selection to reduce residual feed intake. In *Proceedings 7th World Congress on Genetic Applied to Livestock Production*, Montpellier, France. Communication no. 10-22. Edited by Organising committee. 7th WCGALP. August 19-23, Montpellier, France.

Hicks, R.B., Ownes, F.N., Gill, D.R., Martin, J.J., and Strasia, C.A. (1990). Effects of limit feeding on performance and carcass characteristics of feedlot steers and heifers. *Journal of Animal Science* **68**, 233.

Hoffman, L., Baker, A., Foreman, L., and Young, C.E. (2007) "Feed Grains Backgrounder", FDS-07c01, March 2007. Economic Research Service, USDA (http://www.ers.usda.gov) Accessed 19 August 2008

Jarrige, R. (1989). *Ruminant Nutrition: Recommended Allowances and Feed Tables*. INRA publications, Paris, John Libbey Eurotext, London, Paris 389pp.

Kearney, G.A., Knee, B.W., Graham, J.F. and Knott, S.A. (2004). the length of test required to measure liveweight change when testing for feed efficiency in cattle. *Australian Journal of Experimental Agriculture* **44**, 411-414.

Kellner, O. (1909). The Scientific Feeding of Animals. McMillan Co., New York, USA.

Kennedy, B.W., van der Werf, J.H.J. and Meuwissen, T.H.E. (1993). Genetic and statistical properties of residual feed intake. *Journal of Animal Science* **71**, 3239-3250.

Kleiber, M. (1961). "The fire of life: an introduction to animal energetics." John Wiley & Sons Inc. New York, USA.

Koch, R.M., Swiger, L.A., Chambers, D. and Gregory, K.E. (1963). Efficiency of feed use in beef cattle. *Journal of Animal Science* **22**, 486-494

Koots, K.R., Gibson, J.P., and Wilton, J.W. (1994a). Analyses of published genetic parameter estimates for beef production traits. 2. Phenotypic and genetic correlations. *Animal Breeding Abstracts*. **62,** 825-853.

Koots, K.R., Gibson, J.P., Smith, C. and Wilton, J.W. (1994b). Analyses of published genetic parameter estimates for beef production traits. 1. Heritability. *Animal Breeding Abstracts*. **62,** 309-338.

Korver, S., Van Eekelen, E.A.M., Vos, H., Nieuwhof, G.J., and van Arendonk, J.A.M.. (1991). Genetic parameters for feed intake and feed efficiency in growing dairy heifers. *Livestock Production Science* **29**, 49-59.

Linnane, M., Horan, B., Connelly, J., O'Connor, P., Buckley, F., and Dillon, P. (2004): The effect of strain of Holstein-Friesian and feeding system on grazing behaviour, herbage intake and productivity in the first lactation. *Animal Science* **78**, 169-178.

Liu, M.F., Makarechian, M., Price, M.A., and Huedepohl, C. (1995). Factors influencing feed efficiency and back fat thickness in station tested beef bulls. *Journal of Animal Science* **8**, 495-498.

Luiting, P., Scrama, J.W., van der Hel, W., Urff, E.M., Van Boekholt, P.G.J.J., Van Den Elsen, E.M.W., and Vestergen, M.W.A. (1991). Metabolic differences between white leghorns selected for high and low residual feed consumption. In: *Energy Metabolism of Farm Animals*. (Eds. C. Wenk, M. Boessinger) pp. 384-387. European Association of Animal Production, Kartause, Switzerland.

Mason, I., Robertson, A. and Gjelstadt, B. (1957). The genetic connexion between body size, milk production and efficiency in dairy cattle. *Journal of Dairy Research*. **24**, 135-143.

Mathison, G.W., and Engstrom, D. (1995). Ad libitum feeding versus restricted feeding of barley – corn-based feedlot diets. *Journal of Animal Science*. **75**, 637

McCarthy, S., Berry, D.P., Dillon, P.G., Rath, M., and Horan, B. (2007). Influence of Holstein-Friesian strain and feed system on body weight and body condition score lactation profiles. *Journal of Dairy Science* **90**, 1859-1869

McDonagh, M.B., Herd, R.M., Richardson, E.C., Oddy, V.H., Archer, J.A., and Arthur, P.F. (2001). Meat quality and calpain system of feedlot steers following a single generation of divergent selection for residual feed intake. *Australian Journal of Experimental Agriculture*. **41**, 1013-1021.

McKinnon, J.J., Gould, S., Christensen, D.A., Stookey, J., Campbell, J., and Janzen, E. (2001). Limit feeding programs from Western Canada – Are our winters told cold? Pages 278 – 284 in Proceedings of the 22nd Western Nutrition Conference. 25-27 September, Saskatoon, Canada.

Mc Parland, S., Kearney, J.F., Rath, M., and Berry, D.P. (2007). Inbreeding trends and pedigree analysis of Irish dairy and beef cattle populations. *Journal of Animal Science* **85,** 322-331.

Meuwissen, T.H.E., Hayes, B.J., and Goddard, M.E. (2001). Prediction of total genetic value using genome-wide dense marker maps. *Genetics*. **157,** 1819-1829.

Montano-Bermudez, M., Nielsen, M.K., and Deutscher, G.H. (1990). Energy requirements for maintenance of crossbred beef cattle with different genetic potential for milk. *Journal of Animal Science* **68**, 2279-2288.

Moore, K.L., Johnston, D.L., Herd, R.M., and Graser, H.-U. (2003). Genetic and non-genetic effects on plasma insulin-like growth factor-I (IGF-1) concentration and production traits in Angus cattle. *Proceedings of the*

Association for the Advancement of Animal breeding and Genetics. **15**, 222-226.

National Research Council (2001). *Nutrient Requirements of Dairy Cattle.* 7th rev. ed. Natl. Acad. Sci., Washington DC, USA.

Ngwerume, F., and Mao, I.L. (1992). Estimation of residual energy intake for lactating cows using an animal model. *Journal of Dairy Science.* **75**, 2283-2287.

Nieuwhof, G.J., van Arendonk, J.A.M., Vos, H., and Korver, S. (1992). Genetic relationships between feed intake, efficiency and production traits in growing bulls, growing heifers and lactating heifers. *Livestock Production Science* **32**, 189-202.

Nkrumah, J.D., Okine, E.K., Mathison, G.W., Schmid, K., Li, C., Basarab, J.A., Price, M.A., Wang, Z., and Moore, S.S. (2006). Relationship of feedlot efficiency, performance and feed behaviour with metabolic rate, methane production, and energy partitioning in beef cattle. *Journal of Animal Science* **84**, 145-153.

Penning, P.D., Newman, J.A., Parsons, A.J., Harvey, A., and Orr, R.J. (1997). Diet preference of adult sheep and goats grazing ryegrass and white clover. *Small Ruminant Research.* **24**, 175-184.

Richardson, E.C., Herd, R.M., and Oddy, V.H. (2000). Variation in body composition, activity and other physiological processes and their associations with feed efficiency. Feed efficiency in beef cattle. In *Proceedings of the Feed Efficiency Workshop*, pp 46-50, Edited by J.A. Archer, R.M. Herd, and P.F. Arthur. University of New England, Armidale, Australia.

Richardson, E.C., Herd, R.M., Oddy, V.H., Thompson, J.M., Archer, J.A., and Arthur, P.F. (2001). Body composition and implications for heat production of Angus steer progeny of parents selected for and against residual feed intake. *Australian Journal of Experimental Agriculture.* **41**, 1065-1072.

Richardson, E.C., Herd, R.M., Arthur, P.F., Wright, J., Xu, G., Dibley, K., and Oddy, V.H. (1996) Possible physiological indicators for net feed conversion efficiency in beef cattle. *Proceedings of the Australian Society of Animal Production.* **21**, 103-116.

Richardson, E.C., Herd, R.M., Archer, J.A., and Arthur, P.F. (2004). Metabolic differences in Angus steers divergently selected for residual feed intake. *Australian Journal of Experimental Agriculture.* **44**, 441-452.

Richardson, E.C., and Herd, R.M. (2004). Biological basis for variation in residual feed intake in beef cattle. 2. Synthesis of results following divergent selection. *Australian Journal of Experimental Agriculture.* **44**, 431-440.

Robinson, D.L. (2005). Accounting for bias in regression coefficients with example from feed efficiency. *Livestock Production Science.* **95**, 155-161.

Robinson, D.L., Oddy, V.H., Smith, C. (1999). Preliminary genetic parameters for feed intake and efficiency in feedlot cattle. *Proceedings of the Association for the Advancement of Animal breeding and Genetics.* **13**, 492-495.

Roche, J.R., MacDonald, K.A., Burke, C.R., Lee, J.M., and Berry, D.P. (2007). Associations among body condition score, body weight and reproductive performance in seasonal-calving dairy cattle. *Journal of Dairy Science* **90**, 376-391

SCA, (1990). Australian Agricultural Council Ruminants Subcommittee – Feeding Standards for Australian Livestock Ruminants. CSIRO, Rockhampton, Australia.

Scholtz, M.M., Jürgens Y., Bergh, L., van der Westhuizen, J., and Bosman, D.J. (1998) The importance of feed efficiency in the selection of beef cattle in South Africa. In *Proceedings 6ᵗʰ World Congress on Genetic Applied to Livestock Production*, **25**, 89-92. January 11-16, 1998, Armidale, NSW, Australia

Shalloo, L., Dillon, P., Rath, M., and Wallace, M. (2004). Description and validation of the Moorepark Dairy Systems Model. *Journal of Dairy Science.* **87**, 1945-1958.

Sherman, E.L., Nkrumah, J.D., Murdoch, B.M., and Moore, S.S. (2008). Identification of polymorphisms influencing feed intake and efficiency in beef cattle. *Animal Genetics.* **39**, 225-231.

Spicer, L.J., Tucker, W.B., and Adamas, G.D. (1990). Insulin like growth factor-1 in dairy cows: relationships among energy balance, body condition, ovarian activity and estrous behaviour. *Journal of Dairy Science.* **73**, 929-937.

Sprott, L.R., Goehring, T.B., Beverly, J.R., Corah, L.R. (1988). Effects of ionophores on cow herd production: a review. *Journal of Animal Science.* **66,** 1340-1346.

Sutherland, T.M. (1965). The correlation between feed efficiency and rate of gain, a ratio and its denominator. *Biometrics.* **21,** 739-749.

Svendsen, M., Skipenes, P., and Mao, I.L. (1993). Genetic parameters in feed conversion complex of primiparous cows in the first two trimesters. *Journal of Animal Science* **71**, 1721-1729.

Taylor, C.S., Thiessen, R.B., and Murray, J. (1986). Inter-breed relationship of maintenance efficiency to milk yield in cattle. *Animal Production.* **43**, 37-61.

Thompson, J.M. and Barlow, R. (1986). The relationship between feeding and growth parameters and biological efficiency in cattle and sheep. In *Proceedings 3ʳᵈ World Congress on Genetic Applied to Livestock Production*, pp 271-282, Edited by G.E. Dickerson and R.K. Johnson. University of Nebraska, Lincoln, USA.

United Nations, (2004). *World Population Prospects: Analytical Report: the 2002 Revision.* United Nations Department of Economic and Social

Affairs, Population Division, United Nations.

Van Elzakker, P.J.M., and van Arendonk, J.A.M. (1993). Feed intake, body weight and milk production: genetic analysis of different measurements in lactating dairy heifers. *Livestock Production Science* **37**, 37-51.

Van Arendonk, J.A.M., Nieuwhof, G.J., Vos, H., and Korver, S. (1991). Genetic aspects of feed intake and efficiency in lactating dairy heifers. *Livestock Production Science* **29**, 263-275.

Veerkamp, R.F. and Emmans, G.C. (1995). Sources of genetic variation in energetic efficiency of dairy cows. *Livestock Production Science* **44**, 87-97

Veerkamp, R.F., Emmans, G.C., Cromie, A.R. and Simm, G. (1995). Variance components for residual feed intake in dairy cows. *Livestock Production Science* **41**, 111-120.

Venge, O. (1956). Genetic differences in feed utilization in dairy cattle. *Z. Tier. Züchtungsbiol* **67**, 147-168.

Waghorn, G.C., and Dewhurst, R.J. (2007). Feed efficiency in cattle – the contribution of rumen function. In: Meeting the challenges for Pasture-Based Dairying. Proceedings of the Australasian Dairy Science Symposium, September 2007. Melbourne, Australia.

Weller, R.F., and Phipps, R.H. (1986). The effect of silage preference on the performance of dairy cows. *Animal Production.* **42**, 435

Westcott, P.C. (2007). In *Ethanol Expansion in the United States.* FDS-07D-01. USDA Economic Research Service (http://www.ers.usda.gov) Accessed 19 August 2008

5

SAFETY IN THE FOOD CHAIN: BIOSECURITY AND COPING WITH DISEASE OUTBREAKS (with primary reference to the pig industry)

JILL THOMSON

Scottish Agricultural College, Veterinary Services, Edinburgh

Introduction

The subject of biosecurity is very wide-ranging and has played a vital role in intensive farming systems, mainly pigs and poultry, for over 30 years. A wide range of measures is advocated to protect the health status of populations (to keep disease out of farms) and to prevent the dissemination of diseases from known infected sites. The health of animals, hygiene and biosecurity play a vital role in the production of safe, wholesome food. A raft of legislative measures is in existence to support and control farming and transport practices. Most recently, European Union legislation pertaining to Food Chain Information has been introduced to strengthen the farm-to-fork approach to food safety. This chapter outlines the prevalence of food-borne infections, the main approaches to maintaining good biosecurity on farms, and addresses some of the challenges and complexities faced in modern agriculture.

Zoonotic infections in Europe: Trends and figures

The European Food Safety Authority (EFSA) and the European Centre for Disease Prevention and Control (ECDC) provide annual Community Summary Reports on zoonotic infections, antimicrobial resistance and food-borne outbreaks in EU member states and certain non-EU countries. There are a number of important reasons for bringing this information into the public domain. Globally, bacterial food-borne zoonotic infections are the most common cause of human intestinal disease, with Salmonella and Campylobacter accounting for over 90% of reports (Thorns, 2000). In developed countries, it is estimated that one third of populations are affected by food-borne diseases every year, the majority of which are thought to be caused by zoonotic agents (Schlundt *et al*, 2004). Furthermore, it has been predicted that Campylobacter will affect approximately 1% of Europeans annually (O'Brien, 2005). Under the EU Zoonosis Directive (2003) there is a requirement for member states to produce annual data on the main sources of infection, in order to improve prevention through targeting control measures in the food production chain. The latest report presents data on zoonoses from 2006 (EFSA, 2007). The key points in the report on food-borne zoonoses are:

•   Campylobacter infection was the most commonly reported human disease in the EU (175,561 cases). Campylobacter was most commonly detected in fresh poultry meat (on average, 35% of samples were positive); it was also frequently found in live poultry, pigs and cattle.

•   Salmonellosis was second in terms of prevalence (160,649 cases in humans), with the trend showing a significant decrease over the previous 3 years. Fresh poultry and pork meat were the most common sources, with respectively 5.6% and 1% of samples testing positive. There was a significant decrease in the prevalence of salmonella infections in laying hens and in breeding flocks, reflecting the success of control measures.

•   Yersinia infections also showed a slight decrease and affected 8,979 cases in 2006. Pigs are the main source of Yersinia infection.

•   There were 4,916 confirmed human cases of verotoxigenic E.coli infection. This organism was detected mainly in cattle and in bovine products.

•   The number of food-borne listeriosis cases has increased over the past few years, with 1,583 affected in 2006. This is a severe disease with a high mortality rate (approximately 14%) that particularly affects immunocompromised individuals, pregnant women and infants younger than 4 weeks (Koch and Stark, 2006). Sources of infection include ready-to-eat fishery products, certain cheeses and other ready-to-eat products.

In summary, Campylobacter species and Salmonella species are the two most common human food-borne zoonoses in Europe, but the reported cases are believed to represent only a fraction of the true number of cases in the EU (Fisher, 2004).

The importance of good biosecurity on farms

Good biosecurity on farms has wider implications than purely the control of zoonotic infections and safety in the food chain. It is vital for prevention and control of endemic and exotic diseases. Prevention of exotic diseases is dependent on having robust national biosecurity policies and import controls, and strict control of organisms within secure research facilities. However, the arrival of some exotic diseases, for example Blue Tongue and Avian Influenza, can be outwith human control; their introduction to the UK being attributed to insects and wildlife vectors respectively. The system of recognition and rapid reporting of any suspected notifiable disease is vital for national biosecurity, and the success of the system depends on farmers being attuned to recognising signs of notifiable diseases in their animals and adopting a responsible approach to seeking veterinary advice and reporting their suspicions.

The general level of on-farm biosecurity varies considerably between different sectors of the agricultural industry and very much depends on the attitudes and level of importance attributed to herd or flock security by individual farmers. In general, biosecurity is given very high priority in the pig and poultry industries and much less so in the sheep and cattle sectors. Within the intensive livestock industries, the level of biosecurity varies depending on the health status of farms and their position within the supply pyramids. Nucleus herds or flocks and AI stations have extremely high biosecurity requirements that generally apply also to breeding/multiplication farms. 'Commercial farms' that do not supply breeding stock for sale to other farmers apply biosecurity measures according to the will of individual farmers or companies to whom they are contracted. People intending to visit farms for whatever reason should always ensure that they are aware of the biosecurity requirements and any restrictions such as a minimum time interval without contact with specified livestock before visiting the farm.

Prevention of disease introduction onto farms

The major risk factors for introducing disease into farms are as follows:

- Livestock and semen imports into the farm
- Lack of adequate isolation facilities for bought-in stock
- Vehicles of all types entering the farm premises, particularly livestock hauliers with part-loads of animals entering farms for multiple pick-ups or drop-offs
- Poorly designed loading bays and no facility for washing and disinfecting footwear, equipment and ramps used in the loading area
- Visitors, particularly those entering the farm using their own protective clothing and wellington boots (or not using any protective clothing at all)

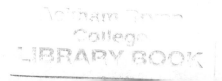

- Equipment shared between farms
- Wildlife, vermin, feral animals and insects
- Proximity to stock on neighbouring farms, particularly if they have known disease problems
- Windborne infection
- Accidents such as flooding
- Lack of secure perimeter fencing allowing strays onto farms
- Bought-in feed and bedding
- Use of common grazing and shared handling facilities.

There are a number of excellent review articles that expand on biosecurity procedures to prevent accidental introduction of diseases onto farms, the value of a risk-based approach to biosecurity, and the importance of ongoing monitoring of on-farm biosecurity measures to ensure the long-term compliance (e.g. Pritchard, Dennis and Waddilove, 2005; Amass, 2005a).

Biosecurity procedures during disease outbreaks on farms

The level of biosecurity required depends upon the significance and severity of the disease involved. In the event of a notifiable disease outbreak, the biosecurity requirements are very stringent and are controlled by Animal Health officers, under the Animal Health Act. The principles of control for a notifiable disease such as foot- and-mouth disease entail:

- Isolation of the farm and personnel
- Declaration of protection and surveillance zones (with radii of 3km and 10km respectively surrounding the infected premises), with movement restrictions imposed
- Elimination of infected animals with safe disposal
- Thorough cleansing and disinfecting of the premises and all equipment using DEFRA-approved disinfectants
- Tracing studies to try and determine the source of infection and any possible spread from the infected premises
- A minimum vacant period before introduction of sentinel animals

Recent outbreaks of notifiable diseases in the UK remind us of the need for vigilance and preparedness. The principles used in fighting such infections can be used in a modified way when dealing with outbreaks of non-notifiable diseases. The role of the veterinary surgeon in advising on outbreak management is vital in order to minimise spread of infection to other susceptible animals on the farm, protect human health if the infection is zoonotic, institute the most effective treatment and vaccination programmes for animals to protect animal health and welfare, and generally, minimise the adverse economic impact for the farmer. The principles include:

- Isolation and treatment of infected animals

- Removal and safe disposal of dead stock

- Establish 'barrier' management of stock whereby different personnel attend to either healthy or diseased stock, with no sharing of equipment, clothing or such like.

- Use footbaths with suitable disinfectant at all access points to stock, both healthy and diseased

- Ensure good stockmanship and care of animals in hospital accommodation

- Remove as much organic matter as possible then thoroughly clean pens, buildings and equipment using a detergent and hot water power washing where possible. This is followed by application of a suitable disinfectant, then allowing a vacant period for pens to dry out before re-filling

- Minimise vehicle access and visitors to the stock as far as possible. Keep visiting vehicles parked on a hard standing at a suitable distance from the stock. Use wheel dips or wash and disinfect wheels of vehicles before departure

- Seek medical assistance if zoonotic infections are involved

- Maintain the treatment register and observe withdrawal periods

- Observe for any spread of infection or re-occurrence in previously infected groups

- Establish a policy for long-term prevention of the disease or suitable control measures in the event of the infection becoming endemic in the herd / flock.

There are excellent review articles that address on-farm disease control procedures in more depth, for example, Amass (2005b)

Biosecurity challenges for modern agriculture

Census data show that there are more than 200,000 livestock holdings in the UK and more than 500,000 people directly involved with farming (DEFRA 2008a). Ensuring adequate awareness of the importance of biosecurity and what this entails on a day-to-day basis are considerable challenges. To this end, DEFRA has issued biosecurity advice through its website (DEFRA, 2008b) with links to relevant legislation, more specific guidance notes (DEFRA, 2003) and a general information leaflet for farmers (DEFRA, 2002).

There are many practical challenges for personnel responsible for implementing biosecurity on farms. Some of the situations and factors to be considered are outlined below:

- Carrier animals, those with subclinical infections or those in the incubation period of a disease process might appear perfectly healthy. Biosecurity procedures for attending to such animals in quarantine or isolation facilities might seem unnecessary to personnel. Suitable training and engagement of personnel in formulating procedures are vital to achieve full understanding and avoidance of accidental disease introduction

- Labour shortages for any reason place increased workload, pressure and responsibilities on others and short-cuts resulting in failure to observe normal biosecurity procedures may result

- Situations might require working at unsociable hours when staff tiredness, and possibly lack of motivation, come into play; for example loading of animals very early in the morning. Likewise, working under adverse weather conditions, such as heavy rain or intense cold, might make staff inclined to speed-up the job by skipping biosecurity procedures

- The cost of materials such as detergents and disinfectants might result in inappropriate use, such as compounds over-diluted or footbaths not changed frequently enough

- Breakdowns of equipment etc. and no back-up facilities or interim provision made for biosecurity procedures would lead to lapses

- Staff might have limited knowledge of which conditions are prevalent on particular farms, whether they change over time and which disinfectants are best to use under different circumstances.

The biosecurity policy and procedures to be used on farms is an important part of staff training and it should form part of the Farm Health Plan which has buy-in by all staff. This is generally well understood, but is implemented variably by both mainstream and so-called 'hobby' farmers. In many countries, including the UK, there has been a great increase in the number of small, usually peri-urban farmers, also referred to as 'hobby farmers'. The exact number of farmers in this category in the UK is unknown, but has been estimated at approximately 78,000 (Conkey, 2008). Such farmers are often involved with organic production, rare breeds or heritage breeds and sell produce directly to consumers through an expanding network of farmer's markets. Although many small farmers have a good understanding of biosecurity issues, others do not and simply do not view themselves as a risk to the wider agricultural sector (Conkey, 2008). They vary considerably in their background experience and general knowledge of farming, and some have little knowledge of exotic diseases, zoonoses, or awareness of regulations such as the ban on swill feeding to pigs. Much of the breeding and movements of poultry by hobby farmers is unregulated, many congregate at exhibitions or shows involving significant movement of birds around the country. It is important that there is industry representation for small farmers, with better engagement on issues of disease control. Mentoring programmes through education nights and on-line tools for health planning are available through agricultural colleges.

Biosecurity challenges for the feed industry

The feed industry is integrally involved with biosecurity issues for the livestock sector, particularly the intensive industries. Deliveries to farms directly from feed mills or via contracted hauliers are a necessary part of the business. Likewise, visits to farms made by nutritionists or representatives of a feed company can pose biosecurity risks. The feed industry should be fully aware of biosecurity requirements of farms and adhere to them at all times.

The role of feed in the expression of disease in farm animals has recently been highlighted through Danish research into feed presentation in relation to the prevalence of salmonella in pig herds (Dahl, 2008). Earlier epidemiological studies had shown that herds using bought-in pelleted feed had on average three-times higher antibody seroprevalence to salmonella compared to herds that used home-mix meal (Dahl 1997, Dahl, Kranker and Wingstrand, 2000). The mechanism behind the apparent protective effect of meal relates to the different physical, chemical and microbiological characteristics of the pigs' stomach contents (Hansen, 2004). Meal feeding was found to increase the viscosity and result in higher numbers in organic acid-producing lactobacilli, higher concentrations of organic acid and reduced numbers of coliforms, including salmonella (Hansen, 2004). Despite these benefits there is an economic downside to meal feeding and many automated feeding systems on farms cannot deliver meal successfully. Other interventions that had variable success in the Danish studies were liquid feeding, providing a pH of <4.5 was achieved, addition of organic acids to finisher diets (0.5 to 1 per cent formic or lactic acid) or using a mixture of 75 per cent pellets and 25 per cent non-heat treated, non-pelleted barley or wheat (Dahl, 2008). Reduction in salmonella carriage on pig farms is the primary aim of zoonosis control programmes in the pig sector of all European countries. The impact of feed-related control strategies is of great importance, along with attempts to prevent introduction of salmonella onto farms and on-farm biosecurity measures to minimise spread of infection on farms. The interaction between feed factors and the prevalence of salmonella infection in pigs has stimulated a new field of research to provide further information on the inter-relationships between feed and enteric infections.

Some modern approaches to food safety issues and food-borne zoonosis prevention

In the UK the Food Safety Act 1990 imposes an obligation on all food suppliers, including farmers, to take all reasonable precautions against contamination with zoonotic infections, and to exercise due diligence at all stages of the production process. More recently, the EU Hygiene Regulations 2006 recognised all primary producers as being part of the whole chain, farm-to-fork food safety process and introduced the requirement for Food Chain Information (FCI). FCI contributes to the slaughterhouse operators' HACCP-based food safety management systems by providing information about animals procured for slaughter. FCI was initially introduced for poultry in 2006, followed by pigs in 2008, with the requirement for cattle and sheep coming into force in 2010. The Food Standards Agency has responsibility for ensuring that legislation relating to FCI is applied through the Meat Hygiene Service. The information supplied relates to the site of production, any health problems and treatments that the animals have had, along with dates and withdrawal periods. FCI information has to accompany each consignment of animals that leave the farm, even if there are several consignments from the site on the same day. For pig farming, details of the latest herd salmonella score tested by meat-juice ELISA under the National Zoonosis Control Plan (ZNCP) should be given (Food Standards Agency, 2007). This information allows the Meat Hygiene Service to apply HACCP-based food safety systems to better control potential zoonotic infections within the processing plant.

Another food safety issue is protecting the health of people visiting farms and working on farms. There has been considerable publicity over the last few years about visitors, for instance, school parties visiting farms and contracting infections such as E.coli O157, cryptosporidiosis and other infections. The Health and Safety Executive provides guidance on procedures to follow, particularly relating to hygiene and avoiding food-borne infections either during or immediately after the visit (HSE, 2008).

Conclusion

In summary, responsibility for biosecurity on farms and food safety lies with everyone involved in agriculture. There is an ongoing quest to improve the health status and welfare of farm animals and effective biosecurity forms a key part of that improvement. Despite the necessity for farmers to comply with ever-increasing amounts of legislation, it is the every-day procedures and practices on-farm that prove whether farmers are successful. The large number of people involved with agriculture all have a duty of care to avoid introduction of infections to farms, and likewise, to take all necessary precautions to avoid spread of disease from an infected premises. Small farmers (or 'hobby' farmers) also play a vital role and their compliance with ensuring good biosecurity and disease control policies will become increasingly important with the buoyant growth in this sector of agriculture.

Amass, S.F. (2005a) Biosecurity: Stop the bugs from getting in. *The Pig Journal*, **55**: 104 – 114.

Amass, S.F. (2005b) Biosecurity: Reducing the spread. *The Pig Journal*, **56**: 78 – 87.

Conkey, H. (2008) Emerging biosecurity implications of peri-urban farming and engagement approaches in USA, Canada, the United Kingdom and Australia. A report for the Australian Government Department of Agriculture, Fish and Forestry.

Dahl, J. (1997) Cross-sectional epidemiological analysis of the relations between different herd factors and salmonella-seropositivity. In: *Procedings of the VIII International Symposium of Veterinary Epidemiology and Economics*. 04.23.

Dahl, J. (2008) Feed related interventions in pig herds with a high salmonella sero-prevalence – The Danish experience. *The Pig Journal*, **61**: 6-11.

Dahl, J., Kranker, S. and Wingstrand, A. (2000) Risk factors for high salmonella sero-prevalence in finishing pigs. In: *Procedings of the 16th International Pig Veterinary Society Congress*. p. 203.

DEFRA (2002) Better biosecurity provides peace of mind, healthy stock and a more viable business. http://www.defra.gov.uk/animalh/diseases/pdf/biosecleaf.pdf

DEFRA (2003) Biosecurity guidance to prevent the spread of animal diseases. http://www.defra.gov.uk/animalh/diseases/pdf/biosecurity-guidance.pdf

DEFRA (2008a) The June Agricultural Survey. http://www.defra.gov.uk/esg/work_htm/publications/cs/farmstats-web/default.htm

DEFRA (2008b) Disease control: biosecurity. http://www.defra.gov.uk/ animalh/diseases/control/biosecurity/index.htm

EFSA (2007) The Community Summary Report on Trends and Sources of Zoonoses, Zoonotic Agents, Antimicrobial resistance and Foodborne outbreaks in the European Union in 2006. www.efsa.eu.int/EFSA/efsa_ locale-1178620753812_1178620767319.htm

Fisher, I. (2004) International trends in Salmonella serotypes 1998 – 2003 – a surveillance report from the Enter-net international surveillance network. *European Surveillance*, **9**: 45 – 47.

Food Standards Agency (2007) Guidance on Food Chain Information for pig slaughterhouses. http://www.food.gov.uk/foodindustry/guidancenotes/ meatregsguid/fcipigslaughter.htm

Hansen, C. (2004) Choice of dry feed influences gastric conditions, incidence of salmonella and performance in growing-finishing pigs. Ph.D.- thesis. The Royal Veterinary and Agricultural University. Copenhagen, Denmark.

HSE (2008) Avoiding ill health at open farms – Advice to farmers. http:// www.hse.gov.uk/pubns/ais23.pdf

Koch, J and Stark, K (2006) Significant increase in listeriosis in Germany – Epidemiological patterns 2001 – 2005. *European Surveillance*, **11**: 85 – 88.

O'Brien, S.J. (2005) Foodborne zoonoses. *British Medical Journal*, **331**: 1217–1218

Pritchard, G., Dennis, I and Waddilove, J. (2005) Biosecurity: reducing disease risks to pig breeding herds. *In Practice*, **27**:230-237

Schlundt, J., Toyofuku, H., Jansen, J., Herbst, S.A. (2004) Emerging food-borne zoonoses. *Revue Scientifique et Technique (International Office of Epizootics)*, **23**: 513-533.

Thorns, C.J. (2000) Bacterial food-borne zoonoses. *Revue Scientifique et Technique (International Office of Epizootics)*, **19**: 226–239.

Zoonosis Directive (2003) European Commission Zoonosis Directive 2003/99/ EC.

6

CAMPYLOBACTER: FARM STRATEGIES FOR CONTROL

V. K. MORRIS AND V. M. ALLEN
Department of Clinical Veterinary Science, University of Bristol, Somerset, BS40 5DU

Campylobacteriosis is the most common cause of bacterial food-borne disease in much of the industrialised world (WHO 2002) and the reduction and/or elimination of campylobacters in the food chain, particularly from chicken products forms a major part in the strategy to control this disease. In 2005 there were more than 46,000 reported cases of human campylobacteriosis in England and Wales (HPA 1990-2000) with over 190,000 cases in the European Union (EFSA, 2006). The provisional data for 2006 indicate there has been little change. The importance placed on the transmission from poultry to humans is reinforced by the Strategic Plan (2005-2010) of the Food Standards Agency (FSA). This is to achieve a 50% reduction in the incidence of UK produced chickens which test positive for *Campylobacter* by the end of 2010 since a survey in 2001 showed that campylobacters were isolated from over half of the retail chicken examined. *Campylobacters* are ubiquitous in the environment in and around broiler houses and these sources are widely believed to be the main route of infection into the flock. Hygiene and biosecurity measures can help control *Campylobacter* infection in the broiler flocks raised under commercial conditions (Gibbens et. al. 2001).

The aim of the current chapter is to summarise several investigations into prevalence, persistence and reduction of *Campylobacter* by on-farm bio-security in standard housed and extensive flocks.

As part of a previous UK Department of Environment, Food and Rural Affairs (Defra)- funded project, a large-scale farm study examined nearly 4,000 samples for *Campylobacter* collected on 130 farm visits. Seventeen of the 26 flocks monitored were found to be *Campylobacter* positive. Of the 26 flocks, 16 underwent thinning and of these flocks 14 (88%) became positive. Of the 10 flocks which did not undergo thinning 3 (30%) became positive. The following describes investigations carried out to identify the risk areas during the thinning process and the application of methods to reduce these risks.

The practice of thinning enables a larger number of chicks to be placed initially and also a wider weight-range of carcasses to be obtained from the flock thereby increasing productivity. The majority of large-scale producers of standard housed flocks in the UK generally thin their flocks at around 35 days of age by removing 10 – 50% of the birds. As farms often have up to for example 6 houses per farm (each holding around 40,000 birds prior to thinning) and due to the processing plant operational schedules, the thinning process can take several nights to complete. Feed is withdrawn from the birds usually 4 – 6 h before thinning begins and water is withheld for a maximum of one hour (mostly 15 min or less) (Allen et. al. 2008).

The significance of flock thinning in the colonisation of broiler chickens by *Campylobacter* has been a matter for debate. In a Danish study of 10 flocks that included separate batches of males and females, Hald et. al. (2001) found that the number of *Campylobacter*-positive batches increased from five to seven for females and from five to 10 for males between thinning and final batch clearance, the females being cleared at five weeks of age in comparison with six weeks for males. From the study, it was concluded that thinning increased the prevalence of infected batches of broilers and *Campylobacter* appeared to gain access to the birds during the thinning process itself. In contrast, Russa et. al. (2005) found no such association between thinning and *Campylobacter* colonisation for Dutch broiler flocks. They investigated 1737 flocks belonging to two integrated poultry companies. Using multivariable modelling, it was found that the difference between thinned flocks and those that were not thinned could be explained by the effects of bird age and season or season alone.

An initial review of existing codes of practices and standard operating procedures was undertaken for large-scale producers in the UK of standard housed table chicken. The review found that no specific recommendations were in use for hygiene and biosecurity during thinning. General guidelines were in place but these mostly related to welfare during catching including bird handling to prevent wing damage and bruising, feed withdrawal and returning houses to pre-catching status. The Assured Chicken Production requirements cover general biosecurity e.g. only essential visitors allowed on site, use of Defra approved disinfectants according to manufacturer's instructions, etc., but nothing that is specific to thinning. Evidence from this and from previous studies (Best et. al. 2003; Hald et. al. 2000; Newell and Fearnley 2003) suggested that the thinning process presented an important risk factor with regard to colonisation of the flock by *Campylobacter*. Thus a 2 year study was set up to investigate the thinning process in detail and quantify the risk factors as this may prove to be a route by which *Campylobacter* reaching the consumer could be reduced.

Materials and methods

A 2-year-study was undertaken whereby microbiological testing (microbiological data published; Allen et. al. 2008) and farm questionnaires were carried out on 51 farms from June-November and the following year from February-September. Between the first and second years it should be noted that the threat of Avian Influenza was heightened and awareness was enhanced by an on-farm biosecurity campaign undertaken by the Food Standards Agency targeted at reducing *Campylobacter* in poultry flocks.

FARM QUESTIONNAIRE

The questionnaire consisted of 136 questions covering 4 main areas: farm and environment, changes pre-thin, the thinning process and post-thin broken down as follows: farm environment, flock health history, house biosecurity, site biosecurity, changes pre-thin, during thinning; catchers, transport lorry, thin itself and post thin. The questionnaire form was designed using SNAP V8 (Snap Surveys, Haymarket, London) and this program as well as the binary logistic regression test on SPSS V12 were used for statistical analysis.

SAMPLING OF FLOCKS

The birds placed in an individual growing house were regarded as a 'flock'. Samples were taken at the stage of feed withdrawal and during the thinning process. Ten caecal samples from culled birds and 30 fresh fecal or caecal droppings were taken. If no *Campylobacter* was isolated from either caecal or faecal samples, sampling of the flock as described continued at one- or two-day intervals, either until the flock was finally cleared for slaughter or became *Campylobacter* positive.

Enumeration of *Campylobacter* at slaughter was carried out from paired caeca which were collected from each of 10 carcasses at the processing plant, both after thinning of the flock and following clearance. This enabled investigation of (i) any increase in numbers during thinning and transport to the plant; (ii) how rapidly the flock had become colonized and (iii) the numbers present in the ceca at slaughter, which could have a bearing on carcass contamination.

SAMPLING OF THE FARM ENVIRONMENT AND PERSONNEL

Samples taken are described in Table 1. Samples 1-11 were taken before and after thinning. Swab samples were taken from each site using a sterile Readiwipe, pre-moistened in a small amount of Maximum Recovery Diluent (MRD: Oxoid, Basingstoke, UK). Gauze overshoes, pre-moistened in a small amount of MRD were used to sample the main driveway and up to the doors of the target house. These were worn over plastic overboots.

Puddle water (20 ml) was collected with the aid of a sterile pipette and transferred to 20 ml of double-strength Exeter broth. All other samples were transferred aseptically to single-strength Exeter broth (Oxoid, Basingstoke, UK and Mast Ltd., Merseyside, UK).

EXAMINATION OF SAMPLES FOR *CAMPYLOBACTER*

Samples from the farm environment and catching personnel were enriched in Exeter broth and incubated at 37°C for 48 h before being used to inoculate modified charcoal cefoperazone desoxycholate agar (mCCDA) (Oxoid Basingstoke, UK), which comprised *Campylobacter* blood-free selective agar base (Oxoid Basingstoke, UK) and *Campylobacter* selective supplement (Oxoid Basingstoke, UK). Plates were incubated at 41.5°C for 48 h under 88% N_2, 5% O_2, 5% CO_2 and 2% H_2 (by volume).

Swabs of fecal or caecal droppings were used for direct inoculation of mCCDA and for enrichment as described above.

Each pair of caeca was opened under aseptic conditions and 2 g of contents added to 20 ml of Exeter broth. Before incubation of the inoculated broth, serial ten-fold dilutions were prepared in MRD and 100 µl of each plated in duplicate on mCCDA. Both broth and plates were then incubated as above.

IDENTIFICATION OF ISOLATES

Presumptive colonies of *Campylobacter* spp. from each positive sample were subcultured onto Blood Agar Base No. 2 which was incubated microaerobically at 41.5°C for 24 h. Then, the following confirmatory tests were carried out: cell morphology, using a wet-mount or Gram-stained preparation for microscopical examination; production of oxidase and failure to grow in air at 25°C after 48h. A selection of isolates was also examined by the Campy Dry Spot test (Oxoid DR 0150M).

Results

MICROBIOLOGICAL TESTING

Of the 51 farms that were studied, 21 were *Campylobacter* positive before thinning, 13 of which were fully colonised. The remaining flocks were negative prior to thinning and became positive in; year one 2-6 days after thinning and in year two 2-10 days after thinning. In year one, 12/24 (50%) flocks sampled were positive and in year two, 9/27 (33.3%) flocks were positive. The reduction in year two followed a general tightening of farm biosecurity measures by the industry as a whole due to the threat of Avian Influenza. At slaughter however caecal samples from all flocks except 2 were positive and contained a mean of $\log_{10}$ 8 cfu / g of *Campylobacter*. Although caecal samples from these two flocks were negative at slaughter, campylobacters had been isolated from faecal and caecal samples on several occasions before clearance of the flock.

Results of the environmental testing are given in Table 1. The catchers, their clothing and equipment, and the transportation modules, crates and trailers were frequently contaminated and therefore potential sources of infection. The contamination rate of all sites was higher in year one than in year two.

Table 1. *Campylobacter*-positive samples (%) from environmental sites and personnel prior to flock thinning on all farms

	Sample	Year one	Year two	Total
1	Main driveway	3/24 (12.5)	2/28 (7.1)	5/52 (9.6)
2	Puddles	9/26 (34.6)	2/41 (4.9)	11/67 (16.4)
3	Exterior of catchers' vehicle	8/26 (30.8)	2/27 (7.4)	10/53 (18.9)
4	Interior of catchers' vehicle	12/26 (46.2)	4/26 (15.4)	16/52 (30.8)
5	Catchers' hands	6/26 (23.1)	2/27 (7.4)	8/53 (15.1)
6	Catchers' footwear	11/26 (42.3)	4/27 (14.8)	15/53 (28.3)
7	Exterior of lorry	11/36 (30.6)	6/30 (20.0)	17/66 (25.8)
8	Interior of lorry	11/36 (30.6)	3/29 (10.3)	14/65 (21.5)
9	Lorry driver's hands	3/36 (8.3)	0/30 (0.0)	3/66 (4.5)
10	Lorry driver's footwear	11/34 (32.4)	4/30 (13.3)	15/64 (23.4)
11	Forklift	6/23 (26.1)	3/27 (11.1)	9/50 (18.0)
12	Empty modules	8/23 (34.8)	6/46 (13.0)	14/69 (20.3)
13	Empty crates	6/23 (26.1)	10/45 (22.2)	16/68 (23.5)
14	Trailer	3/4 (75.0)	2/8 (25.0)	5/12 (41.7)

The vehicles used for thinning, the catcher's minibus and the lorry were frequently positive prior to thinning during both years. *Campylobacter* was recovered from the exterior of the catcher's minibus on 10 occasions before it entered the farm and the organism was isolated from a total of 27 vehicles (exterior of catcher's and lorry) (on 10 of these occasions the vehicle had not visited any other farm that day). The footwear of both the catching teams and the lorry driver's were frequently positive, especially that of theformer. This was contaminated on 15/53 occasions with a reduction from 42% to 15% from year one and year two.

QUESTIONNAIRE RESULTS AND OBSERVATIONS MADE ON SITE

Whilst the questionnaire covered a very wide range of issues, the following section highlights some of that which the research team felt to be the more important farm practices prior to and during catching. The approach in this section is to present the numerical responses to the different questions/issue, split into 'year one' and 'year two'. Year one corresponds to the 'pre-AI' period of concern, year two to the period of 'post-AI' concern, where biosecurity and hygiene measures were increased across the industry. At thin, less environmental samples were positive in year two (15% compared with 34% in year one) while less flocks were positive at this stage (9/27 compared to 12/24).

Statistical analyses were carried out in two ways. Firstly using SPSS V 12.0. Chi squared analysis within Snap 8 which indicated whether there is a relationship or not for changes to biosecurity from year one to year two. The 1% level indicates a very strong relationship, 5% a strong relationship, and 10% a relationship.

In almost all cases, the responses of farm managers to the questionnaire, coupled with the observations made by the research team confirm that there was a widespread and significant strengthening of procedures and practices in year two. Despite this, the responses revealed that considerable scope remained for improving the level of implementation and standards of many of the hygiene and biosecurity measures.

1) Vehicles

There was a significant increase (10% level) in terms of the proportion of vehicles entering sites being disinfected in year two compared to year one and a significant increase ($P<0.05$) in vehicles being disinfected on leaving. Whilst these are encouraging trends, observations made by the research team of vehicle disinfection did reveal very wide variations in the standards achieved, ranging from 'good' (use of pressure washers and thorough cleansing) to 'poor' (use of knapsack sprayer that gives a poor application due to the low volume delivered). It was also reported that the standard of cleaning and disinfection of internal surfaces was variable and in many cases, left scope for improvement (visual assessments). The importance of the vehicles as a potential source of *Campylobacter* infection both inside and outside was confirmed by the microbiological test results (Table 1).

Factors affecting the standards of cleanliness and frequency of cleaning and disinfection of vehicles is largely due to the pressures facing personnel rather than a lack of commitment on behalf of the catchers themselves.

The key constraints were found to be:

- Time pressure to start the catching quickly to meet processing plant requirements
- Lack of adequate facilities for cleaning vehicles – either on board the vehicle or provided on site
- Poorly designed and cluttered cab interiors that make cleaning difficult.

2) Protective clothing and hand washing

Where gloves were used for catching, the questionnaire data suggested that most catchers (> 50%) retained gloves between sites; a practice which might be expected to increase the risk of *Campylobacter* transfer from farm to farm. Less than half the sites visited provided protective gloves for each house, although the vast majority of sites did provide hand sanitisers in the anterooms of the poultry houses. However from the questionnaire responses only 15 farmers stated that they used the hand sanitisers both on entering and exiting the house. Table 1 shows the decrease in positive hand samples from year one to year two (23% to 7%).

3) Provision and use of foot dips and boot brushes

The majority of sites visited provided foot dips for the use of visitors, staff and catchers, although 48/51 were sited within the ante-room. However, most members of catching crews enter the house via the main doors; generally at the end away from the ante-room. The overall incidence of foot dips outside the anteroom increased in year two, from 62% to 81%. The frequency of foot dip disinfectant replacement increased in the second year. Although this trend was significant at the 5% level, it is difficult to draw any conclusions without knowing details of any changes in the type and concentration of the disinfectants used.

The availability of boot brushes for pre-cleaning of boots prior to dipping to remove all organic material for total efficacy of the disinfectant increased significantly (1% level) in year two to 40% of farms providing this equipment. Further, frequently teams had boots that were not suitable to enable efficient cleaning e.g. lace up fronts and not waterproof.

4) Water treatment

A significant (P<0.05) relationship between water treatment and flocks remaining negative up to thinning was found. Most flocks receiving treated water had it continuously but some flocks received treated water for only two or three weeks, and not always during the same period. Interpreting the data is further complicated with two farms reporting that they used Virkon S as water treatment for the birds. This may have been what was used during house cleaning when the flock was cleared, and drinking lines disinfected.

The second method of statistical analysis was carried out using the binary logistic regression in SPSS v.12.0. Data was analysed by classifying the farms on the number of environmental samples which were negative (all 26 samples negative $n=15$ farms in set 1 and a minimum of 11/26 samples positive $n=11$ farms in set 2). Farms which did not fit into either category were not included.

A range of different products were used to treat water with different active ingredients, (chlorine dioxide, organic acids, hydrogen peroxide). A strong trend (P< 0.06) was found where flocks which had water treated with chlorine dioxide were more likely to be negative at thin.

Discussion and conclusions

In this study all flocks which were negative at the thinning process became positive after the process with the lag phase increasing in year two. This increase in lag phase and reduced incidence of positive flocks and environmental samples at thin was due to a general tightening of farm biosecurity measures by the industry as a whole in year two. The isolation of *Campylobacter* on vehicles, equipment and personnel involved with the thinning procedure clearly identified areas of risk.

The recovery of *Campylobacter* from vehicles reduced in year two, however the dilution and correct application of disinfectant was observed to be very variable and 20% of the exterior and 22% of the interiors of lorries were still positive. Similarly the provision of boot dips and hand sanitisers increased in year two and recovery of *Campylobacter* reduced, but 15% of catchers' boots and 7% of hands were still positive. As found for the disinfection of vehicles, the correct application of hand sanitisers and dilution of foot dips was very variable. Whilst the above shows that increased biosecurity and hygiene can be effective in reducing *Campylobacter*, more improvements are needed. These conclusions have led to a series of recommendations that, if followed, should result in significant improvements to hygiene and biosecurity, which should help to reduce the incidence and spread of *Campylobacter* and other types of avian and zoonotic diseases.

Based on the findings from the study, a code of practice was written by the project team (comprised of researchers and poultry company staff) of what were considered best practice procedures before and during thinning. A study is being carried out to evaluate the effectiveness and practicality of the recommendations which focuses on the following key areas:

- Provision of suitable facilities on farm for changing, washing and meal breaks
- Provision of suitable and adequate facilities for cleaning and disinfecting vehicles, personnel and footwear
- Provision of sufficient sets of protective clothing to allow for movement between sites on the same shift

Findings from the study so far show that while many of these things sound simple to implement, thinning is generally carried out at night time and as previously mentioned, is a very time constrained procedure for production schedule and to ensure the birds are not on the lorry for longer than necessary.

The external disinfection of vehicles is carried out after power washing by the research team to remove organic matter. However, this is hampered by large quantities of organic matter sticking to the inside of wheel arches, especially those that have special coatings to prevent road-spray. The interior cleaning of vehicles is difficult to achieve as they are not designed for easy disinfection and wet products are not suitable.

The correct implementation of hand washing, boot washing and sanitisation and disinfection respectively are hampered by on site provision of e.g. hot water, time and cooperation of the teams.

Further work is needed to investigate methods of cleaning, especially vehicles that will travel from farm to farm to reduce the incidence and spread of *Campylobacter* and other types of avian and zoonotic diseases.

References

Allen, V. M., Weaver, H., Ridley, A. M., Harris, J. A., Sharma, M., Emery, J., Sparks, N., Lewis, M. and Edge, S. (2008) Sources and spread of thermophilic Campylobacter spp. during partial depopulation of broiler chicken flocks. *J Food Prot.* **71**(2),264-70

Best, E.L., Powell, E. J., Swift, C., Grant, K. A. and Frost, J. A. (2003) Applicability of a rapid duplex real-time PCR assay for speciation of *Campylobacter jejuni* and *Campylobacter coli* directly from culture plates. *FEMS Microbiol. Lett.* **229**,237-241

EFSA 2005 http://www.efsa.europa.eu/EFSA/efsa_locale-1178620753812_117 8620788301.htm

Gibbons, J., Pascoe, S., Evans, S., Davies, R. and Sayers, A. (2001) A trial of biosecurity as a means to control *Campylobacter* infection of broiler chickens. Prev. Vet. Med. **48**, 85-99

Hald B., A. Wedderkop, and M. Madsen. (2001) Role of batch depletion of broiler houses on the occurrence of *Campylobacter spp.* in chicken flocks. *Lett. Appl. Microbiol.* **32,** 253 – 256

HPA 1990-2006 http://www.hpa.org.uk/webw/HPAweb&HPAwebStandard/HPA web_C/1195733795689?p=1191942152851

Newell, D. G., and Fearnley, C. (2003) Sources of *Campylobacter* colonization in broiler chickens. *Appl. Environ. Microbiol.* **69**,4343 – 4351

Russa, A.D., Bouma, A., Vernooij, J.S., Jacobs-Reitsma, W. and Stegeman. J. A. (2005) No association between partial depopulation and *Campylobacter spp.* colonization of Dutch broiler flocks. *Lett. Appl. Microbiol.* **41**, 280-285

7

BACTERIOPHAGE INTERVENTION TO REDUCE *CAMPYLOBACTER* CONTAMINATION IN POULTRY

A.R. TIMMS, P.L. CONNERTON AND I.F. CONNERTON
Division of Food Sciences, School of Biosciences, University of Nottingham, Sutton Bonington Campus, Loughborough, Leicestershire, LE12 5RD, United Kingdom

Campylobacteriosis

The bacterial genus *Campylobacter* currently comprises 17 species (Korczak, Stieber, Emler, Burnens, Frey and Kuhnert, 2006), isolated from a wide range of wild and domesticated animals, many of which have been associated with human disease. However, worldwide, it is primarily *Campylobacter jejuni* and *Campylobacter coli* that are responsible for the highest number of cases of bacterial gastroenteritis in humans (Adak, Meakins, Yip, Lopman and O'Brien, 2005; Allos, 2001; Mead, Slutsker, Dietz, McCaig, Bresee, Shapiro, Griffin and Tauxe, 1999; Miller and Mandrell, 2005; Tauxe, 2002). In the United Kingdom the most recent full year data, from the United Kingdom Health Protection Agency, give 51,488 laboratory confirmed cases of campylobacteriosis in England and Wales for 2007 (Health Protection Agency, 2008) making it the most commonly identified cause of bacterial infectious intestinal disease (IID). However, under-reporting is a well-recognised phenomenon in the collection of health-related statistics and, for campylobacteriosis in the UK, the number of cases in the community may exceed the number of cases reported to the national surveillance program by up to 8-fold (Wheeler, Sethi, Cowden, Wall, Rodrigues, Tompkins, Hudson and Roderick, 1999). Hence, a more accurate description of *Campylobacter*-related IID may be between 400-500,000 cases per year, representing a significant socio-economic cost to the UK (Roberts, Cumberland, Sockett, Wheeler, Rodrigues, Sethi and Roderick, 2003). The most common clinical manifestations of *Campylobacter* infection are diarrhoea with associated bloody stools and 'stomach' cramps, but infection can range from asymptomatic carriage to more severe systemic illness and bacteraemia or localised topical infection. The vast majority of infections are self-limiting and require no medical intervention, clearing after 7 to 14 days.

However, in some instances, infection leads to the development of serious sequelae including Guillain–Barré syndrome, Miller–Fisher syndrome and reactive arthritis (Nachamkin, 2002; Overell and Willison, 2005; Ternhag, Törner, Svensson, Ekdahl and Giesecke, 2008; Yuki and Koga, 2006), with severe implications for those unfortunate enough to suffer them.

Campylobacter transmission to humans

Numerous factors are associated with contracting campylobacteriosis, however it is the direct handling and consumption of poultry meat or its cross-contamination of uncooked and raw foods, via cooking utensils, that are considered major risks (Lindqvist and Lindblad, 2008; Wingstrand, Neimann, Engberg, Nielsen, Gerner-Smidt, Wegener and Mølbak, 2006). *Campylobacter* colonise and grow easily in the gastrointestinal-tract (GIT) of chickens and they appear to be relatively benign in this host, commonly being regarded as commensal organisms (causing no observable pathogenesis) and forming part of the normal intestinal microflora of the chicken. Once present in the chicken GIT, campylobacters can colonise to high levels and subsequently spread rapidly throughout a flock by horizontal transmission from chicken to chicken, such, that up to 95% of a flock can become infected within 6 days after the organism is first detected (Katsma, De Koeijer, Jacobs-Reitsma, Mangen and Wagenaar, 2007; Van Gerwe, Bouma, Jacobs-Reitsma, van den Broek, Klinkenberg, Stegeman and Heesterbeek, 2005).

The presence of large numbers of campylobacters in chicken caeca, which can be between $\log_{10} 4$ and $\log_{10} 8$ colony forming units (CFU)/g (Rudi, Høidal, Katla, Johansen, Nordal and Jakobsen, 2004), inevitably leads to the physical dissemination of the organism and contamination, or cross-contamination, of many carcasses during slaughter and processing. *Campylobacter* can be recovered from up to 80% of UK retail poultry meat (Corry and Atabay, 2001; Jorgensen, Bailey, Williams, Henderson, Wareing, Bolton, Frost, Ward and Humphrey, 2002; Kramer, Frost, Bolton and Wareing, 2000; Reich, Atanassova, Haunhorst and Klein, 2008) with similar carriage levels observed in other European countries and the USA (reviewed by Wagenaar, Jacobs-Reitsma, Hofshagen and Newell, 2008). Models that assess the quantitative risks for contraction of campylobacteriosis suggest that a reduction of *Campylobacter* numbers on poultry carcasses reaching the consumer, by a factor of 100-fold, would result in up to a 30-fold reduction in human campylobacteriosis (Lindqvist and Lindblad, 2008; Rosenquist, Nielsen, Sommer, Nørrung and Christensen, 2003) representing a significant improvement over the current status quo.

Over the last decade, the routine use of chemical additives and antibiotics in poultry production has been severely curtailed within the European Union;

therefore, other avenues need to be explored to achieve the desired reduction. Various approaches have been proposed to accomplish this, amongst which increased biosecurity and hygienic livestock management, competitive exclusion and bacteriophage therapies are amongst the most prominent (reviewed by Doyle and Erickson, 2006). In practice, because it is so well adapted to life in the chicken GIT, a combination of approaches may be needed to produce the maximum reduction in *Campylobacter* levels.

Bacteriophage as antimicrobial agents

Former Soviet Block countries have exploited the use of bacteriophage for therapeutic, prophylactic and disinfection purposes for many years (reviewed by Alisky, Iczkowski, Rapoport and Troitsky, 1998). However, it is only recently that Western countries have re-examined and reassessed the usage of phage therapy as a means to combat infectious disease; see reviews by Merril, Scholl and Adhya (2003), Sulakvelidze, Alavidze and Morris, Jr. (2001) and Summers (2001). This renewed interest is fuelled by the rise in antibiotic resistance, such that pathogens which had previously been well-controlled are once again becoming serious threats to animal and public health in a variety of contexts (Alanis, 2005; Johnson, Stilwell, Fritsche and Jones, 2006; McDonald, 2006).

The use of bacteriophage to target specific species of bacteria has a number of distinct advantages over traditional chemotherapy treatments including;

1)   The specificity of phage for the target organism means there is less 'collateral' damage to the normal microbial flora of the GIT. Bacterial imbalance or 'dysbiosis' caused by the usage of antimicrobials can lead to a number of ancillary problems which may be difficult to treat and can affect growth rate and yield of animals, phage specificity avoids these side effects.

2)   Phage are both self-replicating and self-limiting, since they will multiply only as long as sensitive bacteria are present and then are gradually eliminated from the animal. In contrast, the routine use of antibiotics and growth promoters commonly led to residues surviving processing and reaching the consumer in foodstuffs or being disseminated to the environment, for example in animal manure and waste water.

3)   Development of phage-resistant mutants does occur *in vivo*; however the molecular basis of bacterial phage resistance is completely different from that involved in development of antibiotic resistance. This removes the inherent problems of selection and dissemination of antibiotic resistance to the general microbial population and specifically to human or animal pathogens.

4) Phage can be selected to target surface receptors that are involved in pathogenesis, so that any population that does develop resistance is usually attenuated in virulence or in their ability to compete with wild type phage sensitive bacteria.

5) Phage are ubiquitous in the environment, or can be ingested through foodstuffs. Indeed, since it is estimated that there may be up to 10^{31} phage in the ecosphere (Hendrix, Smith, Burns, Ford and Hatfull, 1999) they are the most common biological particles on the planet. Hence, the likelihood of side effects (e.g. an allergic response) being associated with phage treatment is remote, as opposed to antimicrobial intervention strategies that carry the risks of sometimes-severe consequences.

6) The cost and time involved in phage 'discovery' is considerably lower than the processes involved in development and production of an antibiotic. Phage can often be co-isolated with their respective target organism and indeed co-evolve with them, thus it is easier to isolate new variants to avoid selection of resistance in the wider population.

SELECTION OF SUITABLE BACTERIOPHAGE

The efficacy and utility of phage therapy or the use of phage as specific agents of disinfection is very much dependent on the selection of the phage to be used. The phage must be virulent and demonstrate high potency against the target bacteria. Virulent phage, such as the T-even phage of *Escherichia coli*, lyse bacterial cells as a consequence of their life cycle. The first stage of the bacteriophage life cycle usually involves absorption to a specific cell surface component, or receptor, of the host bacterium followed by injection of the nucleic acid through the cell wall. The nucleic acid then directs synthesis of further phage nucleic acid and protein capsids using a combination of the host cell and phage encoded biosynthetic apparatus. Once the phage particles have been assembled the cell envelope is ruptured (lysed) to release the phage progeny.

In contrast, lysogenic or temperate phage are generally unsuitable for phage therapy, as they can integrate their DNA into the host DNA and render the host bacterium immune to further infection through the production of a phage-encoded transcriptional repressor. The repressor actively prevents the expression of the genes of the phage and those of other related phage that may subsequently infect a process termed super-infection immunity. Furthermore, lysogenic phage are prone to transduction, the phage-mediated transfer of genetic material from one bacterial host to another. This form of DNA transfer may include the dissemination of pathogenic traits amongst their hosts (Boyd and Brüssow, 2002; Cheetham and

Katz, 1995). For example, Shiga-like toxin-producing strains of *E. coli* which include O157:H7, carry the toxin-encoding genes on lamboid prophage integrated into the host bacterial genome (O'Brien, Newland, Miller, Holmes, Smith and Formal, 1984; Scotland, Smith, Willshaw and Rowe, 1983). The expression of the toxin or toxins is under regulatory control, as if they were phage late gene products, with the consequence that any factor that commits the prophage to excise and initiate lysis will result in the increased expression of the toxin (Smith, Day, Scotland, Gross and Rowe, 1984). Stresses such as antibiotic therapy, infection by resident lambdoid phage populations or the presence of an existing population of susceptible hosts can greatly enhance phage amplification and toxin production in the GIT (Gamage, Strasser, Chalk and Weiss, 2003). Characterisation of phage selected for phage intervention is thus extremely important and demonstration of the lack of transducing ability or the inability to form stable lysogens may be one of the prime issues affecting regulatory approval.

THEORETICAL CONSIDERATIONS

Adoption of phage therapy has been held back by a lack of consistent proof of its efficacy. Previous failures may have been due to a general lack of understanding of the kinetics of phage replication, which is a density-dependent process to which mathematical models can be applied (Bull, Levin, DeRouin, Walker and Bloch, 2002; Levin and Bull, 1996; Payne and Jansen, 2001). However, it is important to develop a suitable theoretical framework for understanding the nonlinear kinetic properties of phages as "self-replicating pharmaceuticals" and to interpret such a framework in terms of therapeutic effect and not purely from an ecological perspective (Payne, Phil and Jansen, 2000). It should be anticipated that any simple model for phage-bacteria interactions will not capture every aspect of a particular combination of phage and bacterial strains, but it is important that models used in designing a phage treatment do provide accurate predictions of parameters such as the inundation and proliferation thresholds, discussed below.

Phage replication is critically dependent on density of susceptible hosts. A consequence of these kinetics is that there will be a threshold above which phage numbers increase and below which they decrease, this theoretical value has been termed the 'phage proliferation threshold' (Payne and Jansen, 2003; Wiggins and Alexander, 1985). The phage concentration will not exhibit net growth unless the host concentration exceeds the appropriate proliferation threshold and, when this occurs, phage proliferation becomes relatively rapid until the phage concentration reaches the 'inundation threshold' (that is the phage concentration above which the rate of infection and cell death exceeds the bacterial growth rate) and begins to suppress the host population. This scenario is considered as phage therapy in an 'active' mode and requires active phage replication. Thus a relatively wide range of initial phage doses should suppress the bacterial population at roughly the same time; this might be particularly important where the timing of phage therapy is relevant such as in agricultural or food safety contexts. Second, at higher doses - those close to or greater than the inundation threshold - the effect of a phage on the bacterial population will change rapidly as the dosage increases; as the initial phage concentration is increased beyond the inundation threshold, the growth of the bacterial population will quickly shift to an exponential decline. In cases where the phage concentration starts substantially above the inundation threshold, phage can be expected to infect all susceptible host cells in a relatively short period of time (phage therapy in a passive mode). When phage are mixed with bacteria at ratios at which they greatly out-number the bacteria (high multiplicity of infection, MOI), then the bacteria may become 'lysed from without'. This occurs because the phage particles interact with the bacteria in large numbers, compromising the integrity of the cell wall and causing the bacterium to swell and burst (Delbrück, 1940). This process may lead to an initial drop in bacterial counts and phage titre, with yet more phage losses occurring as they adhere to bacterial-cell debris rather than to growing bacteria (Rabinovitch, Aviram and Zaritsky, 2003).

The threshold values presume that all the bacteria and phage present are available for infection to occur, but this presumption may not be true *in vivo* where greater rates of phage losses may be encountered and bacteria may become portioned or sequestered from the main population. The later consideration is of particular importance to phage applications against bacteria colonising the intestinal tracts of animals, since the adherence of the target bacteria to the large surface area available and the nature of the mucosa to which they adhere could limit their interaction with phage. The intestinal lumen is a complex environment, where various physical (for example constant flow of material), physiological (for example levels of oxygen), host defences and biochemical factors (such as pH) all influence the populations of colonising bacteria. In addition, the kinetics of phage absorption in the intestine may be quite different from those in laboratory media, due to the viscosity of the mucus layer (Weld, Butts and Heinemann, 2004). For these reasons the effective proliferation threshold may be greater *in vivo*. The outcome of phage therapy will also depend on various other life-history parameters, including the inoculum size, inoculum timing, phage-absorption-rate and burst size (Levin and Bull, 1996; Payne and Jansen, 2001; 2002; Weld *et al.*, 2004). For these reasons, it may be difficult to translate information gained from interaction of homogeneous bacteria and phage populations in a well-mixed and controlled *in vitro* environment to the situation *in vivo*, although general interaction parameters obtained from *in vitro* experiments can serve to inform suitable models.

Bacteriophage intervention in chickens

The two main bacterial zoonoses arising from poultry are *Salmonella* and *Campylobacter*, however bacteria from several other genera including *Listeria, Clostridia, Yersinia, Staphylococcus* and pathogenic *Escherichia* can occasionally be transmitted from poultry to humans if circumstances permit (reviewed by Cox, Richardson, Bailey, Cosby, Cason, Musgrove and Mead, 2005). Use of virulent bacteriophage could provide a practical intervention for reducing the numbers of these pathogenic bacterial species entering the human food chain (Greer, 2005; Hudson, Billington, Carey-Smith and Greening, 2005).

SALMONELLA

There has been a significant decline in the incidence of isolation of *Salmonella* in poultry products since the late 1990s and cases of human infection have fallen concordantly. This is partly due to improvements in the standards of egg production. In particular the implementation of the Lion Code of Practice first introduced in 1998 has had a significant benefit. However, in the UK, there were still approximately 12,000 laboratory confirmed cases of human salmonellosis in 2007 (Health Protection Agency, 2008). *Salmonella* remains a problem in birds raised for meat production and various studies have examined the use of phage to prevent or reduce *Salmonella* colonisation of chickens (Andreatti Filho, Higgins, Higgins, Gaona, Wolfenden, Tellez and Hargis, 2007; Atterbury, Van Bergen, Ortiz, Lovell, Harris, DE, Wagenaar, Allen and Barrow, 2007; Berchieri, Jr., Lovell and Barrow, 1991; Sklar and Joerger, 2001; Toro, Price, McKee, Hoerr, Krehling, Perdue and Bauermeister, 2005). As with *Campylobacter*, to be discussed later, phage treatment did produce a transient decrease in *Salmonella* numbers recovered from chicken caeca (by between $\log_{10} 2$ and $\log_{10} 4$ CFU/g) at 24 h post phage treatment. The degree of reduction was dependent on the specific phage used, some being much more effective than others; however recovery of the *Salmonella* population levels was observed over the following 48 h.

ESCHERICHIA COLI

The genus *Escherichia* contains both commensal and pathogenic members affecting both avian species and humans. In terms of frequency, human infection by poultry-borne pathogenic *Escherichia* is not as significant as for *Salmonella* and *Campylobacter*. *Escherichia* is, however, responsible for a number of pathogenic conditions in poultry and is therefore of economic interest. Phage therapies have been tried for various types of infections including respiratory and septicemic colibacillosis (Barrow, Lovell and Berchieri, Jr., 1998; Huff, Huff, Rath, Balog and Donoghue, 2002; 2003; 2005; Xie, Zhuang, Kong, Ma and Zhang, 2005) with success in decreasing mortality or delaying the progress of disease providing phage were administered rapidly after experimental infection with pathogenic *Escherichia* strains.

CAMPYLOBACTER

The use of phage to control *Campylobacter* in chickens is slightly different from most other phage therapy studies, as campylobacters are considered natural commensals, not pathogens, of poultry species. Reduction in the numbers of campylobacters infecting birds may prove a more feasible proposition than the prevention or eradication of *Campylobacter* from poultry altogether. In the UK, up to 80% of chickens become infected with *Campylobacter*; that is almost certainly due to the prevalence of campylobacters in farm environments and in wildlife reservoirs enabling contamination of domesticated flocks, particularly free range and organic-reared birds (Colles, Jones, Harding and Maiden, 2003; Colles, Jones, McCarthy, Sheppard, Cody, Dingle, Dawkins and Maiden, 2008; Newell and Fearnley, 2003). Different *C. jejuni* strains colonise chickens with variable success (McCrea, Tonooka, VanWorth, Atwill and Schrader, 2006) but most strains will colonise efficiently in the absence of competition. Some progress has been made towards identifying the genetic traits responsible for this and towards identifying some of the virulence factors that may determine pathogenicity of *C. jejuni* strains (Ahmed, Manning, Wassenaar, Cawthraw and Newell, 2002; Hofreuter, Tsai, Watson, Novik, Altman, Benitez, Clark, Perbost, Jarvie, Du and Galan, 2006). However, even where it is possible to produce *Campylobacter*-free chickens, the benefits of this may be negated by cross-contamination from *Campylobacter*-positive flocks at the abattoir (Herman, Heyndrickx, Grijspeerdt, Vandekerchove, Rollier and De, 2003; Reich *et al.*, 2008). Previous work has indicated that there are changes to *Campylobacter* population structure on chicken carcasses during passage through a slaughterhouse (Klein, Beckmann, Vollmer and Bartelt, 2007; Newell and Fearnley, 2003) and the ability to survive stresses during processing was postulated as a potential explanation for these changes. The effective use of bacteriophage to reduce contamination of foods with zoonotic pathogens, such as *Campylobacter,* will require an in-depth understanding of the epidemiology of the pathogen against which the phage preparation is to be used. It also requires the identification of critical intervention points in the processing cycle where phage application will be most beneficial and cost effective.

Previous studies have shown that natural infection with, or the deliberate application of bacteriophage, can reduce the carriage of *Campylobacter* in the GIT of live chickens prior to slaughter or on the surface of raw chicken meat (Atterbury, Dillon, Swift, Connerton, Frost, Dodd, Rees and Connerton, 2005; Atterbury, Connerton, Dodd, Rees and Connerton, 2003b; Goode, Allen and Barrow, 2003; Loc Carrillo, Atterbury, El-Shibiny, Connerton, Dillon, Scott and Connerton, 2005; Wagenaar, Bergen, Mueller, Wassenaar and Carlton, 2005). The incidence of *Campylobacter* phage in intensively-reared chickens, has previously been determined from 22 farms based in the UK (Atterbury *et al.*, 2005). *Campylobacter jejuni* was isolated from 63% (129/205) of the caeca of the birds' sampled and *C. jejuni* specific bacteriophage were isolated from 20% (41/205) of the same samples. Enumeration of campylobacters determined that the mean number in the presence of phage was $\log_{10} 5.1$ CFU/g of caecal contents while it was $\log_{10} 6.9$ CFU/g when phage were absent (Atterbury *et al.*, 2005). This $\log_{10} 1.8$ CFU/g difference was a significant ($P < 0.001$) reduction in numbers comparing caecal counts with or without phage. Clearly the presence of phage already influences the numbers of campylobacters in poultry without any therapeutic intervention.

Campylobacter specific bacteriophage

Campylobacter-specific bacteriophage can readily be isolated from chicken intestinal contents, abattoir effluent and retail poultry meat (El-Shibiny, Connerton and Connerton, 2005; Grajewski, Kusek and Gelfand, 1985; Hansen, Rosenquist, Baggersen, Brown and Christensen, 2007; Loc Carrillo, Connerton, Pearson and Connerton, 2007; Salama, Bolton and Hutchinson, 1989) and they appear to be ubiquitous wherever *Campylobacter* are found. Transmission electron micrographs of a few representative *Campylobacter* phage are shown in Figure 1. Those isolated so far have double stranded DNA genomes and a virion structure consistent with membership of either the *Myoviridae* or *Siphoviridae* families (Atterbury, Connerton, Dodd, Rees and Connerton, 2003a; Sails, Wareing, Bolton, Fox and Curry, 1998; Salama *et al.*, 1989). Compared to the 100 kbp genome size, more typical for other members of the *Myoviridae,* it has previously been noted that *Campylobacter* bacteriophage have unusually large genomes (Sails *et al.*, 1998). Indeed, *Campylobacter* phage commonly fall into one of three genome size ranges, as measured by pulsed-field gel electrophoresis; these include the typing bacteriophage NCTC 12676 and NCTC 12677 which are 320 kbp in size and classified as Group I, although, as shown in Figure 2, in our hands NCTC 12676 would appear to be nearer to 420 kbp. Group II phage with genomes of 180 – 190 kbp and 130 – 140 kbp classified as Group III (Atterbury *et al.*, 2003a; Sails *et al.*, 1998). Precisely what significance the large genome sizes have has

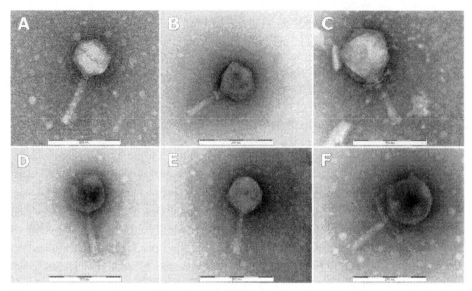

Figure 1. Transmission electron micrographs of *Campylobacter* bacteriophage; A) CP8, B) KW3, C) NCTC 12676 Phage 4, D) KW1, E) CP220 and F) NCTC 12677 phage 12

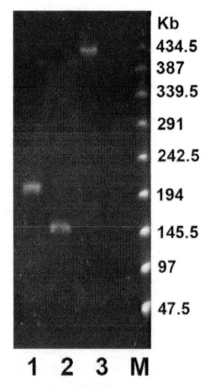

Figure 2. Pulsed Field Gel Electrophoresis of genomic DNA extracted from *Campylobacter* bacteriophage lanes; 1) CP220, 2) CP8, 3) NCTC 12676 and M) molecular weight marker – concatenated phage λ marker.

yet to be determined, but it may be reflected in the wide lytic spectra exhibited against *Campylobacter* strains by some of the larger phages (Frost, Kramer and Gillanders, 1999).

Many of the *Campylobacter* phage thus far isolated have proven to be extremely refractory to genomic analysis. In many cases phage genomic DNA cannot be cut with any of the standard restriction endonucleases, although, *Hha*I has proven to be useful to discriminate some Group III phage (Atterbury *et al.*, 2003a; Loc Carrillo *et al.*, 2007; Sails *et al.*, 1998). Purified DNA has also proven to be very difficult to clone and is extremely refractory to amplification using the Polymerase Chain Reaction, suggesting that the phage DNA may contain unusual nucleotides either incorporated during replication or modified post synthesis (Lunt, Siebke and Burton, 1964; Luria and Human, 1952) and perhaps serving to protect the phage against bacterial endonucleases.

Nevertheless the first phage genomic sequence of a Group II *Campylobacter* phage CP220 has recently been completed at The Welcome Trust Sanger Institute (www.sanger.ac.uk/Projects/Phage/, accessed 22nd August 2008). Preliminary annotation of this 178 kbp sequence has identified the structural proteins that make up the capsid and tail fibres and these have been confirmed from protein sequences derived from phage isolates. The T4-type hallmark protein Gp23 represents the major capsid protein and is clearly recognisable in the *Campylobacter* phage proteome but strangely shows the highest degree of protein sequence similarity with T4-type bacteriophage sequences recovered from marine environments. The genome contains a large number of new reading frames encoding hitherto unrecognised proteins, as well as proteins likely assimilated from a wide variety of bacterial species (Timms,A.R., Scott, A.E., Connerton,P.L. and Connerton,I.F., unpublished observations). As stated previously, the genetic characterisation and understanding of suitable virulent *Campylobacter* bacteriophage is crucial if these bacteriophage are to be utilised to increase food safety.

Decontamination of meat using *Campylobacter* bacteriophage

Phage may be applied directly onto raw produce or onto environmental surfaces in processing facilities, to reduce numbers of food borne pathogens in foods (Sulakvelidze and Barrow, 2005). Application could include phage sprayed onto chicken carcasses after post-chill processing (e.g. after the chlorine wash in "chiller tanks" in the United States, or after processing through air chillers in Europe).

The most effective treatments involve using high doses of phage. Campylobacters are generally believed to be unable to multiply under refrigeration conditions so, unlike *in vivo* therapy, the aim of carcass treatment is not to reduce bacterial numbers through viral replication, but to kill them rapidly through passive inundation or 'lysis from without' or to prevent bacterial out-growth should suitable conditions for bacterial growth occur, i.e. when food is incorrectly stored or contaminated food is consumed. As such, there would be little or no opportunity for growth of phage-resistant or insensitive sub-populations on the surface of the product. Additionally, there is limited recycling of phage in the environment, reducing the possibility of resistance developing in the wider *Campylobacter* population.

Bacteriophage have been successfully applied as a decontamination technique to reduce *C. jejuni* and *Salmonella enterica* on poultry meat under experimental conditions. Goode *et al.* (2003) demonstrated that spraying chicken skin, contaminated with 10^4 CFU/cm^2 of *C. jejuni* C222, with 10^6 plaque forming units (PFU)/cm^2 of phage NCTC 12673 reduced *Campylobacter* recovery by 95%. A $\log_{10}$ 1 CFU reduction of *C. jejuni* NCTC 12662 was also observed by Atterbury *et al.* (2003b) using phage NCTC 12674 that found a combination of phage application and freezing led to a synergistic reduction in *Campylobacter* numbers ($\log_{10}$ 2.5 CFU) compared to the reductions observed when these methods were applied separately. As such, phage treatment could be particularly useful in countries such as Iceland, that routinely freezes *Campylobacter*-positive birds (Stern, Hiett, Alfredsson, Kristinsson, Reiersen, Hardardottir, Briem, Gunnarsson, Georgsson, Lowman, Berndtson, Lammerding, Paoli and Musgrove, 2003). Atterbury *et al.* (2003b) suggested that the observed reduction in *Campylobacter* contamination was most likely to result from the phage adsorbing to their hosts and then initiating replication during the recovery phase on agar plates.

The ability of phage to survive processing is an important aspect of their potential use in the biocontrol of *Campylobacter* in poultry production. Procedures have been developed to recover *Campylobacter* bacteriophage from chilled and frozen retail poultry, and have been validated using a characterised *Campylobacter* phage NCTC 12674 (Atterbury *et al.*, 2003b). Survival experiments demonstrated that bacteriophage can be recovered for up to ten days following inoculation, thus phage could conceivably provide protection throughout the stated shelf life of the product.

Demonstrating efficacy in laboratory trials is only the starting point in the process of making phage treatment of food surfaces viable and many important additional issues will need to be addressed before phages can be used to improve food safety in real-life settings (Greer, 2005). For example, phage preparations added to foods must meet stringent requirements for purity, which requires the development of commercially-viable protocols for large-scale phage production that avoid carry over of bacterial antigens or toxins (Greer, 2005).

Campylobacter specific bacteriophage intervention *in vivo*

There are a number of practical considerations that need to be addressed before any application of phage therapy with perhaps one of the most important being the method of delivery. Phage have the advantage that they are fairly robust in nature and therefore can simply be added to drinking water or encapsulated in feed, provided that the intended targets are intestinal bacteria. However, some phage may be sensitive to the low pH encountered in the stomach or proventriculus (El-Shibiny, Scott, Timms, Metawea, Connerton and Connerton 2008; Leverentz, Conway, Alavidze, Janisiewicz, Fuchs, Camp, Chighladze and Sulakvelidze, 2001; Verthé, Possemiers, Boon, Vaneechoutte and Verstraete, 2004). This particular problem can be overcome through the use of antacid or by selection of appropriate low-pH-tolerant phage. Antacids such as Maalox (aluminium and magnesium hydroxide) or calcium carbonate have been used to improve the ability of phage to survive low acidity in digestive systems (Koo, Marshall and DePaola, 2001; Smith, Huggins and Shaw, 1987a; Verthé *et al.*, 2004).

Phage treatment of chickens was first reported by Wagenaar *et al.* (2005). In a series of experiments the authors compared the effects of both therapeutic and preventative treatment of broiler chickens using two of the phage used in the phage typing scheme of Frost *et al.*, (1999). The administration of phage NCTC 12671 with a dose of approximately $\log_{10}$ 10 PFU/chicken on each of six consecutive days to birds that had been infected 5 days earlier with *C. jejuni* C356 (a strain of *Campylobacter* isolated from a broiler chicken), resulted in a $\log_{10}$ 3 CFU/g decline in caecal counts of *C. jejuni* within 48 h, compared to the non-phage treated controls. After 5 days the *Campylobacter* counts in the treated birds had recovered, but remained approximately $\log_{10}$ 1 CFU/g below controls. Preventative phage treatment using phage NCTC 12671, where doses between $\log_{10}$ 9.7 and $\log_{10}$ 10.3 PFU were given each day to chicks from 7 days of age, delayed but did not prevent the onset of *C. jejuni* colonisation in young birds. Colonisation levels were initially up to $\log_{10}$ 2 lower than seen in the control group, however, *Campylobacter* numbers eventually stabilised at a level $\log_{10}$ 1 lower than the control group. In both applications, the colony forming units and phage forming units rose and fell over time, and were out of phase with each other that is typical of predator-prey populations in nature. In a third experiment, birds were infected with *Campylobacter* at 32 days of age and subsequently treated with a cocktail of phages (NCTC 12669 and NCTC 12671) at 39 days of age at doses between $\log_{10}$ 9.7 and $\log_{10}$ 11.6 PFU, for four consecutive days. Birds of this age were used in order to mimic the age at which broiler chickens approach the optimum size for slaughter thus reproducing the ideal time to administer the treatment in a commercial environment. *Campylobacter* counts in this experiment decreased by $\log_{10}$ 1.5 CFU/g caecal contents compared to controls but rose slightly after four days remaining approximately $\log_{10}$ 1 CFU/g lower than the counts in the control birds. No adverse effects of phage treatment were observed on the birds.

Loc Carrillo *et al.* (2005) performed phage therapy experiments using bacteriophage and *C. jejuni* host strains isolated from broiler chickens. A large number of phages were characterised but only those that showed a broad lytic spectrum were selected for the phage intervention experiments. To evaluate the efficacy of phage therapy, low passage phage-sensitive *C. jejuni* isolates (HPC5 and GIIC8 isolated from UK broiler chickens) were selected on the basis of their ability to reproducibly colonise 20 to 22 day old broilers. Birds of this age were selected to parallel the first detection of colonisation often observed in commercial broiler chickens (Newell and Fearnley, 2003). Chickens at 20 days of age were dosed with the *C. jejuni* strains at a dose of $\log_{10} 8$ CFU, with maximal colonisation achieved within 48 h. These levels were shown to be maintained over the 9 day period of the trial (chickens of 22-30 days of age) without any evidence for the excursion of the organisms from the GIT (for example none were detected in the liver, pancreas, heart or kidney). Phage intervention was carried out using bacteriophage administered as a single treatment to 25 day old birds pre-colonised with *Campylobacter*. Phage were administered at three different doses, $\log_{10} 9$, $\log_{10} 7$ and $\log_{10} 5$ PFU in an antacid suspension. All the experimental bacteriophage treatments of *C. jejuni* colonised birds resulted in the phage persisting in the chicken GIT implying that the phage administered were delivered to the intestinal sites colonised by *C. jejuni* and were able to replicate within this environment. It became apparent that the optimum dose for phage therapy was $\log_{10} 7$ PFU with the higher ($\log_{10} 9$ PFU) and lower doses ($\log_{10} 5$ PFU) of phage being generally less effective (Loc Carrillo *et al.*, 2005). The reason for the highest dose being less effective was unclear but it may have been due to the fact that higher phage densities are prone to phage aggregation and non-specific association with digesta or non-host bacteria (Rabinovitch *et al.*, 2003). Alternatively, it could be due to an initial phage concentration above the inundation threshold, discussed earlier, resulting in a depletion of bacteria, possibly by "lysis from without" and subsequent loss of phage from the system. For the lower dose ($\log_{10} 5$ PFU) the numbers surviving ingestion may simply be insufficient to cause an effect within the experimental time frame.

The success of phage treatment in reducing *Campylobacter* numbers depended on the bacteriophage and on the colonising strain. Some phage, for example CP8, were very effective with one strain (GIIC8) but ineffective with another (HPC5). The bacteriophage-treated birds showed a marked reduction in numbers of campylobacters particularly for the first 48 h after treatment. The reduction in caecal *C. jejuni* numbers varied from phage to phage ranging from $\log_{10} 2$ to $\log_{10} 5$ (per g of caecal contents) compared to untreated controls. The success of treatment was dependant on the bacteriophage and the colonisation strain used with some bacteriophage being considerably more virulent than others. The reductions observed in *Campylobacter* colonisation levels following phage administration were between $\log_{10} 1.5$ and $\log_{10} 5$ CFU/g of intestinal contents. The greatest reductions recorded in the caecal *Campylobacter* counts were observed between 24 and 72 h post-phage treatment in all three sample sites (upper intestine, caecum and lower intestine), after which the *Campylobacter* counts began to recover. The single treatment regime appeared to be effective over 48 h, which would give a window of opportunity to catch and transport the birds for slaughter. In these trials, optimisation of dose and selection of appropriate phage were found to be the key elements in the use of phage therapy to reduce campylobacters in broiler chickens.

Recently a Group II *Campylobacter* bacteriophage, CP220 with a genome size of 180 kbp, was found to be effective against both *C. jejuni* and *C. coli in vitro*. Administration of CP220 to both *C. jejuni* and to *C. coli* colonised birds resulted in reduction of *Campylobacter* counts. A $\log_{10}$ 2 CFU/g decline in caecal *Campylobacter* counts was observed after 48 h in birds colonised with *C. jejuni* HPC5 administered with a single $\log_{10}$ 7 PFU dose of CP220. The level of phage resistance developing upon exposure to virulent phage in chickens was determined for this bacteriophage and found to be at a low level (0.02) indicating that resistance to bacteriophage causes a decrease in *Campylobacter* fitness. To achieve a similar reduction in numbers in *C. coli* OR12 colonised birds, a $\log_{10}$ 9 PFU dose of CP220 was required (El-Shibiny *et al.*, 2008).

The selection of resistant bacteria has always been perceived as a potential drawback to phage therapy and has been reported following phage treatments of experimental animals colonised by *Escherichia coli* (Sklar and Joerger, 2001; Smith and Huggins, 1982; Smith, Huggins and Shaw, 1987b). However for *C. jejuni* colonising broiler chickens, phage resistance can be correlated with a reduced ability to compete against phage sensitive types in the same environment (Scott, Timms, Connerton, El-Shibiny and Connerton, 2007; Scott, Timms, Connerton, Loc, Adzfa and Connerton, 2007). The numbers of phage resistant campylobacters present in the experimental birds following bacteriophage therapy was determined and found to be less than four per cent (Loc Carrillo *et al.*, 2005), comparable to that observed with CP220 phage. Interestingly these resistant isolates appeared to be compromised in their ability to colonise a further set of experimental birds, rapidly reverting back to a phage sensitive phenotype in the absence of phage selection. In contrast, when phage resistant isolates were obtained by mixing host and phage *in vitro* and culturing on laboratory media, the frequency of resistance was found to be 11% and the resistant phenotype was stable on subculture (Loc Carrillo *et al.*, 2005). This frequency of mutation means that phage resistant types soon dominate phage challenged laboratory cultures but this is not observed in equivalent experiments *in vivo*. Other studies have noted decreased fitness when bacteria acquire phage resistance through mutation (Park, Shimamura, Fukunaga, Mori and Nakai, 2000; Smith *et al.*, 1987b). This is often because phage have evolved to target essential structures present on the bacterial outer surface to gain entry to the cell. If bacteria alter these structures through mutation, it may prevent phage entry but can also be detrimental to their fitness such that they do not survive in competitive or challenging environments. Chickens subject to environmental challenge will encounter diverse *Campylobacter* genotypes and, under these conditions, it is therefore more likely that succession of phage-insensitive genotypes is responsible for the recovery of the *Campylobacter* numbers rather than *de novo* development of resistance. The implication from this work was that, while campylobacters like other bacteria can mutate to become resistant to phage, this may have negative consequences in terms of fitness.

PHAGE COCKTAILS

Clearly chickens reared outdoors will be exposed to a wider variety of *Campylobacter* genotypes and bacteriophages than those reared in barns where biosecurity measures are employed to limit the exposure of the birds to biological agents that will affect their welfare or market value. To ensure the effectiveness of phage therapy against as wide a selection of *Campylobacter* strains as possible and to prevent the selection of phage resistant or insensitive types in mixed populations, it has been suggested that phage be applied as a mixture or 'cocktail' to cover a broader range of hosts (Kudva, Jelacic, Tarr, Youderian and Hovde, 1999; Sklar and Joerger, 2001). In practice cocktails of phages having different receptor specificities are preferred as development of cross-resistance becomes less problematic. Using cocktails will assist in the efficacy of the phage preparation, but will require that the individual components are produced and tested individually to ensure their contribution to extending the host range spectrum of the phage mix. Another important quality-control issue is that older phage stocks may become less effective, despite retaining high titres in laboratory tests (Weld *et al.*, 2004). For these reasons limited phage cocktails may be preferred, allowing for individual components to be easily refreshed with new phages and with the possibility of cycling their use to retain their efficacy.

Regulatory issues

There are many restrictions on the types of additives and processing aids which can be used in food production. Therefore, it was important to establish that *Campylobacter*-specific phage could be found naturally associated with poultry meat (Rees and Dodd, 2006). However government regulatory bodies may yet require that phage used for bio-control purposes must be removed from the final product or inactivated (Rees and Dodd, 2006). Atterbury *et al.* (2003b) found that freezing chicken skin inoculated with *Campylobacter* phage led to an appreciable loss of phage recovery, suggesting that physical methods could be used after treatment to inactive the phages if required. One possible method to do this would be crust-freezing which minimises damage to the appearance of the carcass (James,

James, Hannay, Purnell, Barbedo-Pinto, Yaman, Araujo, Gonzalez, Calvo, Howell and Corry, 2007).

In 2006 the United States Food and Drug Administration (FDA) approved a cocktail of six phages for the control of *Listeria monocytogenes* on ready-to-eat meats (United States Food and Drug Administration, 2006). There are several companies in the US and Europe working towards the commercial use of bacteriphage to control food-borne pathogens and in July 2008 it was announced that the United States Department of Agriculture, Food Safety and Inspection Service had issued a 'no objection' letter for use of Salmonella-targeted phage on the feathers of live poultry before processing. This may represent the beginning of the approval process whereby phage treatments are licensed for use in food production.

However the use of bacteriophage in the EU would be subject to directive 89/107/EEC (Food Additives and Processing Aids) that states that the use of any chemical or substance in food preparation or processing is banned unless it is explicitly authorised by the EU (http://ec.europa.eu/food/fs/sfp/addit_flavor/flav07_en.pdf, accessed 21st August 2008). An additional problem is that the use of phage to decontaminate poultry could fit the definition of both a food additive and a processing aid. Although the use of phage treatments is being debated amongst the EU Member States, the bureaucratic nature of the organisation means that approval for such treatments is unlikely to materialise in the immediate future.

Bacteriophage Intervention has been shown to be effective in a number of 'proof of principle' trials for a range of different pathogenic organisms. For *Campylobacter*, the efficacy appears to be enough to achieve a reduction in bacterial load of $\log_{10} 2$ at the pre-slaughter stage that, if carried through the processing cycle to the consumer, should be commensurate with a significant reduction in human cases of campylobacteriosis.

References

Adak, G.K., Meakins, S.M., Yip, H., Lopman, B.A. and O'Brien, S.J. (2005) Disease risks from foods, England and Wales, 1996-2000. *Emerg.Infect. Dis.*, **11**, 365-372.

Ahmed, I.H., Manning, G., Wassenaar, T.M., Cawthraw, S. and Newell, D.G. (2002) Identification of genetic differences between two *Campylobacter jejuni* strains with different colonization potentials. *Microbiology*, **148**, 1203-1212.

Alanis, A.J. (2005) Resistance to antibiotics: are we in the post-antibiotic era? *Arch.Med.Res.*, **36**, 697-705.

Alisky, J., Iczkowski, K., Rapoport, A. and Troitsky, N. (1998) Bacteriophages show promise as antimicrobial agents. *J.Infect.*, **36**, 5-15.

Allos, B.M. (2001) *Campylobacter jejuni* Infections: update on emerging issues and trends. *Clin.Infect Dis.*, **32**, 1201-1206.

Andreatti Filho, R.L., Higgins, J.P., Higgins, S.E., Gaona, G., Wolfenden, A.D., Tellez, G. and Hargis, B.M. (2007) Ability of Bacteriophages Isolated from Different Sources to Reduce *Salmonella enterica* Serovar Enteritidis *In Vitro* and *In Vivo*. *Poult.Sci.*, **86**, 1904-1909.

Atterbury, R.J., Connerton, P.L., Dodd, C.E., Rees, C.E. and Connerton, I.F. (2003a) Isolation and characterization of *Campylobacter* bacteriophages from retail poultry. *Appl.Environ.Microbiol.*, **69**, 4511-4518.

Atterbury, R.J., Dillon, E., Swift, C., Connerton, P.L., Frost, J.A., Dodd, C.E., Rees, C.E. and Connerton, I.F. (2005) Correlation of *Campylobacter* bacteriophage with reduced presence of hosts in broiler chicken ceca. *Appl. Environ.Microbiol.*, **71**, 4885-4887.

Atterbury, R.J., Van Bergen, M.A., Ortiz, F., Lovell, M.A., Harris, J.A., DE, B.A., Wagenaar, J.A., Allen, V.M. and Barrow, P.A. (2007) Bacteriophage therapy to reduce *Salmonella* colonization of broiler chickens. *Appl.Environ. Microbiol.*, **73**, 4543-4549.

Atterbury, R.J., Connerton, P.L., Dodd, C.E.R., Rees, C.E.D. and Connerton, I.F. (2003b) Application of host-specific bacteriophages to the surface of chicken skin leads to a reduction in recovery of *Campylobacter jejuni*. *Appl.Environ. Microbiol.*, **69**, 6302-6306.

Barrow, P., Lovell, M. and Berchieri, A., Jr. (1998) Use of lytic bacteriophage for control of experimental *Escherichia coli* septicemia and meningitis in chickens and calves. *Clin.Diagn.Lab Immunol.*, **5**, 294-298.

Berchieri, A., Jr., Lovell, M.A. and Barrow, P.A. (1991) The activity in the chicken alimentary tract of bacteriophages lytic for *Salmonella typhimurium*. *Res Microbiol.*, **142**, 541-549.

Boyd, E.F. and Brüssow, H. (2002) Common themes among bacteriophage-encoded virulence factors and diversity among the bacteriophages involved. *Trends in Microbiology*, **10**, 521-529.

Bull, J.J., Levin, B., DeRouin, T., Walker, N. and Bloch, C. (2002) Dynamics of success and failure in phage and antibiotic therapy in experimental infections. *BMC Microbiology*, **2**, 35

Cheetham, B.F. and Katz, M.E. (1995) A role for bacteriophages in the evolution and transfer of bacterial virulence determinants. *Mol.Microbiol.*, **18**, 201-208.

Colles, F.M., Jones, K., Harding, R.M. and Maiden, M.C.J. (2003) Genetic diversity of *Campylobacter jejuni* isolates from farm animals and the farm environment. *Appl.Environ.Microbiol.*, **69**, 7409-7413.

Colles, F.M., Jones, T.A., McCarthy, N.D., Sheppard, S.K., Cody, A.J., Dingle, K.E., Dawkins, M.S. and Maiden, M.C. (2008) *Campylobacter* infection of broiler chickens in a free-range environment. *Environ.Microbiol.*, **10**, 2042-2050.

Connerton, P.L., Loc Carrillo, C.M., Swift, C., Dillon, E., Scott, A., Rees, C.E.D., Dodd, C.E.R., Frost, J. and Connerton, I.F. (2004) Longitudinal study of *Campylobacter jejuni* bacteriophages and their hosts from broiler chickens. *Appl.Environ.Microbiol.*, **70**, 3877-3883.

Corry, J.E.L. and Atabay, H.I. (2001) Poultry as a source of *Campylobacter* and related organisms. *Symp.Ser.Soc.Appl Microbiol.*, **30**, 96S-114S.

Cox, N.A., Richardson, L.J., Bailey, J.S., Cosby, D.E., Cason, J.A., Musgrove, M.T. and Mead, G.C. (2005) Bacterial contamination of poultry as a risk to human health. In *Food safety control in the poultry industry,* **pp** 21-43. Edited by G.C. Mead. Woodhead Publishing, Cambridge.

Delbrück, M. (1940) The Growth of Bacteriophage and Lysis of the Host. *J Gen. Physiol*, **23**, 643-660.

Doyle, M.P. and Erickson, M.C. (2006) Reducing the carriage of foodborne pathogens in livestock and poultry. *Poult Sci.*, **85**, 960-973.

El-Shibiny, A., Connerton, P.L. and Connerton, I.F. (2005) Enumeration and diversity of Campylobacters and bacteriophages isolated during the rearing cycles of free-range and organic chickens. *Appl.Environ.Microbiol.*, **71**, 1259-1266.

El-Shibiny, A., Scott, A.E., Timms, A.R., Metawea, Y., Connerton, P.L. and Connerton, I.F. (2008) A class II *Campylobacter* bacteriophage to reduce *C.jejuni* and *C.coli* in poultry production. Submitted for publication.

Frost, J.A., Kramer, J.M. and Gillanders, S.A. (1999) Phage typing of *Campylobacter jejuni* and *Campylobacter coli* and its use as an adjunct to serotyping. *Epidemiol.Infect.*, **123**, 47-55.

Gamage, S.D., Strasser, J.E., Chalk, C.L. and Weiss, A.A. (2003) Nonpathogenic *Escherichia coli* can contribute to the production of Shiga toxin. *Infect. Immun.*, **71**, 3107-3115.

Goode, D., Allen, V.M. and Barrow, P.A. (2003) Reduction of experimental *Salmonella* and *Campylobacter* contamination of chicken skin by application of lytic bacteriophages. *Appl.Environ.Microbiol.*, **69**, 5032-5036.

Grajewski, B.A., Kusek, J.W. and Gelfand, H.M. (1985) Development of a bacteriophage typing system for *Campylobacter jejuni* and *Campylobacter coli. J Clin.Microbiol.*, **22**, 13-18.

Greer, G.G. (2005) Bacteriophage control of foodborne bacteria. *J.Food Prot.*, **68**, 1102-1111.

Hansen, V.M., Rosenquist, H., Baggersen, D.L., Brown, S. and Christensen, B.B. (2007) Characterization of Campylobacter phages including analysis of host range by selected Campylobacter Penner serotypes. *BMC.Microbiol.*, **7**, 90.

Health Protection Agency (2008) Recent trends in selected gastrointestinal infections. *Health Protection Report*, **2**, No. 28.

Hendrix, R.W., Smith, M.C., Burns, R.N., Ford, M.E. and Hatfull, G.F. (1999) Evolutionary relationships among diverse bacteriophages and prophages: All the world's a phage. *PNAS*, **96**, 2192-2197.

Herman, L., Heyndrickx, M., Grijspeerdt, K., Vandekerchove, D., Rollier, I. and De, Z.L. (2003) Routes for *Campylobacter* contamination of poultry meat: epidemiological study from hatchery to slaughterhouse. *Epidemiol.Infect.*, **131**, 1169-1180.

Hofreuter, D., Tsai, J., Watson, R.O., Novik, V., Altman, B., Benitez, M., Clark, C., Perbost, C., Jarvie, T., Du, L. and Galan, J.E. (2006) Unique features of a highly pathogenic *Campylobacter jejuni* strain. *Infect Immun.*, **74**, 4694-4707.

Hudson, J.A., Billington, C., Carey-Smith, G. and Greening, G. (2005) Bacteriophages as biocontrol agents in food. *J.Food Prot.*, **68**, 426-437.

Huff, W.E., Huff, G.R., Rath, N.C., Balog, J.M. and Donoghue, A.M. (2002) Prevention of *Escherichia coli* infection in broiler chickens with a bacteriophage aerosol spray. *Poult.Sci*, **81**, 1486-1491.

Huff, W.E., Huff, G.R., Rath, N.C., Balog, J.M. and Donoghue, A.M. (2003) Bacteriophage treatment of a severe *Escherichia coli* respiratory infection in broiler chickens. *Avian Dis.*, **47**, 1399-1405.

Huff, W.E., Huff, G.R., Rath, N.C., Balog, J.M. and Donoghue, A.M. (2005) Alternatives to antibiotics: utilization of bacteriophage to treat colibacillosis and prevent foodborne pathogens. *Poult.Sci.*, **84**, 655-659.

James, C., James, S.J., Hannay, N., Purnell, G., Barbedo-Pinto, C., Yaman, H., Araujo, M., Gonzalez, M.L., Calvo, J., Howell, M. and Corry, J.E. (2007) Decontamination of poultry carcasses using steam or hot water in combination with rapid cooling, chilling or freezing of carcass surfaces. *Int.J Food Microbiol.*, **114**, 195-203.

Johnson, D.M., Stilwell, M.G., Fritsche, T.R. and Jones, R.N. (2006) Emergence of multidrug-resistant *Streptococcus pneumoniae*: report from the SENTRY Antimicrobial Surveillance Program (1999-2003). *Diagn.Microbiol.Infect. Dis.*, **56**, 69-74.

Jorgensen, F., Bailey, R., Williams, S., Henderson, P., Wareing, D.R., Bolton, F.J., Frost, J.A., Ward, L. and Humphrey, T.J. (2002) Prevalence and numbers of *Salmonella* and *Campylobacter* spp. on raw, whole chickens in relation to sampling methods. *Int.J Food Microbiol.*, **76**, 151-164.

Katsma, W.E., De Koeijer, A.A., Jacobs-Reitsma, W.F., Mangen, M.J. and Wagenaar, J.A. (2007) Assessing interventions to reduce the risk of *Campylobacter* prevalence in broilers. *Risk Anal.*, **27**, 863-876.

Klein, G., Beckmann, L., Vollmer, H.M. and Bartelt, E. (2007) Predominant strains of thermophilic *Campylobacter* spp. in a german poultry slaughterhouse. *Int.J.Food Microbiol.*, **117**, 324-328.

Koo, J., Marshall, D.L. and DePaola, A. (2001) Antacid increases survival of *Vibrio vulnificus* and *Vibrio vulnificus* phage in a gastrointestinal model. *Appl Environ.Microbiol.*, **67**, 2895-2902.

Korczak, B.M., Stieber, R., Emler, S., Burnens, A.P., Frey, J. and Kuhnert, P. (2006) Genetic relatedness within the genus *Campylobacter* inferred from *rpoB* sequences. *Int.J Syst.Evol.Microbiol.*, **56**, 937-945.

Kramer, J.M., Frost, J.A., Bolton, F.J. and Wareing, D.R. (2000) *Campylobacter* contamination of raw meat and poultry at retail sale: identification of multiple types and comparison with isolates from human infection. *J Food Prot.*, **63**, 1654-1659.

Kudva, I.T., Jelacic, S., Tarr, P.I., Youderian, P. and Hovde, C.J. (1999) Biocontrol of *Escherichia coli* O157 with O157-Specific Bacteriophages. *Appl.Environ. Microbiol.*, **65**, 3767-3773.

Leverentz, B., Conway, W.S., Alavidze, Z., Janisiewicz, W.J., Fuchs, Y., Camp, M.J., Chighladze, E. and Sulakvelidze, A. (2001) Examination of bacteriophage as a biocontrol method for *Salmonella* on fresh-cut fruit: a model study. *J Food Prot.*, **64**, 1116-1121.

Levin, B.R. and Bull, J.J. (1996) Phage Therapy Revisited: The Population Biology of a Bacterial Infection and Its Treatment with Bacteriophage and Antibiotics. *Am.Nat.*, **147**, 881-898.

Lindqvist, R. and Lindblad, M. (2008) Quantitative risk assessment of thermophilic *Campylobacter* spp. and cross-contamination during handling of raw broiler chickens evaluating strategies at the producer level to reduce human campylobacteriosis in Sweden. *Int.J Food Microbiol.*, **121**, 41-52.

Loc Carrillo, C., Atterbury, R.J., El-Shibiny, A., Connerton, P.L., Dillon, E., Scott, A. and Connerton, I.F. (2005) Bacteriophage therapy to reduce *Campylobacter jejuni* colonization of broiler chickens. *Appl.Environ. Microbiol.*, **71**, 6554-6563.

Loc Carrillo, C.M., Connerton, P.L., Pearson, T. and Connerton, I.F. (2007) Free-range layer chickens as a source of *Campylobacter* bacteriophage. *Antonie Van Leeuwenhoek*, **92**, 275-284.

Lunt, M.R., Siebke, J.C. and Burton, K. (1964) Glucosylated nucleotide sequences from T2-bacteriophage deoxyribonucleic acid. *Biochem.J*, **92**, 27-36.

Luria, S.E. and Human, M.L. (1952) A nonhereditary, host-induced variation of bacterial viruses. *J Bacteriol.*, **64**, 557-569.

McCrea, B.A., Tonooka, K.H., VanWorth, C., Atwill, E.R. and Schrader, J.S. (2006) Colonizing capability of *Campylobacter jejuni* genotypes from low-prevalence avian species in broiler chickens. *J Food Prot.*, **69**, 417-420.

McDonald, L.C. (2006) Trends in antimicrobial resistance in health care-associated pathogens and effect on treatment. *Clin.Infect.Dis.*, **42 Suppl 2**, S65-S71.

Mead, P.S., Slutsker, L., Dietz, V., McCaig, L.F., Bresee, J.S., Shapiro, C., Griffin, P.M. and Tauxe, R.V. (1999) Food-related illness and death in the United States. *Emerg.Infect.Dis.*, **5**, 607-625.

Merril, C.R., Scholl, D. and Adhya, S.L. (2003) The prospect for bacteriophage therapy in Western medicine. *Nat.Rev.Drug Discov.*, **2**, 489-497.

Miller, W.G. and Mandrell, R.E. (2005) Prevalence of *Campylobacter* in the food and water supply: incidence, outbreaks, isolation and detection. In Campylobacter: *Molecular and Cellular Biology*, **pp** 101-163. Edited by J.M. Ketley and M.E. Konkel. Horizon Bioscience, Norfolk VA.

Nachamkin, I. (2002) Chronic effects of *Campylobacter* infection. *Microbes Infect.*, **4**, 399-403.

Newell, D.G. and Fearnley, C. (2003) Sources of *Campylobacter* colonization in broiler chickens. *Appl.Environ.Microbiol.*, **69**, 4343-4351.

O'Brien, A.D., Newland, J.W., Miller, S.F., Holmes, R.K., Smith, H.W. and Formal, S.B. (1984) Shiga-like toxin-converting phages from *Escherichia coli* strains that cause hemorrhagic colitis or infantile diarrhea. *Science*, **226**, 694-696.

Overell, J.R. and Willison, H.J. (2005) Recent developments in Miller Fisher syndrome and related disorders. *Curr.Opin.Neurol.*, **18**, 562-566.

Park, S.C., Shimamura, I., Fukunaga, M., Mori, K.I. and Nakai, T. (2000) Isolation of bacteriophages specific to a fish pathogen, *Pseudomonas plecoglossicida*, as a candidate for disease control. *Appl Environ.Microbiol.*, **66**, 1416-1422.

Payne, R.J. and Jansen, V.A. (2002) Evidence for a phage proliferation threshold? *J Virol.*, **76**, 13123-13124.

Payne, R.J. and Jansen, V.A. (2003) Pharmacokinetic principles of bacteriophage therapy. *Clin.Pharmacokinet.*, **42**, 315-325.

Payne, R.J., Phil, D. and Jansen, V.A. (2000) Phage therapy: the peculiar kinetics of self-replicating pharmaceuticals. *Clin.Pharmacol.Ther.*, **68**, 225-230.

Payne, R.J.H. and Jansen, V.A.A. (2001) Understanding bacteriophage therapy as a density-dependent kinetic process. *Journal of Theoretical Biology*, **208**, 37-48.

Rabinovitch, A., Aviram, I. and Zaritsky, A. (2003) Bacterial debris--an ecological mechanism for coexistence of bacteria and their viruses. *Journal of Theoretical Biology*, **224**, 377-383.

Rees, C.E. and Dodd, C.E. (2006) Phage for rapid detection and control of bacterial pathogens in food. *Adv.Appl Microbiol.*, **59**, 159-186.

Reich, F., Atanassova, V., Haunhorst, E. and Klein, G. (2008) The effects of *Campylobacter* numbers in caeca on the contamination of broiler carcasses with *Campylobacter*. *Int.J Food Microbiol.*, In Press. doi:10.1016/j.ijfoodmicro.2008.06.018

Roberts, J.A., Cumberland, P., Sockett, P.N., Wheeler, J., Rodrigues, L.C., Sethi, D. and Roderick, P.J. (2003) The study of infectious intestinal disease in England: socio-economic impact. *Epidemiol.Infect.*, **130**, 1-11.

Rosenquist, H., Nielsen, N.L., Sommer, H.M., Nørrung, B. and Christensen, B.B. (2003) Quantitative risk assessment of human campylobacteriosis associated with thermophilic *Campylobacter* species in chickens. *Int.J Food Microbiol.*, **83**, 87-103.

Rudi, K., Høidal, H.K., Katla, T., Johansen, B.K., Nordal, J. and Jakobsen, K.S. (2004) Direct real-time PCR quantification of *Campylobacter jejuni* in chicken fecal and cecal samples by integrated cell concentration and DNA purification. *Appl Environ.Microbiol.*, **70**, 790-797.

Sails, A.D., Wareing, D.R., Bolton, F.J., Fox, A.J. and Curry, A. (1998) Characterisation of 16 *Campylobacter jejuni* and *C. coli* typing bacteriophages. *J.Med.Microbiol.*, **47**, 123-128.

Salama, S., Bolton, F.J. and Hutchinson, D.N. (1989) Improved method for the isolation of *Campylobacter jejuni* and *Campylobacter coli* bacteriophages. *Lett Appl Microbiol.*, **8**, 5-7.

Scotland, S.M., Smith, H.R., Willshaw, G.A. and Rowe, B. (1983) Vero cytotoxin production in strain of *Escherichia coli* is determined by genes carried on bacteriophage. *Lancet*, **2**, 216.

Scott, A.E., Timms, A.R., Connerton, P.L., El-Shibiny, A. and Connerton, I.F. (2007) Bacteriophage influence *Campylobacter jejuni* types populating broiler chickens. *Environ.Microbiol.*, **9**, 2341-2353.

Scott, A.E., Timms, A.R., Connerton, P.L., Loc, C.C., Adzfa, R.K. and Connerton, I.F. (2007) Genome Dynamics of *Campylobacter jejuni* in Response to Bacteriophage Predation. *PLoS.Pathog.*, **3**, e119.

Sklar, I.B. and Joerger, R.D. (2001) Attempts to utilize bacteriophage to combat *Salmonella enterica* serovar Enteritidis infection in chickens. *J Food Safety*, **21**, 15-30.

Smith, H.R., Day, N.P., Scotland, S.M., Gross, R.J. and Rowe, B. (1984) Phage-determined production of vero cytotoxin in strains of *Escherichia coli* serogroup O157. *Lancet*, **1**, 1242-1243.

Smith, H.W. and Huggins, M.B. (1982) Successful treatment of experimental *Escherichia coli* infections in mice using phage: its general superiority over antibiotics. *J Gen.Microbiol.*, **128**, 307-318.

Smith, H.W., Huggins, M.B. and Shaw, K.M. (1987a) Factors influencing the survival and multiplication of bacteriophages in calves and in their environment. *J Gen Microbiol.*, **133**, 1127-1135.

Smith, H.W., Huggins, M.B. and Shaw, K.M. (1987b) The control of experimental *Escherichia coli* diarrhoea in calves by means of bacteriophages. *J.Gen. Microbiol.*, **133**, 1111-1126.

Stern, N.J., Hiett, K.L., Alfredsson, G.A., Kristinsson, K.G., Reiersen, J., Hardardottir, H., Briem, H., Gunnarsson, E., Georgsson, F., Lowman, R., Berndtson, E., Lammerding, A.M., Paoli, G.M. and Musgrove, M.T. (2003) *Campylobacter* spp. in Icelandic poultry operations and human disease. *Epidemiol.Infect.*, **130**, 23-32.

Sulakvelidze, A. and Barrow, P. (2005) Phage therapy in animals and agribusiness. In *Bacteriophages: Biology and Applications*, **pp** 335-380. Edited by E. Kutter and A. Sulakvelidze. CRC Press, Boca Raton.

Sulakvelidze, A., Alavidze, Z. and Morris, J.G., Jr. (2001) Bacteriophage Therapy. *Antimicrob.Agents Chemother.*, **45**, 649-659.

Summers, W.C. (2001) Bacteriophage Therapy. *Annual Review of Microbiology*, **55**, 437-451.

Tauxe, R.V. (2002) Emerging foodborne pathogens. *Int.J Food Microbiol.*, **78**, 31-41.

Ternhag, A., Törner, A., Svensson, Å., Ekdahl, K. and Giesecke, J. (2008) Short- and long-term effects of bacterial gastrointestinal infections. *Emerg.Infect. Dis.*, **14**, 143-148.

Toro, H., Price, S.B., McKee, A.S., Hoerr, F.J., Krehling, J., Perdue, M. and Bauermeister, L. (2005) Use of bacteriophages in combination with competitive exclusion to reduce *Salmonella* from infected chickens. *Avian Dis.*, **49**, 118-124.

United States Food and Drug Administration (2006) Food Additives Permitted for Direct Addition to Food for Human Consumption; Bacteriophage Preparation. *Federal Register*, **71**, 47729-47732.

Van Gerwe, T.J.W.M., Bouma, A., Jacobs-Reitsma, W.F., van den Broek, J., Klinkenberg, D., Stegeman, J.A. and Heesterbeek, J.A.P. (2005) Quantifying transmission of *Campylobacter* spp. among broilers. *Appl.Environ. Microbiol.*, **71**, 5765-5770.

Verthé, K., Possemiers, S., Boon, N., Vaneechoutte, M. and Verstraete, W. (2004) Stability and activity of an *Enterobacter aerogenes*-specific bacteriophage under simulated gastro-intestinal conditions. *Appl Microbiol.Biotechnol.*, **65**, 465-472.

Wagenaar, J.A., Bergen, M.A., Mueller, M.A., Wassenaar, T.M. and Carlton, R.M. (2005) Phage therapy reduces *Campylobacter jejuni* colonization in broilers. *Vet.Microbiol.*, **109**, 275-283.

Wagenaar, J.A., Jacobs-Reitsma, W.F., Hofshagen, M. and Newell, D.G. (2008) Poultry Colonization with *Campylobacter* and its control at the primary production level. In *Campylobacter* 3rd Edition, **pp** 667-678. Edited by I. Nachamkin, C.M. Szymanski and M.J. Blaser. ASM Press.

Weld, R.J., Butts, C. and Heinemann, J.A. (2004) Models of phage growth and their applicability to phage therapy. *Journal of Theoretical Biology*, **227**, 1-11.

Wheeler, J.G., Sethi, D., Cowden, J.M., Wall, P.G., Rodrigues, L.C., Tompkins, D.S., Hudson, M.J. and Roderick, P.J. (1999) Study of infectious intestinal disease in England: rates in the community, presenting to general practice and reported to national surveillance. The Infectious Intestinal Disease Study Executive. *BMJ*, **318**, 1046-1050.

Wiggins, B.A. and Alexander, M. (1985) Minimum bacterial density for bacteriophage replication: implications for significance of bacteriophages in natural ecosystems. *Appl.Environ.Microbiol.*, **49**, 19-23.

Wingstrand, A., Neimann, J., Engberg, J., Nielsen, E.M., Gerner-Smidt, P., Wegener, H.C. and Mølbak, K. (2006) Fresh chicken as main risk factor for campylobacteriosis, Denmark. *Emerg.Infect.Dis.*, **12**, 280-285.

Xie, H., Zhuang, X., Kong, J., Ma, G. and Zhang, H. (2005) Bacteriophage Esc-A is an efficient therapy for *Escherichia coli* 3-1 caused diarrhea in chickens. *J Gen.Appl Microbiol.*, **51**, 159-163.

Yuki, N. and Koga, M. (2006) Bacterial infections in Guillain-Barré and Fisher syndromes. *Curr Opin Neurol.*, **19**, 451-457.

8

GLOBAL SUPPLIES AND TRENDS IN COMMODITIES

ANGELA BOOTH
Commercial Services Director, AB Agri Ltd, Oundle Road, Peterborough PE2 9PW

During the last few years, agricultural commodity prices have seen substantial increases accompanied by a significant expansion in volatility. For the purpose of this chapter, agricultural commodities will be defined as those bulk feed materials used to manufacture compound pig, poultry and ruminant feeds. Equally, although global trends will be discussed, prices will be mentioned in the context of the UK market only, and in relation to the time of writing (August 2008). Figure 1, which relates to the wheat futures price on the LIFFE market, demonstrates the significant rise in wheat prices over the last 18 months, which is a typical example of the pattern of recent commodity prices.

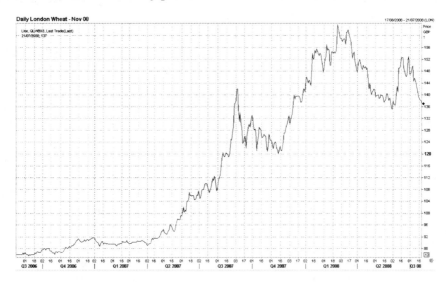

Figure 1. LIFFE wheat futures (Courtesy of Reuters)

147

Protein sources have shown substantial increases also, as is seen in Figure 2. This shows the Chicago soya meal price over the last two years and demonstrates the rapid price increase that has been experienced with this commodity.

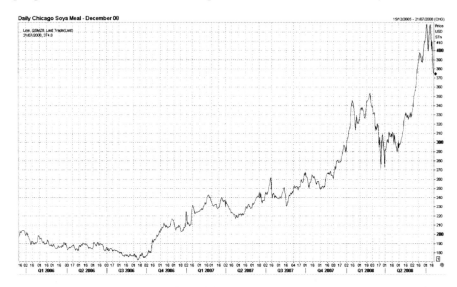

Figure 2. Chicago soya meal futures (Courtesy of Reuters)

Commodity prices are fundamental to any feed compounder, as his role is to balance the cost of the feed input against the value of the animal output and maximise the difference. Understanding and being able to predict commodity prices enables the feed compounder to minimise the price of his purchases and to buy the most cost-effective range of commodities. In the past, to a large extent, commodity prices have been influenced principally by the fundamental factors of supply and demand. Threats to food security have led to governments in various parts of the globe creating measures that are also manipulating this supply and demand scenario. In addition, over the last 5 years, the commodity futures markets have been a favourite investment area for speculators. Whilst still reacting to supply and demand, this pure investment involvement would seem to have exacerbated the increased volatility that is present today. Figure 3 indicates the change in volatility over the last ten years. The upper part of the chart shows the market price for soyabean meal and the lower part of the chart describes the implied volatility.

Inevitably the rising price of oil (Figure 4) has had an effect on the price of agricultural commodities, particularly with the link with biofuel production, which will be discussed later in this chapter. However, it is interesting to compare the relativity between the prices of food, agricultural commodities and oil over time. Whilst these showed a close relationship over 10 years ago, that relationship has

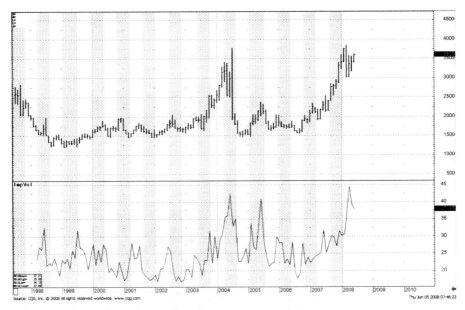

Figure 3. Market volatility (Source CQG Inc)

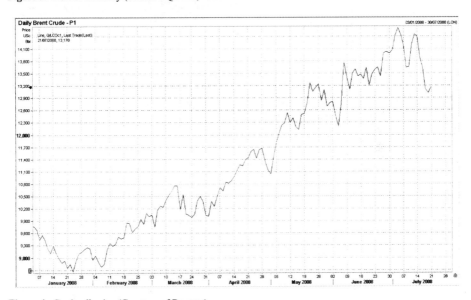

Figure 4. Crude oil price (Courtesy of Reuters)

now changed, and some might argue that the price of agricultural commodities and food should be higher. Comparing the price index for food with the index for all commodities and that for oil, shows that whilst the food commodity index has risen 98%, that of all commodities has increased by 286% and the oil index escalated by a startling 547%.

Commodity supply

CEREALS

Current world cereal production of approximately 2 billion tonnes is dominated by corn (maize), wheat and rice, which constitute 39%, 30% and 20% of the total respectively. Corn and wheat are the commodities of interest to the animal feed industry. The split of total cereal supply is shown in Figure 5.

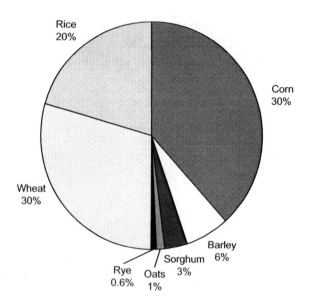

Figure 5. World cereal production by type 2007/8 (Source USDA)

CORN

Both the global area used for corn production and the yield has been increasing steadily but slowly over the last twenty years, and are now the highest ever in both respects (Figure 6). Corn production is dominated by the quantity grown in USA, which amounts to over 300 million tonnes. This is more than twice that of the next largest corn producer, China (Figure 7). During recent years a growing area has been devoted to corn at the expense of soyabean for the biofuels market; this battle for area depends on the relative profitability of the two options and on weather conditions at the time of planting.

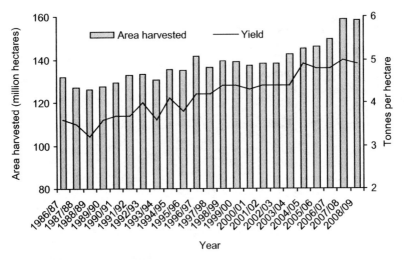

Figure 6. World corn harvest (Source USDA)

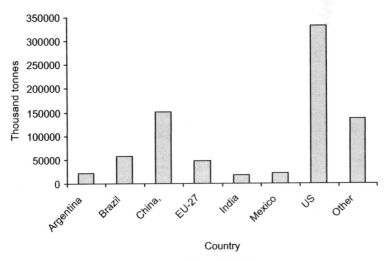

Figure 7. World corn production (2007/8) by country (Source USDA)

WHEAT

The area used for wheat production on a global basis shows little sign of increasing and is lower now than it was in the mid 1990s. Average wheat yield has increased only gradually and at the current yield of 3 tonne/ha still has significant potential to fulfil. The pattern of this change can be seen in Figure 8. Unlike corn production, global wheat production is spread across a number of countries (Figure 9), although the EU-27, China, India and USA predominate.

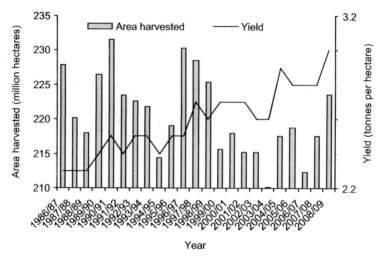

Figure 8. World wheat harvest (Source USDA)

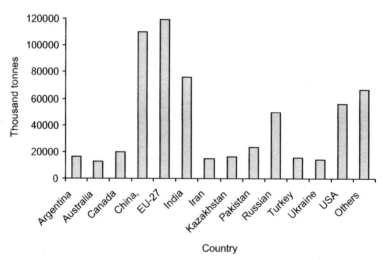

Figure 9. World wheat production 2007/8 (Source USDA)

For the last two years the global wheat crop has suffered as a consequence of weather; the Australian crop was virtually halved due to drought and similarly the EU crop was reduced by approximately 10% (Table 1). Conditions are currently looking good for this year and hence an increase in production is predicted to over 650 million tonnes, which is likely to be the highest ever production.

Table 1. Australia and EU-27 Wheat Production (thousand tonnes) 2004/5 to 2008/9 (Source USDA)

	2004/5	2005/6	2006/7	2007/8	2008/9
Australia	21,905	25,173	10,641	13,100	24,000
EU-27	146,886	132,356	124,783	119,481	140,000

OILSEEDS

As regards oilseeds, nearly 60% of the total oilseeds production is soyabeans (Figure 10). 218 million tonnes of soyabeans were produced in 2007/8 and this is anticipated being higher in 2008/9. Rapeseed and cottonseed are the second largest, but a long way behind at 12% of total production. USA, China, India, Brazil and Argentina are the main soyabean growing counties of the world, with Brazil and Argentina in particular, increasing steadily the production of beans over the last few years, as depicted in Figure 11 which shows the growth in production from exporting countries. China and India use their production for their own domestic consumption and hence export little. With the USA also increasing the amount grown, global soyabean production has been rising over the last few years until last year (2007/8) when it was 218 million tonnes compared to 236 million tonnes in the previous year. This was mainly due to USA reducing the area planted with soyabean from 30 million hectares to 25 million hectares as a consequence of farmers switching land into corn production due to demand from the ethanol industry. However, the balance has changed again this year and total soyabean production is expected to reach a record 240 million tonnes.

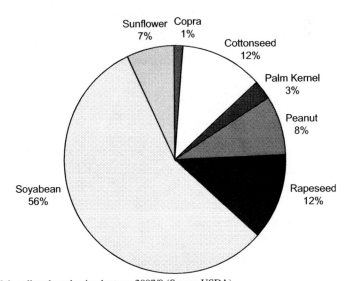

Figure 10. Major oilseed production by type 2007/8 (Source USDA)

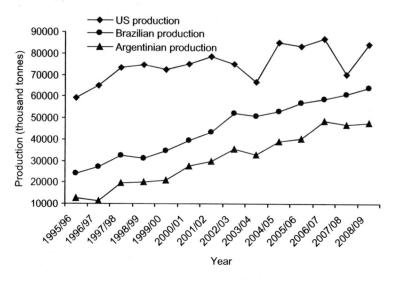

Figure 11. Soyabean production in major exporting countries (Source USDA)

Factors affecting supply

The stability of food prices over the last two decades led to a feeling of complacency, which resulted in situations such as the Common Agricultural Policy paying arable farmers not to grow food crops; and similar programmes existed in the USA. At the same time, government and institution research programmes relating to maximising crop production were reduced substantially. Near-market research by private companies continued, but this was more likely to be investigating cost reduction rather increasing crop yield. As supply and demand start to put pressure on global stocks, the negative impact of these decisions is being seen.

WEATHER AND NATURAL DISASTERS

As is inevitable with an agricultural crop, weather plays a significant role in the supply equation, and this can be seen in situations detailed already. However in recent times there has been a catalogue of events that have affected crop production globally; for example, extremely cold weather in China, cyclone in Pakistan, floods in USA, earthquake in China. Although general variations in frost, rainfall and temperature have always been relevant, some people suggest that adverse weather and natural effects are becoming more pronounced. The ability to predict them is low, and the effects are inevitably substantial.

ASYNCHRONOUS AUTHORISATION

A further complication exists in the EU in relation to legislation, which unless changed will impact upon feed materials imported into the EU from 2009 onwards. 'Asynchronous GM (genetic modification) authorisation' refers to genetic modification traits that have been approved outside the EU, but are not approved within the EU. Legislation in the EU has zero tolerance on the presence of feed material containing an unauthorised genetic trait; hence it cannot be present. This 'zero tolerance' approach means that importers will not risk importing feed materials into the EU if there are GM varieties being grown in exporting countries. The most likely feed materials to be affected are soyabean meal and corn co-products such as corn gluten. There are already a number of varieties of soyabean approved in the US by the Food and Drug administration and US Department of Agriculture (for example Round-up Ready [RR11/Mon-89788], which are being grown for seed to harvest in autumn 2008 but are not authorised in the EU. These will be in commercial production for harvest in 2009. DGAGRI in their own report state that in the worst case scenario, EU pig and poultry production could fall by 29% in 2009 and 44% in 2010, and feed expenditure rising by 600% in 2010 is a possibility. Lobbying on this subject has been extensive within the EU, with the livestock industry seeking a faster approach to approval and changing the 'zero tolerance' approach. As regards the last point, the EU is currently seeking a technical solution to the problem.

POLITICAL INTERVENTION

The concern over food security has led to numerous exporting countries protecting their internal market and, on the other side of the equation, changes in policy from importing countries. Protection policy measures exist as different types. Export taxes are present in several cases; for example, Argentina created a substantial export tax on soya exports, China increased the tariff for exported grains, Russia and Kazakhstan applied an export tax on wheat, whilst Malaysia acted similarly with regard to palm oil. In another scenario, India imposed a minimum export tax for basmati rice. Elsewhere, governments reduced the volume of exports allowed or have banned them completely; Argentina banned maize exports, China, Egypt and Vietnam banned rice exports and India did the same with non-basmati rice. Importing countries were also taking action; some, such as Bolivia, India and El Salvador, decreased or removed import tariffs. In other situations subsidies were available on the commodities to help the consumer; Bangladesh provided subsidies on rice and Senegal on wheat. A further tactic was to subsidise the inputs needed to grow the crops; hence China initiated subsidies on machinery, fuel and fertiliser, and Malawi did likewise for fertiliser. Decisions were also taken to increase stock piles, as happened in India. Finally, some countries took atypical actions; for example, Iran imported from the USA. In short, exporting countries have attempted to reduce supplies whilst importers have less opportunity and want to buy more.

Commodity demand

In the long term, demand for agricultural commodities continues to strengthen for several reasons and constantly challenges supply. A recent report from the Economic Research Unit of the USDA describes how there has been only one year since 2000 when global demand for cereals and oilseeds has not exceeded production. Consequently stocks of both have declined sharply, with the 'stocks-to-use' ratio falling from 30% to less than 15%. This is ably demonstrated by Figures 12 and 13, which show the end stocks of corn and wheat at their lowest in 2007/8, with hopefully a slight improvement in this harvest year. Global stocks of soyabean also showed a decrease in 2007/8 (Figure 14).

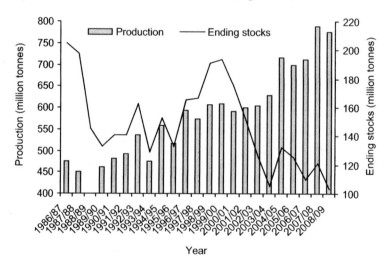

Figure 12. Global corn production and ending stocks (Source USDA)

POPULATION GROWTH AND INCREASING WEALTH

Demand for agricultural commodities is partly being driven by population growth, although this is slowing. Figure 15 shows the predicted change in population growth rate over the next 10 years which, although declining in comparison to previous

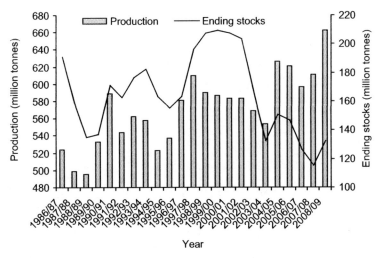

Figure 13. Global wheat production and ending stocks (Source USDA)

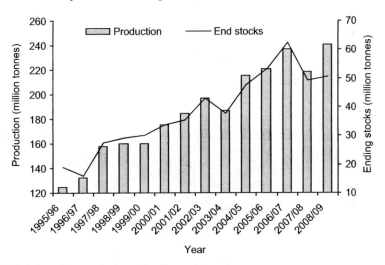

Figure 14. Global soyabean production and ending stocks

years, will result in a substantially increased global population. However, increasing wealth in developing countries is a major factor for the growing demand for livestock products. This is further exacerbated by the migration of rural populations to urban areas and consequently a change in diet.

Figure 16 shows the varying rates of GDP growth in different parts of the world. The former Soviet Union, China and India are predicted to maintain high rates of wealth creation. China has historically had the highest growth rate in Asia with figures over 10% in the last few years. Whilst this is expected to reduce, it will nevertheless exceed 8%. India is expected to be not far behind China. This

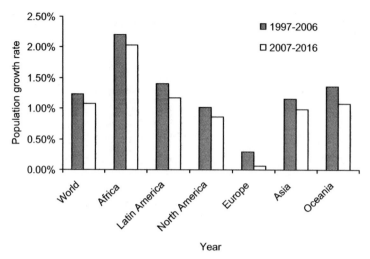

Figure 15. Comparative population growth (Source UN 2004)

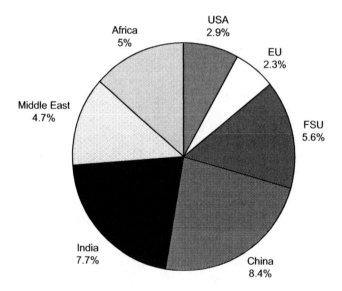

Figure 16. Global real GDP growth assumptions 2008-2017 (Source USDA)

ultimately results in a change of diet with staple foods being replaced by more meat, dairy, fruit, vegetables and processed foods. The increase in meat consumption per capita is an important factor to consider in the supply and demand balance for agricultural commodities. Figure 17 shows how consumption of meat in China, Russia and Ukraine is expected to increase significantly in the next 10 years, whereas meat consumption in the European Union and in the USA will remain almost static. The population of China currently exceeds 1.3 billion: an increase

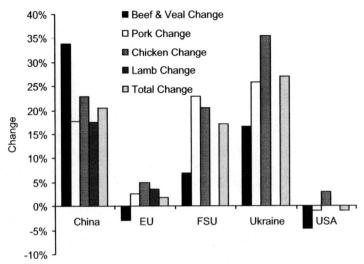

Figure 17. Meat consumption per capita change 2007-2017 (Source FAPRI Agriculture 2008 Outlook)

in total meat consumption of 10kg per capita would result in a requirement for an additional 13 million tonnes of meat in China alone and a consequential increase in demand for agricultural commodities to feed that livestock.

The migration of rural population to urban areas is likely to have a further effect. In this scenario, more reliance is placed upon longer distribution chains, with much greater emphasis placed upon activities where costs are energy dependent. Hence food price is affected increasingly by changes in energy prices rather than the base commodity price and conversely, affected decreasingly by changes in the base commodity price. This means that as commodity prices rise or fall there is less response in terms of demand. Also, as food costs comprise a smaller proportion of expenditure, the impact of higher food prices becomes less.

However, food security is a global issue rather than one related to individual countries. For example, the UK government has published a report (July 2008) entitled 'Food Matters – Towards a Strategy for the 21st Century', which states the actions to be taken "- both in the UK and globally – to ensure our long-term food security, the sustainability of food production and consumption, and the promotion of public health". Concern that the era of cheap and stable food prices is over is a global problem that cannot be tackled in isolation.

BIO-FUELS

A major change in the supply and demand balance for cereals and oilseeds since 2000 is the emergence of the bio-fuels market. This brings a completely different perspective with a new market that is not connected to food or feed and is effectively a fossil fuel substitute. Global demand for oil continues to strengthen due to the global economic activity and especially as a result of meeting the needs of heavily energy-dependent industrial growth in developing countries such as India and China. The effect on oil price of this demand pressure was highlighted earlier in this chapter. Equally, governments across the world, for a number of reasons, have introduced legislation to insist upon the use of renewable energy sources, or financial incentives to encourage it. For example, in the UK the Renewable Transport Fuel Obligation (RTFO) requires 2.5% (by volume) of transport fuel to be delivered from renewable sources by 2008/9, rising to 5.75% by 2010/11. This was decided to be the most effective means for the UK to meet its commitment to the Kyoto Protocol. Also, EU directive 2003/30EC necessitates member states to put in place measures to enable, by 2010, 5.75 % of the EU transport fuels being provided by bio-fuels. The UK also created its own targets in the 2003 Energy White Paper, of a 20% reduction in CO_2 emissions by 2010 and a 60% carbon saving by 2050. Similarly in the USA, the Energy Policy Act of 2005 demanded that by 2012 the use of renewable fuels should achieve 7.5 billion gallons. There were also significant incentives for bio-fuels provided by federal tax laws in the USA.

Bio-fuels exist in two forms; bio-ethanol and bio-diesel. Bio-ethanol originates from a starch substrate such as wheat, maize or sugar, which is ground and then subjected to saccharification followed by yeast fermentation. The end products are bio-ethanol, distillers grains and solubles, and carbon dioxide. Bio-diesel originates from oilseeds such as palm, rape and soya, which are used to extract oil that then undergoes esterification with methanol to produce bio-diesel and glycerine. The outline of these processes is shown in Figure 18. The potential yield of bio-fuels varies significantly (Table 2). For ethanol production, yield in terms of litres per hectare from sugar cane and sugar beet is far higher than other sources and, as regards cereal crops, corn has the most efficient yield per hectare. It is no surprise, therefore, that Brazil using sugar cane and the USA using corn are currently the two most important global producers of ethanol. The use of corn for ethanol has seen major growth in the USA during recent years and the USA dominates the world production of ethanol from cereals. USA and Brazil are predicted to continue to be the major players in this market (Figure 19). According to the OECD–FAO Agricultural Outlook 2008-17, in 2005, 46 million tonnes of wheat and coarse grains were used globally for ethanol production and, of that total, 41 million tonnes were used in the USA, which amounted to 14% of USA corn production. In 2007, the USA usage of corn for ethanol had doubled to 81 million tonnes in comparison to a global usage of 93 million tonnes. Ultimately, approximately 33% of the USA corn crop is predicted to be directed to ethanol production, with 125-130 million tonnes of corn being used in this way by 2017. This inevitably will continue to put pressure on the supply and demand balance.

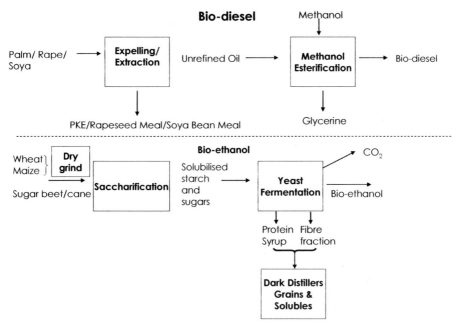

Figure 18. Bio-fuel processing

Table 2. Feedstock options

Carbohydrate crops

		Barley	*Maize*	*Wheat*	*Sugarbeet*	*Sugarcane*	*Cassava*
Yield	Tonnes per hectare	2.5	4.7	2.8	43.2	65.3	10.9
Ethanol	Yields						
	Litres per tonne	360	430	400	100	70	180
	Litres per hectare	910	2020	1140	4320	4570	1960

Oilseed crops

		Oil palm fruit	*Rapeseed*	*Soyabean*	*Sunflower*
Yield	Tonnes per hectare	13.4	1.7	2.3	1.2
Ethanol	Yields				
	Litres per tonne	240	440	200	480
	Litres per hectare	3220	760	460	600

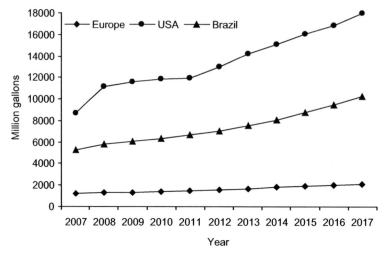

Figure 19. Ethanol production 2008-2017 (Source FAPRI 2008 Agricultural Outlook)

When considering oilseeds, palm produces four times more yield per hectare than other oilseeds (Table 2). Europe currently leads production of bio-diesel, but with the efficiency factor to be gained from the use of palm, bio-diesel production is likely to expand in Asia. Current predictions for bio-diesel production growth during the next ten years are shown in Figure 20. World usage of vegetable oil increased by 9 million tonnes (approximately 10%) between 2005 and 2007 and half of that additional demand was due to bio-diesel. OECD-FAO Agricultural Outlook predicts that demand for vegetable oil for bio-diesel will double by 2017 to 21 million tonnes. This increase of 12 million tonnes accounts for approximately one third of the predicted increase in global demand for vegetable oil between 2007 and 2017. The remainder of that significant increase will be driven by food demand.

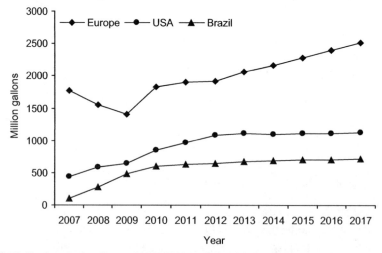

Figure 20. Biodiesel production (Source FAPRI 2008 Agricultural Outlook)

Supply and demand

It can be seen clearly from the previous discussions that demand for agricultural commodities, in terms of cereals and oilseeds, is projected to remain strong in the future. Population growth and increasing wealth will have inevitable consequences for continuation of existing trends. However, although escalation in demand is driven largely by requirements for food and feed, there is a significant contribution from the bio-fuels market. The magnitude of the expected increase in demand from the bio-fuels market does depend on political support for this activity and the absence of 'second generation' bio-fuel feedstocks, e.g. using cellulose-based materials rather than existing agricultural commodities. China, for example, has already banned any further use of corn for ethanol production and there would appear to an elevated level of discussion on whether this type of energy generation should be encouraged and supported. As regards the second factor, it is unlikely that 'second generation' feedstocks will be used commercially in the next 10 years.

It is generally predicted that global agriculture will increase production to meet demand for both cereal and oilseeds, and this will probably be delivered by higher yields rather than increased land use. The demand originating in developing countries also suggests that the increase in production will be proportionately higher in developing countries than in the developed world. However China, for example, will probably have to be a net importer of corn in the future. Future weather patterns are an uncertainty; climatic conditions have been responsible for significant issues in the last few years and there remains no firm view as to whether climate change factors exist and will increase the frequency of these events.

The rise in prices seen as an outcome of this supply and demand situation has concerning consequences. Inevitably those people with low incomes in importing countries become subjected to higher food prices and difficulties in supply; hence the vulnerable become more vulnerable. Food security is a global issue demanding participation by all. This is being recognised; the FAO held a Food Security Summit in June 2008 to highlight and seek solutions for this issue. Equally, the same point was made in the UK government publication, 'Food Matters – Towards a Strategy for the 21st Century'.

SPECULATOR INVOLVEMENT IN AGRICULTURAL COMMODITIES

Futures markets in soyabeans, wheat and corn have always played a key role in commodity markets and traditionally allowed agricultural commodity traders to manage risk. Futures prices are used as the 'market price' and hence are the focal point of many decisions. Recently though, the level of participation from investors with no interest in the physical commodity market has increased. These investors, which include index and hedge funds, are purely buying a position and hoping to see the market rise and make a profit. Hence they tend to always hold 'long' positions (a commitment to buy) and are prepared to maintain the positions for long periods. Figure 21 shows the positions being held by funds in the Kansas wheat market since 2002 (as at 21/07/08) and the '% of open interest'. It can be seen clearly that it predominates as a 'long' position with funds taking a commitment to buy and that their involvement has increased significantly in the last 3 years. In this particular example, the funds have at the highest level of involvement held over 40% of the open interest. There is a view that this involvement, which does not take action based on the fundamental factors normally used by agricultural commodity traders, distorts the market. It is likely that prices rise much higher than the underlying value of the commodity and then drop suddenly, resulting in the increased volatility seen in recent times. The Gallagher Review in July 2008 suggested that this could be a factor in food price rises and should be investigated by the UK treasury.

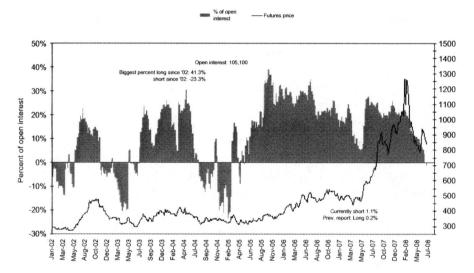

Figure 21. Weekly KC wheat fund positions as percent of open interest (excluding commodity index funds)

EFFECTS ON OTHER COMMODITIES

Although interest usually focuses on commodities such as cereals and oilseeds, which are used for both food and feed and constitute a large proportion of livestock diets, some of the factors described already have had major impacts on other livestock feed materials that may be used in lower quantities, but are nevertheless important. An example of this is the feed phosphate market. Strong prices for cereals have encouraged arable farmers to increase inputs to achieve maximum yields, which resulted in a much higher demand for phosphate fertiliser. Of the phosphate mined, 90% is used for fertiliser and 5% is used for animal feed phosphates. The increase in use for fertiliser drastically reduced supply for the animal feed market with, in some situations, a third of the quantity contracted not being available. This put immense pressure on the price of feed phosphates. For example, the price of dicalcium phosphate in December 2007 was £250/tonne and in July 2008 was in excess of £700/tonne.

Conclusion

Increasing global demand for agricultural commodities is without doubt a feature for the future, with that demand being driven by both food and non-food needs. The belief is currently that production will just manage to keep pace with need; hence there is unlikely to be any significant rise in end-stocks and the stocks to usage ratio will continue to fall. Developing countries, which will experience the highest demand growth, are likely also to be the ones with the greatest capability for increases in production. Prices, although there may be some relief from the extreme levels seen recently, will continue in an elevated range and with high volatility. Food security will be discussed as a global issue, particularly with the concern over the vulnerability of the lower income sectors of the population in developing countries. Emphasis will be placed on improving production in developing countries. However, the key uncertainties of level of political intervention, unusual weather patterns and the use of second generation bio-fuel substrates still remain.

9

DEVELOPMENTS IN THE RUSSIAN LIVESTOCK INDUSTRIES: IMPLICATIONS FOR EUROPEAN PRODUCERS AND THE FEED INDUSTRY

TON SAS
Provimi B.V., Rotterdam, The Netherlands

Introduction

After the collapse of the Soviet Union in 1991 an economic crisis occurred in the Russian Federation. The agricultural sector also suffered this crisis, leading to many farms becoming bankrupt. The number of animals decreased sharply during the early nineties. The economy reached its lowest point in August 1998, with a strong devaluation of the Russian Rouble and a major reduction in Gross Domestic Product (GDP). The Russian economy recovered strongly after the crisis and, since 2000, the annual growth in GDP averaged 5 – 8 % per year (Figure 1). In 2007 the GDP reached $ 10,640 per capita.

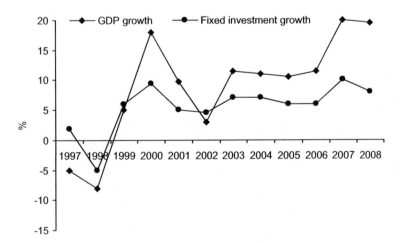

Figure 1. Annual Growth of GDP in Russia (Berkum *et al.*, 2007, Goskomstat, 2008).

During the past several years Russia's trade balance has shown a significant increase in trade surplus, which has been also positively influenced by high oil and gas prices. In 2007 the Russian trade surplus was estimated at approximately $ 150 billion.

Russian Federation

The Russian Federation (Russia) has 141 million inhabitants. In recent years the number of inhabitants has decreased. It is expected, however, that this number will increase in the near future due to Government incentives, for example special financial support for home renovation and for education of children in families with more than 1 child.

The land surface of Russia is approximately 17 million square km, making Russia the largest country in the world. Russia includes 11 time zones. The country is divided into 7 Federal Districts, named: Far East Federal District (F.D.), Siberian F.D., Urals F.D., North West F.D., Central F.D, Privolsky F.D., and South F.D. (Figure 2). Arable farming and animal husbandry are carried out in mainly the latter 4 Federal Districts, which are in the European part of Russia (west of the Ural Mountains). Approximately 75 % of the animal husbandry takes place in this part of Russia. The remaining 25 % of animal husbandry in the Asian part of Russia, this is mainly carried out in the southern parts of the Urals F.D. and the Siberian F.D. In these Federal Districts the farms with animal husbandry are mainly located in the neighbourhood of the big cities.

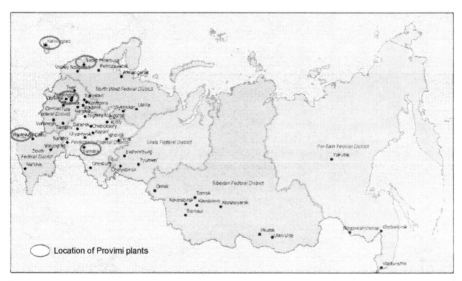

Figure 2. Map of Russia

The agricultural sector

In Russia the size of farms varies substantially. There are several farms of 50,000 to 1,000,000 hectares, the so called "agro-holdings". These farms focus on arable farming, mainly the production of grains, sunflower and sugar beet (Figure 3). In the past three to four years these agro-holdings have also started animal production, in particular poultry and pig production. Besides these activities, the agro-holdings have also built their own feed production plants, slaughterhouses and meat processing plants. In this way the agro-holdings have become totally vertically-integrated.

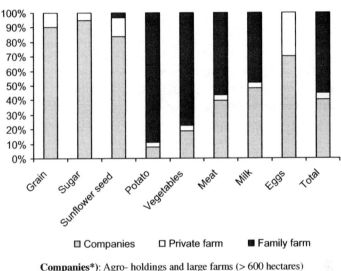

Companies*): Agro- holdings and large farms (> 600 hectares)
Private farm*): Average size 70 - 100 hectares
Family farm*): Back yard farms

*Subdivision adjusted by author

Figure 3. Share of business forms (Berkum *et al.*, 2007)

At the same time there are in Russia also many "back yard farms", usually less than 0.5 hectares in size. About 50 % of both pigs and cattle are kept as back yard farming.

Animal husbandry

As shown in Table 1, during the period 2000 – 2007 the total number of cattle decreased by about 25 %. The number of dairy cattle decreased by a similar percentage. This is due mainly to the low profitability of cattle farming.

Table 1. Changes in the number of animals between 2000 – 2007, in million head (Goskomstat, 2008)

	2000	*2005*	*2006*	*2007*
Number of cattle	28.0	24.5	21.5	21.3
of which dairy cattle	12.6	10.2	9.4	9.3
Number of sheep	15.1	18.2	19.7	20.2
Number of pigs	15.7	15.5	15.8	16.2
Number of poultry	348.8	334.7	350.6	363.6
of which broilers	188	179	190.8	202.7
layers	155	150	154	155
other	5.8	5.7	5.8	5.9

The number of pigs remained fairly constant until 2007. From 2007 onwards the number of pigs increased as a result of newly-built farms.

For poultry, the number of broilers increased by about 8 % during this period, and the number of layers remained about the same.

Table 2. Animal production per animal species in million metric tons *) (Goskomstat, 2008)

	2000	*2005*	*2006*	*2007*
Cow milk	31.9	310.	31.4	31.2
Beef and veal	1.9	1.8	1.8	1.8
Sheep and goat	0.14	0.15	0.15	0.16
Pork	1.6	1.5	1.6	1.9
Poultry meat	0.8	1.4	1.6	1.9
Eggs	1.8	2.1	2.1	2.1

*) metric ton = 1,000 kg

Although the number of dairy cattle decreased by about 25 %, the total quantity of milk produced remained nearly the same (31.9 versus 31.2 million metric tons).

Pork production increased during 2007, as a result of more pigs and better performance by these animals. Broiler meat production more than doubled during 2000 to 2007, while egg production remained the same in the last 3 years.

Future developments of Russian agricultural production

Given the aim set by the Russian Federation, to become less dependent on imports of e.g. meat and milk products, the Russian Government approved several projects, aiming at developing animal production.

One of these projects is the "Agro-industrial Complex Development" project, approved by the Russian Government in 2005. Within this project farms could borrow money with low interest rates, and/or purchase imported animals and equipment with decreased import tariffs. Leasing agreements provided farms with better payment facilities.

In 2007 the Russian Government approved a new 5-year programme: "The State Program for Development and Regulation of Food and Agricultural Markets during 2008 – 2012". The total budget for this programme is about USD 44.3 billion (Euro 30 billion). Within this programme, newly built farms get financial support through subsidized credits for the required investments. The relevant subsidies are paid 50 % by the Russian Federal Government and 50 % by the Regional Federal Government.

Animal production

DAIRY SECTOR

The dairy sector is poorly developed. In 2007 average milk production was only 3,460 kg per cow per year (Goskomstat, 2008), although some farms had a high milk production, exceeding 7,000 kg per cow per year. The main reasons for this low average production are:

*   50 % of cattle are kept in back yard farms
*   lack of good management and skilled farm staff
*   poor quality roughages

It is expected that the number of dairy cattle will increase to 10.5 million by 2015 (Table 3). It is also expected that average milk production per cow will increase to 4,143 kg per cow per year (Table 3).

Table 3. Forecast of Dairy Production (Goskomstat 2008).

Year	Number of dairy cows (Million head)	Milk production (Million metric tons)	Average milk production (kg/cow/year)
2010	9.6	36.4	7,792
2012	9.8	39.2	4,000
2015	10.5	43.5	4,143

BEEF SECTOR

Beef production is expected to increase slightly during the coming years to 1.8 million metric tons in 2010, 1.9 in 2012, and 2.0 in 2015 (Goskomstat 2008).

PIG SECTOR

Pig farms always produce pigs from farrowing to slaughter weight. In the past the entire production took place on the same site, or even in the same building with separated sections (birth to 25 kg and 25 kg to slaughter). Nowadays, in newly built farms, production is carried out on 3 or 4 sites, allowing better bio-security to be realized.

Current technical performance varies strongly per farm. The average number of slaughter pigs varies from 12 to 23 per sow per year. In future, pork production is expected to increase (Table 4) both by an increase of the number of large pig farms and by better technical performance (in terms of daily gain) of the pigs. It is expected that several new farms with 15,000 – 30,000 sows will be established.

Table 4. Forecast of Pork Production (Goskomstat , 2008)

| Year | Quantity (million metric tons) | |
	Minimum	Maximum
2008	1.94	1.98
2010	1.96	2.07
2012	2.00	2.17
2015	2.15	2.28

POULTRY SECTOR

The poultry sector is the best developed sector. Several Agro-holdings own large, completely integrated farms with skilled management. Although the number of broilers hardly increased (Table 1), the output of broiler farms increased considerably during recent years (Table 2). The main reason is a substantial increase in technical performance. Daily gain currently varies from 42 to 58 g. For the coming years further growth in broiler meat production and egg production are expected (Table 5).

Table 5. Forecast of Poultry production (Goskomstat, 2008)

	2007	2010	2015
Broiler meat (million metric tons)	1.89	2.59	3.52
Eggs (billions)	39.5	43.0	48.0

Human food consumption in Russia

During recent years meat consumption has increased (Table 6) and this tendency is expected to continue in the near future. As Russia's inhabitants gain more purchasing power, there is a resulting higher demand for more luxurious foods, especially meat.

Table 6. Food consumption per capita, kg (Goskomstat 2008).

Year	2005	2007	2010
Beef	16.5	17.5	18.0
Pork	18.0	18.6	22.5
Poultry	18.5	22.3	24.8
Total meat	53.0	58.4	65.3
Milk*	230	250	270
Eggs	14.6	14.7	15.2

* including milk products

Self-sufficiency

The consumption per capita (Table 6) and the forecast of production levels for meat, milk and eggs (Tables 3, 4 and 5) will result in an increase in self-sufficiency in Russia (Table 7).

Table 7. Expected self-sufficiency (%) in Russia in 2010 and 2015

Year	2010	2015
Beef	72	80
Pork	63	70
Broiler meat	74	100
Milk	85	114
Eggs	122	136

Egg production reached self-sufficiency of 100 % in 2007. Table 7 shows that Russia may become an exporting country for several animal products, including eggs, milk and broiler meat during the coming years.

Feed industry

During 2007 a total of about 38 million metric tons of animal feed was produced. Of this total, 16 million metric tons was produced in feed plants (animal feed industry and in feed plants of integrated farms). With the likely increase in animal production, a higher demand for high quality industrial feed is expected. The increase in animal production is primarily expected to take place in newly-built large farms. This expected increase in demand for feed will either be met by the feed industry or will be produced in the relevant integrated farms. It is not expected that back yard farming will increase. Based on the expected increase in animal production, the total quantity of feed required is estimated to increase to 50 million metric tons in 2015. Of this total, 28 million metric tons of feed is expected to be produced by the feed industry or in the feed plants of integrated farms.

Table 8. Feed production, million metric tons

	2007	*2015*
Dairy cattle feed	8.1	10.9
Beef cattle feed (incl. young stock)	4.9	5.6
Pig feed	10.0	11.4
Broiler feed	6.0	11.2
Layer feed	7.0	8.5
Others	2.0	2.3
Total	38.0	50.0

SWOT analysis

Russian animal husbandry will increase in the near future. A SWOT analysis is given, analyzing the animal production in Russia.

Strengths

• Own cheap grain production.
• Vertical integrations

- Own energy sources
- Much land is available

In Russia the main grain sources are wheat and barley. Production of maize is increasing, but it is still a minor part of total grain production due to the climatic conditions. With the availability of much land and an expected increase in grain production per hectare, Russia has a sufficient quantity of grains to meet its own demand.   Russia has its own sources of gas and oil.

Weaknesses

- Lack of high quality protein sources
- Climatic conditions
- Infrastructure
- High bureaucracy
- Lack of well skilled farm staff
- Low efficiency

Due to the climate in the country, the main protein sources for the feed industry are sunflower meal and rapeseed meal. It is expected that production of sunflower seed and rapeseed will increase. In the southern part of Russia soya is cultivated, but the area under cultivation is limited. Therefore high quality protein sources, like soyabean meal and fish meal, have to be imported.

Infrastructure suffers from under investment. Roads have to be improved; water ways are hardly used and also during several months of the year are frozen-over and unusable. Rail roads are excellent. Much transport of feed ingredients and compound feeds takes place by rail. Rail transport is, however, limited by the availability of sufficient rolling-stock. In many farms there is a shortage of skilled labour, in particular to do the practical work properly.

Opportunities

- Financial support by Russian government
- Increase in purchasing power of Russian consumers
- High demand for luxury foods
- Increasing world population
- Low prices for land

The Russian government took measures to support development of the agricultural sector. A portion of the investments will be returned by the Russian government. In the past two to three years average salaries increased by 20 to 30 % per year, resulting in more purchasing power. As the world population increases, demand for food in the world will increase. This will provide export opportunities for meat, milk and eggs from Russia in the future.

Threats

•   Investors are from outside the agricultural sector

•   Increase in grain prices

•   Shortage of highly skilled labour

•   Bureaucracy

Many newly established farms are built by investors from outside the agricultural sector, such as investors from the oil industry. The return on investment in the agricultural sector, i.e. animal production, is currently significantly lower than in the oil industry. When returns on investment do not meet the expectations of investors, in future they may invest less or even withdraw from animal production. The increase in grain prices world-wide will have a negative influence on profitability of farms. In nearly all farms, including the recently established farms, there is a shortage of skilled persons for the practical work. The high level of bureaucracy may act as a constraint to people trying to start up at business.

Conclusions

Animal husbandry in the Russian Federation improved a lot during the last 5 years and will increase further during the coming years. Between 2007 and 2015, production of milk will increase by 35%, beef by 14%, pork by 14 %, broiler meat by 86%, and eggs by 22%. At the moment self-sufficiency of egg production is 100 %. Self-sufficiency for broiler meat production will reach 100 % in 2015. Self-sufficiency for milk will be reached around 2012. Only for beef and pork will Russia stay dependent on imports after 2015. Russia offers good opportunities for starting up new farms. At the same time it will be necessary to set up education and/ or training centres regarding the practical work on the farms. Technical performance of animals and the efficiency of farms have to be improved to be competitive on the world market.

Because animal husbandry will increase, particularly on newly built farms, the feed industry will increase as well. In 2007 a quantity of 16 million metric tons of compound feeds was produced by the feed industry. This quantity will increase to 28 million metric tons in 2015. The higher demand for feeds will require an adequate development of the animal feed industry.

Acknowledgements

The author wishes to thank Nikolay Nesterov, marketing director Provimi LTD, Russia for his data input and for providing information personally.

References

Berkum, S.van, Roza P. and Belt J. (2007) Long-term perspectives for the Russian agri-food sector and market opportunities for the Dutch agribusiness. LEI, The Hague, The Netherlands, report 5.07.03.
Goskomstat (2008) The State Committee for Statistics, Russia.

10

USING InraPorc TO REDUCE NITROGEN AND PHOSPHORUS EXCRETION

JAAP VAN MILGEN[1,2], LUDOVIC BROSSARD[1,2], ALAIN VALANCOGNE[1,2] AND JEAN-YVES DOURMAD[1,2]
[1]INRA, UMR1079, F-3500 Rennes, France
[2]Agrocampus Ouest, UMR1079, F-35000, Rennes, France

Introduction

InraPorc is a model and software tool designed to evaluate the response of pigs to different nutritional strategies. The model concepts have been described for sows by Dourmad, Étienne, Valancogne, Dubois, van Milgen and Noblet (2008) and for growing pigs by van Milgen, Valancogne, Dubois, Dourmad, Sève and Noblet (2008). The software is available for free for educational organisations and at a moderate cost for commercial purposes (see www.rennes.inra.fr/inraporc/ for details).

The purpose of the current chapter is to illustrate how models, like InraPorc, can help in controlling the environmental impact of pig production while ensuring animal performance. Because the reliability of the outcome of a simulation depends on the concepts used in the model, it is essential that model users have some knowledge about the model structure and the limitations of its use. The discussion will focus only on the feed and growing pig modules of InraPorc. The concepts used for the sow module are similar to those used for growing pigs.

General description of the growing pig module of InraPorc

To realize a simulation with InraPorc, the user has to provide a feed sequence plan, a feed rationing plan and an animal profile. In a feed sequence plan the user indicates, through a series of rules, the feeds that are used in a simulation. For example, a two-phase feed sequence plan can be defined where the use of a grower diet is followed by a finisher diet. The user has to indicate the condition that triggers the change of diets (e.g., number of days, amount of feed, body weight). The feed rationing plan is conceptually similar to a feed sequence plan, but here the user defines the quantity of feed or energy that will be distributed during different periods.

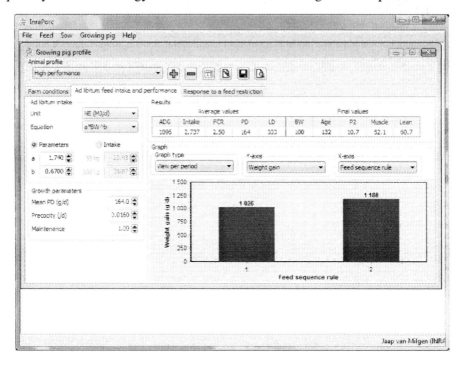

Figure 1. The phenotypic potential of the animal is described in this window of InraPorc. Model parameters for ad libitum feed intake and protein deposition (growth) are given on the left-hand side of the window and results of the simulation are given on the right-hand side.

The animal profile is the core of the InraPorc model and describes the phenotypic potential of the growing pig in terms of feed intake capacity and growth. Within the software, most of the required information is grouped together in the tab-sheet "Ad libitum feed intake and performance" (Figure 1). Parameter values are given in the left-hand panel whereas results of the simulation are given numerically or graphically in the right-hand panel. Body weight is assumed to be the driving force for ad libitum feed intake (as a phenotypic trait) but it is left to the user to decide whether ad libitum feed intake is controlled metabolically (e.g., by Net Energy (NE) or Metabolisable Energy (ME) supply) or by gut capacity (e.g., by Dry Matter (DM) or Digestible Energy (DE)). Depending on the type of feed provided, the mechanisms controlling voluntary feed intake may vary. It is important to realize that the response of InraPorc to diets differing in energy content depends on the choice made here.

InraPorc works internally by describing the change in protein and lipid mass, used as state variables. Other traits such as body weight and backfat thickness are calculated by empirical equations from these state variables. The protein deposition (PD) curve can be parameterized by modifying the model parameters "mean PD" and "precocity" (Figure 1). These parameters are used in the construction of a Gompertz function describing PD (see van Milgen *et al.* (2008) for details). There are two methods in using the Gompertz function to describe growth. The first one (used in InraPorc) is using the Gompertz function as a differential equation describing PD. In the second method, the differential equation is integrated analytically leading to time being the driving force for PD, rather than the current state of the animal. The choice of the method has implications on how the animal deals with compensatory growth. When the current state of the animal is the driving force for PD, a nutrient deficiency will not have an impact on the potential PD and compensatory growth will remain possible (although perhaps not completely). If time is the driving force for PD, growth retardation may result in a situation where the growth potential of the animal will be lost (because time has passed), making compensatory growth without compensatory feed intake virtually impossible.

At first hand, it may seem difficult to find these parameters for a given phenotype. However, if information can be obtained concerning the average feed intake and growth for two separate periods (e.g., for the grower and finisher phases), it is not too difficult to find model parameters that predict this situation. In the help file of the software, a numerical example is given that will show how to do this.

Nitrogen utilization and excretion

Most nitrogen (N) in animal feeds originates from protein and thus from amino acids. Amino acids contain an amino group that can form a peptide bond with the carboxyl group from an adjacent amino acid. Although it is generally assumed that "crude" protein contains 160 g N/kg, it is known to vary with the origin of the protein. Dairy protein contains on average 157 g N/kg whereas soy protein contains 174 g N/kg. The reason for this difference is two-fold. First, the side chain of amino acids varies considerably in length. For example, glycine is a relatively simple amino acid with only hydrogen as side chain, whereas amino acids such as tyrosine and phenylalanine have relatively complex carbon-ring structures as side chains. As these amino acids only contain N in the amino group, the N content of these amino acids varies greatly. Secondly, some amino acids contain one (Lys, Trp, Gly, Asp), two (His) or even three (Arg) additional N atoms. As a result, the N content of protein depends of the amino acid content (Figure 2).

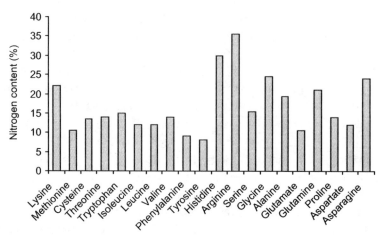

Figure 2. Nitrogen content of amino acids.

All N ingested by the animal but not retained will be excreted. In InraPorc, the potential of an animal to retain N (as body protein) is determined by three factors. The first is the potential PD of the pig when feed is offered ad libitum and the change of this potential during growth. The potential PD of the animal is determined by the Gompertz function described above. The second factor is the reduction in PD due to a reduction in feed intake. It is known that a reduction in feed intake not only changes lipid deposition, but that it also can affect PD. The response of the animal to a change in feed intake is determined by a single, user-defined parameter called "BW PDmax", which corresponds to the body weight beyond which the animal will not reduce its PD when feed intake is marginally reduced (by default, this value is set to 70 kg). The relevance of this parameter is limited when feed is offered ad libitum throughout growth. However, it becomes important when specific feed rationing strategies are applied (e.g., reducing feed intake at the end of the finishing phase to reduce carcass fatness). The third factor is the supply and the balance between amino acids. Amino acids supplied in excess of requirements are deaminated and the resulting ammonia, if not used for the synthesis of non-essential amino acids, will be converted to urea and excreted by the animal. The concept of ideal protein refers to a situation where all amino acids are equally limiting. If the composition of dietary protein differs from that of the ideal protein, PD will be determined by the most limiting amino acid. In InraPorc, the use of amino acids is based on a concept similar to that of ideal protein. Twelve amino acids (including arginine) and total N are considered to be potentially limiting for PD. The model requires that the amino acid supply is given on a standardized ileal digestible (SID) basis. Consequently, amino acids not digested prior to the terminal ileum will be lost, including the specific endogenous losses. Part of SID amino acid supply will be used for maintenance purposes. This includes the use of amino acids and N used for the integumentary system (i.e., the synthesis and renewal of skin, hair and nails), amino acids lost during the minimal turnover of body protein and the basal endogenous losses. The first two are assumed to depend on the body weight of the animal using values proposed by Moughan (1998). The basal endogenous losses are assumed to vary with DM intake using the values of INRA/AFZ (Sauvant, Perez and Tran, 2002). It is also assumed that there is maximum efficiency of amino acid and N utilization when these are actually limiting PD. This maximum efficiency can also be interpreted as a minimum, or obligatory, oxidation of amino acids. Maximum efficiencies differ between amino acids and are calculated from the ideal amino acid profile (van Milgen *et al.*, 2008). Maximum efficiencies for Lys and N utilization are assumed to be 0.72 and 0.85, respectively. The amino acids and N required for maintenance plus those required for growth (i.e., potential amino acid or protein retention divided by the maximum efficiency) determine the requirement by the animal.

The partitioning of nutrients discussed above allows calculation of N retention and excretion. The N excretion can be further separated in urinary and faecal N excretion. Urinary N mainly originates from urea. Due to the presence of bacterial urease, urea can be rapidly converted to ammonia. Faecal N on the other hand is mostly composed of bacterial protein and is therefore less "volatile". The distinction between faecal and urinary N is realized by subtracting the faecal indigestible N excretion from total N excretion. Although faecal digestibility is considered constant in InraPorc, it is known that the presence of fermentable fibre in the hindgut can stimulate the transfer of ammonia from the blood to the intestine (Dourmad and Jondreville, 2007). Consequently, the partitioning of excreted N between faecal and urinary N has to be interpreted with caution.

The environmental impact of animal production can be minimized if the supply of nutrients is close to the requirements. The protein and amino acid requirements expressed by kg feed intake will mainly depend on the ratio between the PD curve and the feed intake curve. As indicated above, the PD under ad libitum conditions varies according to a Gompertz function, which in most cases will resemble an asymmetric bell-shaped curve. Ad libitum feed intake is a power function of body weight. This means that the protein and amino acid requirements (per kg of feed) will typically decline during growth. The N content of the diet should ideally follow this trend in order to reduce N excretion.

The remainder of this section will illustrate the usefulness of tools like InraPorc in evaluating different feeding strategies on performance and nutrient excretion. The strategies were tested using the "high performance" animal profile available in InraPorc. This profile describes the growth of a pig between 27 and 100 kg body weight having an average feed intake of 2.74 kg/d and growing at a rate of 1.10 kg/d (Le Bellego, van Milgen and Noblet, 2002). Although InraPorc does not allow least-cost feed formulation, it can be used to calculate the chemical and

Table 1. Composition (g/kg) and relative price of diets formulated on a least-cost basis

Item	Diet 1	Diet 2	Diet 3	Diet 4	Diet 5	Diet 6	Diet 7
Relative price[1]	100.0	89.9	80.3	109.8	88.0	101.6	81.6
Wheat	561	836	663	-	657	558	676
Maize	222	-	-	611	-	222	-
Barley	-	45.1	312	-	67.4	-	298
Peas	-	-	-	55.6	241	-	-
Soyabean meal	176.3	87.7	-	293.2	14.2	176.9	-
Soya oil	4.81	-	-	10.37	-	5.60	-
L-Lys HCl	3.70	3.86	3.32	-	-	3.69	3.33
L-Threonine	1.24	1.20	0.81	-	-	1.23	0.81
DL-Methionine	0.61	0.41	0.11	-	-	0.62	0.11
Phytase (0-250 IU/kg)[2]	0.05	0.05	0.05	0.05	0.05	-	-
Phytase (250-500 IU/kg)[2]	0.05	0.05	0.05	0.05	0.023	-	-
Phytase (500-750 IU/kg)[2]	0.05	0.05	0.028	0.05	-	-	-
Calcium carbonate	15.0	13.8	12.4	14.8	12.1	10.1	7.9
Dicalcium phosphate	7.67	3.54	-	7.09	-	13.99	5.93
Salt	3.0	3.0	3.0	3.0	3.0	3.0	3.0
Vitamin and mineral mixture	5.0	5.0	5.0	5.0	5.0	5.0	5.0

[1]Relative price of diets using diet 1 as a reference. Prices of feed ingredients are those of May 2008 given by Ifip (http://www.ifip.asso.fr/newsletters/sommaire_lettres.htm).
[2]Different digestible P levels were attributed to account for the diminishing phytase activity with increasing phytase level. Digestible P levels were assumed to be 10000, 5000, 2600, 1400 g/kg for phytase levels 0-250, 250-500, 500-750 and 750-1000 IU/kg respectively, and each level could be included at a maximum rate of 0.05 g/kg. It was economically not feasible to include the phytase level providing 750-1000 IU/kg in the diets.

nutritional composition of a feed based on the composition of feed ingredients. The feeds listed in Table 1 are formulated using an external least-cost feed formulation program using feed ingredients from the Inra/AFZ database (Sauvant *et al.*, 2002). This data base is also available within InraPorc and was used to calculate the composition of the diets. Microbial phytase was included as a separate ingredient depending on the inclusion level to account for the diminishing efficacy of phytase with increasing inclusion level. Each incremental increase in phytase level was attributed a diminishing digestible P content and "each phytase" could be incorporated at a maximum rate of 0.05 g/kg (Jondreville and Dourmad, 2005). As all diets are to be used as pellets, the effect of endogenous phytase was not considered. Diets were formulated on a least-cost basis using feed ingredient prices of May 2008 and contained 10 MJ NE/kg. Differences between diets originate from different constraints on SID Lys and digestible P, and the inclusion or not of crystalline amino acids and microbial phytase.

Diet 1 was formulated to contain 9.2 g SID Lys and 30 g digestible P/kg. These levels are 10% higher than the requirement of the animal at the start of the simulation. This higher requirement was used to cover the requirement of a population of these animals (see section below "Dealing with a population of animals"). Diets 2 and 3 were formulated with lower SID Lys and P levels corresponding to the population requirement at approximately 60 kg BW (diet 2) and at the end of the finisher period (diet 3). These three diets were then used in three different feeding strategies: single-phase feeding with diet 1 (strategy 1), two-phase feeding with diets 1 and 2 and changing diets at 60 kg BW (strategy 2), and multiphase-feeding replacing diet 1 gradually with diet 3 (strategy 3). In InraPorc a "comparison of simulations" can be used to evaluate these strategies. As diets were formulated to exceed the requirement, the animal was able to express its phenotypic potential with all three feeding strategies. Total N intake decreased from 4.79 kg for strategy 1 to 3.86 kg for strategy 3 (Table 2). Because N retention was equal for the three strategies, N excretion decreased from 3.01 kg for strategy 1 to 2.08 kg for strategy 3. Most of the N was excreted via the urine. The small differences in the faecal N excretion originated from differences in faecal N digestibility between feed ingredients. Apart from the reduction in N excretion, adapting the diet to the requirement of the animal also reduced total feed cost. The feed cost for the two-phase and multiphase feeding strategies were respectively 0.946 and 0.892 of that of the single-phase feeding strategy.

It is theoretically possible to reduce further the N content and thus N excretion. To obtain an in-depth analysis of N use, a "single simulation" can be used in InraPorc. Dietary N was most efficiently used with strategy 3 and with this strategy, 0.13 of the total N supply was digested and absorbed prior to the terminal ileum, whereas 0.17 of the total N supply was used for other physiological functions (i.e., basal endogenous fraction, maintenance, and minimal oxidation), all of which can be considered as obligatory. More than 0.24 of the N supply was given in excess of requirement, but part of this was due to the fact that the diet was formulated to provide Lys 0.10 above the requirement of the individual animal. The excess supply of N can be reduced if the amino profile of the diet would match more closely the requirement of the animal. When the supply and requirement curves

Table 2. Effect of different feeding strategies on N and P utilisation and excretion simulated by InraPorc

Strategy	1	2	3	4	5	6
Feeding strategy	Single-phase	Two-phase	Multi-phase	Multi-phase	Multi-phase	Single-phase
Diets[1]	1	1 and 2	1 and 3	4 and 5	6 and 7	2
Include crystalline AA	Yes	Yes	Yes	No	Yes	Yes
Include phytase	Yes	Yes	Yes	Yes	No	Yes
SID Lys (g/kg diet)	9.2	9.2-7.5	9.2-5.2	9.2-5.2	9.2-5.2	7.5
Digestible P (g/kg diet)	3.0	3.0-2.4	3.0-1.8	3.0-1.8	3.0-1.8	2.4
Relative feed cost[2]	100	94.1	89.2	97.8	90.8	90.8
Average daily gain	1.10	1.10	1.10	1.10	1.10	1.09
Nitrogen						
Content (g/kg diet)	25.9	25.9-21.9	25.9-16.8	31.0-21.2	25.8-16.8	21.9
Intake (kg)	4.79	4.34	3.86	4.73	3.86	4.10
Retention (kg)	1.78	1.78	1.78	1.78	1.78	1.77
Excretion (kg)[3]	3.01	2.56	2.08	2.95	2.08	2.33
Faeces (kg)	0.69	0.64	0.62	0.73	0.62	0.61
Urine (kg)	2.32	1.92	1.46	2.22	1.46	1.72
Ileal indigestible (kg)	0.60	0.53	0.51	0.69	0.50	0.50
Other (kg)[4]	0.65	0.65	0.64	0.64	0.64	0.68
Excess (kg)[5]	1.77	1.38	0.93	1.61	0.93	1.15
Phosphorus						
Content (g/kg diet)	5.08	5.08-4.12	5.08-3.18	5.12-3.38	6.40-4.42	4.12
Intake (g)	940	830	746	769	982	770
Retention (g)	378	379	379	378	379	365
Excretion (g)	562	451	367	391	603	405
Indigestible (g)	384	343	313	337	549	321
Maintenance (g)	42	42	42	42	42	42
Excess (g)[6]	135	66	11	12	11	42

[1]See Table 1 for the diets used.

[2]Relative to the cost of strategy 1.

[3]N excretion can be partitioned between the routes of excretion (faeces or urine) or according to physiological origin.

[4]Including minimum oxidation, basal endogenous losses and maintenance.

[5]Compared with a situation where N supply equals the requirement and no amino acid limits performance.

[6]Compared with a situation where digestible P supply equals the requirement.

of the individual amino acids are evaluated, it appears that Trp (Figure 3) and Val are close to limiting (for the population) during the early phase of growth, whereas Ile is close to limiting at the end of the finishing phase. L-Tryptophan is available as a crystalline amino acid but the other two amino acids are not. Consequently, to reduce N excretion further, other feed ingredients may have to be used (which would occur at a greater cost).

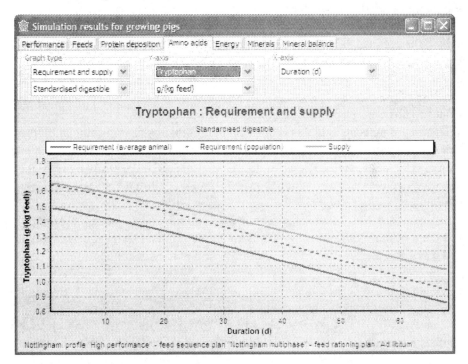

Figure 3. Simulated change in tryptophan supply and requirement of an individual pig and of a population of pigs using a multi-phase feed strategy where diet 1 is gradually replaced by diet 3 (see Table 1 for the composition of the diets).

The availability of crystalline amino acids has been very important in reducing N excretion. Diets 4 and 5 were formulated using the same constraints as diets 1 and 3 respectively, but without using crystalline amino acids (here: L-Lys, DL-Met, and L-Thr). Apart from being almost 10% more expensive, strategy 4 provided 23% more crude protein than strategy 3 (Table 2). In addition, N excretion was 42% greater when no crystalline amino acids were used (2.95 vs 2.08 kg). Most of this difference was caused by differences in urinary N excretion due to the excess supply of N, but also the faecal N excretion was lower for the diet including crystalline amino acids (because of the lower protein content of the diet).

Phosphorus utilization and excretion

The approach to P utilization is relatively simple in InraPorc. Feeds and feed ingredients are characterized by the total and apparently digestible P contents, the phytic acid fraction and the (endogenous or microbial) phytase activity. As heat treatment during pelleting destroys endogenous phytase activity, the digestible P content depends on whether the feed is given as mash or pellets. Microbial phytase can be used as a feed ingredient and should be attributed a digestible P value. The phytase included in the feed database of InraPorc assumes that 500 IU has a digestible P value of 0.8 g, but others types of phytase can be added by the end user. Because P digestibility (and thus the digestible P content) is not a linear function of the phytase activity, it will be useful to attribute different digestible P values to different phytase inclusion levels (e.g., see Table 1).

As for amino acids and N, it is possible to visualize the P utilisation in InraPorc. Only the apparently digestible P supply will be metabolically available to the animal. The maintenance P requirement is assumed to be 0.01 of body weight and potential P retention is a combined function of daily gain and body weight. Using a multiphase feed sequence plan with diets 1 and 3 (strategy 3), 0.88 of the digestible P supply was retained, the remainder being used for maintenance (0.13) or given in excess of the requirement (0.03). Despite the efficient utilization of digestible P, 0.42 of the total P supply was indigestible and thus excreted in the faeces. In the current model and in contrast to amino acids, a deficient P supply will limit P retention, but will not limit growth. Moreover, no compensatory P retention is possible when P supply exceeds the requirement after a period of deficiency. In a future version of the software, it is likely that the pool of total body P will be explicitly represented as a state variable, as currently is done for body protein and lipid, and that this will affect P absorption. This will allow the body P pool to vary independently of protein and lipid mass, and would allow simulating different phases of P deficiency (e.g., an initial phase of bone weakening while maintaining performance, followed by a phase of growth reduction) and compensatory bone mineralization. The important role of the intestines in P metabolism and excretion justifies the interest in developing specific models of P digestion and metabolism (e.g., Fernández, 1995; Schulin-Zeuthen, Lopes, Kebreab, Vitti, Abdalla, Haddad, Crompton and France, 2005; Létourneau-Montminy, Jondreville, Lescoat, Meschy, Pomar, Bernier and Sauvant, 2007).

InraPorc allows visualizing the total P balance, but without separating urinary and faecal P. As with the crystalline amino acids, the availability of microbial phytase allows for an important reduction in P excretion. Comparing feeding strategy 3 (with phytase) with strategy 5 (without phytase) indicates that the P excretion can be reduced by almost 40% (367 vs 603 g) by using microbial phytase. Due to the high cost of mineral phosphate, it is also economical to include phytase and limit the use of phosphate. With the price context of feed ingredients in May 2008, feeding strategy 3 was less expensive and has a considerable smaller impact on the environment than strategy 5. Because the efficacy of phytase diminishes with the level of inclusion, it was more economical for diet 1 to include mineral phosphate than to include a higher (fourth) level of phytase having a relatively low digestible P value.

Utilization and excretion of other minerals

InraPorc does not include recommendations concerning requirements for other macro- or trace-elements, but allows calculation of mineral balances for calcium, potassium, copper and zinc. The contribution of the different feed ingredients to the mineral content of compound feeds can be graphically evaluated. Calcium is mainly provided by supplements such as calcium carbonate or calcium phosphate, whereas potassium is provided by feed ingredients such as soybean meal and, to a lesser extent, cereals. The trace-elements copper and zinc are mainly provided by vitamin and mineral premixes. When InraPorc is used to evaluate trace mineral excretion, it is important that the appropriate mineral composition of the premix is provided (especially for the copper and zinc contents of the premix).

The availability of copper to the animal is known to vary with the copper source and requirement (Hill and Spears, 2008). Copper serves metabolically as an activator of several enzymes. The liver is the major site of copper storage and copper homeostasis is maintained both by absorption and biliary excretion of copper (Jondreville, Revy, Jaffrezic and Dourmad, 2002). There is little information concerning the copper requirements in pigs. The recommended NRC (1998) requirement for copper ranges from 3 ppm for finishing pigs to 6 ppm for post-weaned piglets while INRA (1989) and the British Society of Animal Science (2003) recommend 10 and 6 ppm throughout, respectively. Copper has been used for a long time as a growth-promoting agent at pharmacological concentrations (> 125 ppm). In the European Union, this use of copper is now banned for pigs over 12 wks of age and the maximum level of copper is now 25 ppm (Dourmad and Jondreville, 2007). In InraPorc, copper retention is assumed to be a quadratic function of body weight and in most cases will not exceed 0.5 ppm. This means that more than 90% of the ingested copper will be excreted into the environment. Because of the metabolic role of copper, the low retention of copper should not be interpreted as a requirement. Given the copper content of feed ingredients (especially soybean meal), copper inclusion in premixes does not seem to be necessary in order to attain 6 ppm of copper in the diet.

Like copper, zinc has been used in the past at pharmacological doses as a growth-promoting agent. Current European regulations allow 150 ppm zinc in complete feeds (Dourmad and Jondreville, 2007). The NRC (1998) suggests zinc requirements ranging from 50 ppm for finishing pigs to 100 ppm for post-weaned piglets and the British Society of Animal Science (2003) suggests similar values. Phytate can bind zinc in the intestine thereby lowering its availability. Revy, Jondreville, Dourmad and Nys (2006) confirmed the zinc requirement of around 90 ppm in post-weaned piglets, but indicated that this requirement could be 0.35 lower if phytase is included in the diet, which illustrates the complexity of the digestive process in the availability of trace-elements for the animal. Zinc, like copper, plays a role in numerous functions (e.g., as part of metalloenzymes) and its requirement is driven more by these functions than by storage of zinc in body tissue per se. In InraPorc, zinc retention is assumed to be a linear function of empty body weight (21 mg/kg; Dourmad, Pomar and Massé, 2002). Expressed per kg feed intake, zinc retention is then approximately 10 ppm during the early phases of growth and decreases with body weight. Although InraPorc can be used to quantify the excretion of trace-elements, it cannot indicate how this excretion can be minimized.

Dealing with a population of animals

The first version of the InraPorc software was released in April 2006 and several (minor) releases have been available since. Although the model and software is useful in evaluating how an animal uses its nutrient supply, practical application is somewhat limited because the concepts apply to a single, average animal. In reality, decisions are made for groups of animals.

It is known that the average response of a population does not necessarily correspond to the response of the average animal of that population (e.g., Pomar, Kyriazakis, Emmans and Knap, 2003). The amino acid requirements provided by InraPorc (expressed in g/kg feed) are rather low compared to standard practice and this value should not be used to formulate feeds for a population of animal. The reason for the low predicted requirement is that there is variation in feed intake and growth between animals. If all animals were fed according to the requirement of the average animal, approximately 0.50 of the population would receive more than required and these animals would perform according to their potential. The other 0.50 would receive a diet below their requirement thereby penalizing their performance. Consequently, the average performance of the population will be below the performance of the average animal.

Modelling the response of a population of animals to nutrients is rather difficult. In certain decision support tools, variation between individuals is taken into account by first predicting traits for the average animal, and then adding random variation to these traits. An approach is currently being used where individual pigs within a population are characterized by model parameters used by InraPorc in order to analyze the relationships between these model parameters. For example, it is likely that an animal that eats more also grows more than other animals, or that an animal that eats "early" also grows "early" (Brossard, van Milgen, Lannuzel, Bertinotti and Rivest, 2006). Once the relationship between model parameters is known (i.e., variance-covariance matrix), this information can be used to create virtual populations of pigs based on the profile of average pig. Random variation can then be included to all model parameters but accounting for the relationships between these parameters. It is then possible to perform simulations concerning the population. This will allow finding the most appropriate period to switch diets from an economic and environmental perspective or find the most suitable slaughter strategy given the payment grid for carcasses (e.g., all-in-all-out versus slaughter during one or more weeks). A research version of the software allows simulation of the performance of a population of pigs in a batch procedure using the characteristics of the individual animals (Brossard, Dourmad, van Milgen and Quiniou, 2007). Different feeding strategies were tested for a population of pigs involving phase feeding with 1, 2, 3 or 10 different diets and varying the Lys supply between 0.70 and 1.30 of the average requirement of the population. It appeared that a Lys supply at 1.10 of the average requirement was sufficient to cover the requirement for most animals, independent of the feeding strategy. The 10-phase feeding strategy required the smallest quantity of Lys (and N) but was also the most sensitive to a Lys deficiency, potentially leading to increased heterogeneity within the population.

These simulations with different levels of nutrients imply that the nutrient requirement is not always met for all animals throughout a simulation. Periods of nutrient deficiency may be followed by periods of nutrients excess, allowing for some compensatory gain. The way InraPorc deals with compensatory growth can easily be evaluated. For example, in feeding strategy 6, only diet 2 is used. This diet covers the requirement (of the population) at 60 kg of BW, but will be deficient in nutrient supply during the early phase of growth. When a single simulation is performed with this strategy using the "high performance animal" offered feed ad libitum, it appears that the supply of several amino acids (Met, Lys, Val, Thr, Ile, Met+Cys, Trp, and Leu) are limiting performance of the animal, with methionine being the first-limiting amino acid. At approximately 45 kg of body weight, the feed intake capacity of the pigs had increased sufficiently so that the requirement for all amino acids could be met. This strategy can be compared with strategy 2 (two-phase feed sequence plan). Both strategies result in almost identical curves of PD beyond 45 kg of body weight when PD is plotted against body weight. However, when it is plotted against age, InraPorc predicts that (a very marginal) compensatory PD occurs during the last part of the finishing phase, but that this was accompanied by a lower PD immediately following the nutrient deficiency (due to the lower body weight and feed intake). Consequently, there was no overall compensatory gain. The nutrient deficiency resulted overall in a slightly lower daily gain (1086 vs 1102 g/d) and PD (161 vs 164 g/d) combined with a similar lipid deposition (342 vs 343 g/d). Consequently, pigs were slightly fatter at slaughter. However, total feed cost was 0.04 lower for strategy 6 compared with strategy 2. Quiniou, Brossard, Gaudré, van Milgen and Salaün (2007) performed such a simulation for a population of pigs and concluded that the reduction in feed cost was outweighed by the decreased carcass value. It was confirmed that it was economically most advantageous to feed a population at 1.10 of the average nutrient requirement, and that an ever greater margin may be required when feed ingredients are very expensive.

Conclusion

Tools such as InraPorc can be used to evaluate different feeding strategies for growing pigs and sows from both a nutritional and environmental perspective. Knowledge of how PD evolves over time in relation to feed intake is essential if N excretion is to be reduced. The amino acid profile in the diet should resemble as much as possible to amino requirement of the animal at a given stage of growth. The availability of crystalline amino acids combined with a modelling approach to find the most appropriate feeding strategies offer an opportunity to go "from crude protein to precision protein" (title of Forum Bioscience seminar held in 2002).

The P digestibility varies widely between feed ingredients and depends to a large extent on the phytate and endogenous phytase contents. This, combined with the fact that approximately 0.50 of the total dietary P supply can be retained, underlines the importance to formulate diets on a digestible P basis. The use of microbial phytase allows minimizing P excretion considerably.

References

British Society of Animal Science (2003). *Nutrient Requirement Standards for Pigs*. British Society of Animal Science, Penicuik.

Brossard, L., Dourmad, J., van Milgen, J. and Quiniou, N. (2007) Analyse par modélisation de la variation des performances d'un groupe de porcs en croissance en fonction de l'apport de lysine et du nombre de phases dans le programme d'alimentation. *Journées de la Recherche Porcine en France*, **39**, 95-102.

Brossard, L., van Milgen, J., Lannuzel, P.Y., Bertinotti, R. and Rivest, J. (2006) Analyse des relations entre croissance et ingestion à partir de cinétiques individuelles : implications dans la définition de profils animaux pour la modélisation. *Journées de la Recherche Porcine en France*, **38**, 217-224.

Dourmad, J.Y., Étienne, M., Valancogne, A., Dubois, S., van Milgen, J. and Noblet, J. (2008) InraPorc: a model and decision support tool for the nutrition of sows. *Animal Feed Science and Technology*, **143**, 372-386.

Dourmad, J.Y., Pomar, C. and Massé, D. (2002) Modélisation du flux de composés à risque pour l'environnement dans un élevage porcin. *Journées de la Recherche Porcine en France*, **34**, 183-194.

Dourmad, J.Y. and Jondreville, C. (2007) Impact of nutrition on nitrogen, phosphorus, Cu and Zn in pig manure, and on emissions of ammonia and odours. *Livestock Science*, **112**, 192-198.

Fernández, J. (1995) Calcium and phosphorus metabolism in growing pigs. III. A model resolution. *Livestock Production Science*, **41**, 255-261.

Hill, G.M. and Spears, J.W. (2008) Trace and ultratrace elements in swine nutrition. In *Swine Nutrition*, pp 229-261. Edited by A.J.Lewis and L.L.Southern. CRC Press, Boca Raton.

INRA (1989). *L'Alimentation des Animaux Monogastrique: Porc, Lapin, Volailles*. INRA, Paris.

Jondreville, C. and Dourmad, J.Y. (2005) Le phosphore dans la nutrition des porcs. *INRA Productions Animales*, **18**, 182-192.

Jondreville, C., Revy, P.S., Jaffrezic, A. and Dourmad, J.Y. (2002) Le cuivre dans l'alimentation du porc: oligo-élément essentiel, facteur de croissance et risque potentiel pour l'Homme et l'environnement. *INRA Productions Animales*, **15**, 247-265.

Le Bellego, L., van Milgen, J. and Noblet, J. (2002) Effect of high temperature and low-protein diets on the performance of growing-finishing pigs. *Journal of Animal Science*, **80**, 691-701.

Létourneau-Montminy, M.P., Jondreville, C., Lescoat, P., Meschy, F., Pomar, C., Bernier, J.F. and Sauvant, D. (2007) First step of a model of calcium and phosphorus metabolism in growing pigs: Fate of ingested phosphorus in the stomach. *Livestock Science*, **109**, 63-65.

Moughan, P.J. (1998) Protein metabolism in the growing pig. In *A Quantitative Biology of the Pig*, pp 299-331. Edited by I.Kyriazakis. CABI Publishing, Oxon, UK.

NRC (1998). *Nutrient Requirements of Swine*. National Academy Press, Washington, DC.

Pomar, C., Kyriazakis, I., Emmans, G.C. and Knap, P.W. (2003) Modeling stochasticity: Dealing with populations rather than individual pigs. *Journal of Animal Science*, **81** (**E. Suppl. 2**), E178-E186.

Quiniou, N., Brossard, L., Gaudré, D., van Milgen, J. and Salaün, Y. (2007) Optimum économique du niveau en acides aminés dans les aliments pour porcs charcutiers. Impact du contexte de prix des matières premières et de la conduite d'élevage. *TechniPorc*, **30**, 25-36.

Revy, P.S., Jondreville, C., Dourmad, J.Y. and Nys, Y. (2006) Assessment of dietary zinc requirement of weaned piglets fed diets with or without mircobial phytase. *Journal of Animal Physiology and Animal Nutrition*, **90**, 50-59.

Sauvant, D., Perez, J.-M., and Tran, G. (2002). *Tables de Composition et de Valeur Nutritive des Matières Premières Destinées aux Animaux d'Élevage. Porcs, Volailles, Bovins, Ovins, Caprins, Lapins, Chevaux, Poissons.* INRA Editions, Paris.

Schulin-Zeuthen, M., Lopes, J.B., Kebreab, E., Vitti, D.M.S.S., Abdalla, A.L., Haddad, M.D., Crompton, L.A. and France, J. (2005) Effects of phosphorus intake on phosphorus flow in growing pigs: Application and comparison of two models. *Journal of Theoretical Biology*, **236**, 115-125.

van Milgen, J., Valancogne, A., Dubois, S., Dourmad, J.Y., Sève, B. and Noblet, J. (2008) InraPorc: A model and decision support tool for the nutrition of growing pigs. *Animal Feed Science and Technology*, **143**, 387-405.

11

GUT HEALTH, MICROBIOTA AND IMMUNITY

I. MULDER, B. SCHMIDT, R. AMINOV AND D. KELLY,
Rowett Institute of Nutrition & Health, University of Aberdeen, Greenburn Road, Bucksburn, Aberdeen AB21 9SB

Introduction

The mammalian gastrointestinal tract contains an immense number of micro-organisms, collectively known as the microbiota. In fact, bacterial cells outnumber host cells in the body by a factor of ten. Formation of the microbiota starts shortly after birth and quickly expands into a complex and dynamic ecosystem that fulfils important roles in promoting health of the host. Principal functions include degrading dietary compounds and providing essential nutrients, protecting against invading pathogens, and stimulating gut morphology as well as immune development and maintenance (Falk *et al.*, 1998; Salminen *et al.*, 1998).

This chapter will focus on the progress made in understanding the factors that influence the acquisition and succession of the commensal microbiota in the pig gut. The role of the microbiota in both promoting health and preventing disease and its manipulation to benefit the host will also be discussed.

Development of the commensal microbiota

The microbiota of the gastrointestinal tract represents an open ecosystem, that is not only in contact with the outside environment, but also a relatively stable community that has successfully established during the period between birth and adulthood. The processes involved in the acquisition, establishment, succession and stabilisation of microbial community structure are complex, and integrate both microbial and host factors that eventually result in a dense and stable microbial population inhabiting specific regions of the gut.

ACQUISITION OF THE INTESTINAL MICROBIOTA AFTER BIRTH

Colonisation and succession of the gut microbiota is shaped by both external and internal host-related factors. External factors include the microbial load of the immediate environment, diet, and the composition of the maternal microbiota. Internal factors include host physiology, nutrient availability in the gastrointestinal tract, and the presiding microbiota (Mackie *et al.*, 1999). Microbial succession during the first few weeks of life in the gastrointestinal tracts of humans, pigs, chickens and cows is surprisingly similar (Mackie *et al.*, 1999).

Prior to birth, the gastrointestinal tract of the piglet is sterile (Kelly and King 2001). From the moment the piglet passes through the birth canal, it is exposed to a wide variety of microbes originating from the maternal vagina, faeces and skin as well as the environment (Mackie *et al.*, 1999). In this very early stage, the gastrointestinal microbiota is heterogeneous (Fanaro *et al.*, 2003). Colonising aerobic and facultative anaerobic bacterial populations alter local environmental conditions within the gut by consuming and depleting the available molecular oxygen. As a consequence, the primary colonising aerotolerant bacteria are gradually replaced by strict anaerobic bacteria, which are now able to grow in the oxygen-depleted gut environment (Swords *et al.*, 1993). Bacterial groups such as lactobacilli and streptococci become the dominant bacteria throughout the suckling period, due to their ability to utilise milk substrates. *Clostridium*, *Bacteroides*, *Bifidobacterium*, *Eubacterium* and *Streptococcus* genera are also present at this stage, but in lower abundance (Mackie *et al.*, 1999).

The second major phase in gut microbial community succession occurs at weaning with the introduction of solid food, and the switch to complex carbohydrates as the main energy source rather than the lipid-rich milk diet of the pre-weaning phase. The gut microbial community grows to be more diverse and becomes dominated by *Bacteroidetes* and *Firmicutes*, bacterial divisions that remain prevalent throughout adult life (Swords *et al.*, 1993; Mackie *et al.*, 1999).

THE ADULT MICROBIOTA

The normal adult microbiota is characteristic to each individual, and inhabits specific regions of the gut with an increasing gradient of microbes from the upper to the lower gastrointestinal tract (Zoetendal *et al.*, 1998).

The stomach and small intestine contain low numbers of bacteria. Only bacterial groups that can overcome colonisation limitations (such as acid, bile and rapid flow of digesta) inhabit this part of the gastrointestinal tract. The jejunal and ileal luminal microbiota consists of mostly facultative anaerobes, such as lactobacilli, streptococci, enterococci, gamma-proteobacteria, and bacteroides (Hayashi *et al.*, 2005). The caecum and colon are the main sites for bacterial colonisation in the gut, and the microbiota in this region forms an increasingly complex ecosystem. High substrate availability, slow passage rate and higher pH create a favourable environment for diverse and stable colonisation of bacteria, with numbers reaching up to 10^{12} colony-forming units/g of digesta (Pryde *et al.*, 1999). The majority of culturable bacteria include gram-positives such as streptococci, lactobacilli, peptostreptococci and clostridia, and gram-negative bacteria affiliated with prevotella and bacteroides. Comparative phylogenetic analysis of 16S ribosomal RNA (rRNA) genes from the microbial community with data generated by culture-based methods indicates that 60 to 80% of the micro-organisms in the total microbiota have not been cultivated previously (Suau *et al.*, 1999; Salzman *et al.*, 2002; Leser *et al.*, 2002; Eckburg *et al.*, 2005; Ley *et al.*, 2008).

In terms of composition of the gastrointestinal microbiota, most current knowledge has been derived from analyses of faecal samples. Little attention has been paid to potential differences between the specific anatomical sites within the gut. For example, surface-adherent and luminal microbial populations, the latter reflecting faecal diversity, may be distinct and may fulfil different roles within the ecosystem (Pryde *et al.*, 1999; Zoetendal *et al.*, 2002). The analysis of biopsy samples by Zoetendal *et al.* (2002) revealed that the predominant bacterial communities from different locations within the colon are similar to each other, but differ significantly from those recovered from faecal samples of the same subject. Furthermore, although bacterial communities adherent to the different mucosal sites within an individual show little variation, communities from different individuals show a high degree of variation (Green *et al.*, 2006), indicating the potential importance of the host genotype as a determinant of microbial diversity within the gastrointestinal tract.

Effects of the commensal microbiota on the host

The gut microbiota, which has been shaped by the long co-evolutionary history of symbiotic host–microbe interaction, plays an important role in maintaining health. Recent work suggests that the commensal microbiota influences processes as complex as pathogen colonisation, nutrient partitioning and lipid metabolism (Backhed *et al.*, 2004; Ley *et al.*, 2006), immune development and homeostasis, inflammation, repair and angiogenesis (Rakoff-Nahoum *et al.*, 2004; Kelly *et al.*, 2004; Stappenbeck *et al.*, 2005).

HOST-MICROBE INTERACTION: STRUCTURE AND DEVELOPMENT OF THE IMMUNE SYSTEM

The intestinal epithelial lining defines the barrier between the host and the environment and protects the body against invasion and systemic dissemination of both pathogens and commensal micro-organisms. The mucosal immune system in the gastrointestinal tract incorporates both organised and diffuse tissues. The organised tissues of the intestinal immune system include the Peyer's patches and the mesenteric lymph nodes. Pigs have two types of Peyer's patch. A large ileocaecal patch is present in the terminal ileum of young animals, which involutes at one year of age. This Peyer's patch is a primary source of B cells. Approximately 25-35 small Peyer's patches are found in the jejunum and proximal ileum that persist throughout life (reviewed by Dvorak *et al.*, 2006).

A wide variety of antigens, including those of dietary and bacterial origin, are present in the gut, and are found on both on the mucosal surface and in the lumen. Jejunal Peyer's patches are involved in directly sampling antigens from the lumen. Antigens are taken up across the follicle-associated epithelium of the Peyer's patches through specialised M cells (microfold cells) or via the paracellular route. Antigens are then sampled by dendritic cells (DCs) in the Peyer's patch. Migration of DC cells to the mesenteric lymph nodes and contact with naïve T cells results in T cell activation, relocation and initiation of immune responses in the follicle. A second way of antigen sampling is direct sampling of luminal antigens by DC subsets lying just beneath the intestinal epithelium. These DCs extend their dendrites through the epithelium by manipulation of tight-cell junctions (Rescigno *et al.*, 2001; Macpherson and Uhr, 2004). Following antigen acquisition, mucosal dendritic cells travel to the mesenteric lymph nodes, where they can present antigen to T cells (Huang *et al.*, 2000).

The diffuse lymphoid tissue consists of the epithelium and the lamina propria. Leukocytes are present within the intestinal epithelium, predominantly expressing the CD8 co-receptor (Bailey *et al.*, 2005). The lamina propria in the pig intestine shows a high level of organisation. Antigen-presenting cells expressing MHC II are present in large numbers in the lamina propria of adult pigs (Wilson *et al.*, 1996) and they have been characterised as functional, immature dendritic cells (Haverson *et al.*, 2000). Dendritic cells are also present in large numbers within the villi and co-localise with T cells expressing the CD4 co-receptor. In addition to active antigen sampling by the organised lymphoid tissue, this cluster of MHC class II+ dendritic cells, endothelium and CD4+ T cells could act as a complex antigen-presenting zone in a site frequently exposed to antigens from the environment (Bailey *et al.*, 2005). Antibody-producing cells (mostly immunoglobulin A) are mainly found around the intestinal crypts (Bailey *et al.*, 2005). This complex system of antigen recognition, sampling and presentation is underdeveloped in the newborn and develops with constant antigen exposure, particularly antigens of microbial origin.

Immune responses in the pig do not differ substantially from those seen in humans and mice. However, the porcine gastrointestinal tract is heavily biased toward immunological non-responsiveness and oral tolerance (Dvorak *et al.*, 2006). Development of the mucosal immune system takes place with age, but is strongly influenced by environmental factors including microbial colonisation and exposure to specific antigens. In the neonatal pig, mucosal development takes place in four phases (Table 1; Bailey *et al.*, 2005). By week seven the architecture of the intestine is comparable to that of a mature animal.

Table 1. Stages of mucosal immune system development within the pig (Bailey *et al.*, 2005)

Stage 1	The newborn pig	Rudimentary Peyers patches, small numbers of mucosal APCs and T-cells
Stage 2	1 day - 2 weeks	Non-specific expansion of Peyers patches and B-cells. Appearance of some conventional, activated, CD4+ T-cells, influx of MHCII+ cells
Stage 3	2 weeks - 4 weeks	Appearance of mature CD4+ T-cells
Stage 4	4 weeks - 6 weeks	Expansion of B-cell repertoire, appearance of CD8+ T-cells

Microbial colonisation of the intestine drives the development of the immune system in several ways, and although much of it is antigen-specific, it appears that important antigen-independent effects also occur. These antigen-independent effects are driven by recognition events involving pattern-recognition receptors (PRRs) and microbial products, referred to as pathogen associated microbial patterns (PAMPs) (Butler *et al.*, 2000). It has recently become clear that these interactions are important for mucosal immune development, but also for the development of the systemic immune system. Cross-talk between (mucosa-associated) commensal bacteria and the gut immune system is facilitated by PRRs referred to as Toll-like receptors (TLRs) (Medzhitov and Janeway, 1997) and NOD-like receptors, which are expressed on numerous cell lineages including dendritic cells, macrophages and epithelial cells. Careful regulation of this communication is critical to mucosal immune homeostasis, as the immune system in the gut needs to be able to mount adequate immune responses against potential pathogens, whilst at the same time maintaining tolerance to commensal bacteria. This is made more complicated by the fact that many commensal bacteria possess PAMPs similar to those found on pathogenic bacteria. It is still unclear what factors are important in determining whether a tolerance response or an active immune response is mounted as a result of antigen and/or PAMP recognition.

When commensal bacteria are not properly recognized as harmless by the mucosal immune system, inappropriate immune responses can be mounted, triggering damaging inflammatory and allergic reactions. Conversely, inadequate immune responses to specific pathogens can lead to enhanced disease susceptibility. Attempts to explain the increased incidence of immune-mediated disorders, particularly in Westernised countries, have led to the development of the so-called "Hygiene Hypothesis". This hypothesis states that allergy and autoimmune diseases are consequences of reduced infectious stresses during early childhood (Strachan, 1989). Factors such as the high-hygiene status of western lifestyle, decreased infection rates and reduced bacterial load as a result of widespread vaccine and antibiotic use provide a direct causal relationship with the increased incidences of both autoimmune and allergic diseases (Wills-Karp *et al.*, 2001). Animal models have provided some insight into immune-disease aetiology: animals susceptible to autoimmune disease have an increased incidence and severity of disease when bred under germ-free conditions, whereas disease is prevented when the animals are exposed to bacteria (Bach, 2005). In this context, the "Hygiene Hypothesis" suggests that appropriate bacterial loading is a major factor in protection of the human population from immune-related disorder. This notion extends the "Hygiene Hypothesis" beyond the protective effects of both natural infections and pathogen exposure, to include the protective effects of the normal commensal microbiota. The relevance of the "Hygiene Hypothesis", originally formulated to explain the rising incidence of human immune-mediated diseases, to animal health is currently speculative. Analogies can be drawn, however, between the hygienic lifestyle of westernised human populations and intensively-farmed animals, where susceptibility to disease should be demonstratively greater than that of organically-farmed animals (Pluske *et al.*, 2007).

IMPORTANCE OF MICROBIOTA FOR IMMUNE DEVELOPMENT - EVIDENCE FROM GERM-FREE ANIMALS STUDIES

Major limiting factors in studying interactions of the gastrointestinal microbiota with the host are both the complexity and potential variation in bacterial populations between individuals. Defined-flora and germ-free animal models have been developed and used successfully to study the effects of the microbiota on host physiology and immunity.

Maturation of the gut is directly influenced by the presence of commensal bacteria. Germ-free animals have little development of the mucosal immune system. Gross-morphological defects include a reduction in intestinal thickness and length due to reduced number of lymphocytes, plasma cells and mononuclear cells and an enlarged caecum filled with undegraded mucus (Wostmann *et al.*, 1996). The number of intraepithelial T lymphocytes is significantly reduced in both the jejunum and ileum of germ-free pigs (Rothkötter *et al.*, 1999). At the histological level, the villi-crypt ratio is increased (Umesaki *et al.*, 1993), indicating a direct link between the commensal microbiota and cell turnover rate in the intestinal epithelium (Alam *et al.*, 1994). Indeed, several studies suggest that the microbiota can influence cell fate in the gut epithelium. For example, secretory cells such as mucus-secreting goblet cells are less abundant in the gut epithelium of germ-free rats (Sharma and Schumacher, 1995).

These studies not only find that the germ-free animal remains morphologically underdeveloped, but also demonstrate that the introduction of intestinal contents or faeces of conventional mice into germ-free mice (a process known as conventionalisation) restores normal physiological and immunological characteristics. This provides compelling evidence of the importance of the normal commensal microbiota in gut development (Matsumoto *et al.*, 1992; Umesaki *et al.*, 1993; Okada *et al.*, 1994).

Mono-association studies show that introduction of single bacterial strains can effectively restore aspects of immunological development in a strain-specific manner. Segmented filamentous bacteria (SFB) increase the number of ß intraepithelial lymphocytes (IELs), the mitotic activity and ratio of number of columnar cells to goblet cells, and induce MHC class II in small intestinal epithelial cells (Umesaki *et al.*, 1995). Moreover, SFB interact with intraepithelial mononuclear cells in Peyer's patches (Meyerholz *et al.*, 2002) and stimulate IgA production (Klaasen *et al.*, 1993; Talham *et al.*, 1999). In addition it was demonstrated recently, that a single bacterial molecule, namely the Zwitterionic polysaccharide A of the commensal bacterium *Bacteroides fragilis*, directs cellular and physical maturation of the immune system by correcting systemic T-cell deficiency and restoring the T helper cell (Th1/Th2) balance in germ-free animals (Mazmanian *et al.*, 2005).

The effects of the commensal microbiota on immune development are specific to both the bacterial strain and the responsive region of the intestine. For example, mono-colonisation with SFB results in improved immune development in the small intestine but not in other gut segments. Conversely, immunological development in the large intestine was restored by colonisation with clostridia, a common bacterial group of the large intestine. In the presence of both SFB and clostridia, almost the same level of development of the gut immune system occurs as observed after conventionalisation (Umesaki *et al.*, 1999). This demonstrates not only, that different commensal species exert their immune-stimulating effects in different locations within the gut, but also the complexity by which the commensal microbiota modulates the host's immune system.

ANALYSIS OF HOST-MICROBE INTERACTIONS IN THE PIG - NEW ADVANCES WITH MOLECULAR APPROACHES

Substantial efforts have been directed towards characterising the intestinal microbiota of humans and animals, with a view to identifying compositional shifts in the commensal microbiota in both the healthy and disease state and to establishing the modulating influences of nutrition and environment. This work has been undertaken using microbiological methods based on one of two different techniques: culture-based enumeration and phylogenetic analysis of 16S rRNA genes (Russell, 1979). A major drawback of the culturing method is the fact that a large proportion of the microbiota is unculturable, leading to bias towards the description and functional analyses of culturable bacterial strains. More detailed knowledge of the microbial community composition in natural systems has been gained recently from the phylogenetic analysis of 16S rRNA sequences obtained by PCR amplification, cloning, and sequencing. The highly conserved regions of 16S rRNA can serve as primer binding sites for polymerase chain reactions. The more variable sequence regions can be applied for species-specific hybridisation probes. The use of 16S rRNA library techniques have now been applied to analysis of the intestinal bacterial community in a wide variety of mammals (Leser *et al.*, 2002; Eckburg *et al.*, 2005; Ley *et al.*, 2008) and shows the great complexity of those populations within the gastrointestinal system. Leser *et al.* (2002) have used 16S rRNA sequencing to describe the microbiota of the pig gastrointestinal tract. Sequencing of 4,270 16S genes revealed that 83% of the phylotypes were unknown, with less than 97% similarity to previously identified species. The majority of identified phylotypes (around 81%) belonged to the low-G+C gram-positive division (*Streptococcus, Staphylococcus, Bacillus, Clostridium, Lactobacillus*), and 11.2 % belonged to *Bacteroides* and *Prevotella* groups.

In order to assess the host response to microbial colonisation different platforms for porcine expression profiling are now available and have been described by Tuggle and co-authors (2007). A first generation Affymetrix porcine GeneChip® containing over 23,000 transcripts has been applied to study the gene expression response in pig intestinal tissue to the gut microbiota. Wang *et al.* (2007) assessed the transcriptomic response in mesenteric lymph nodes to the pathogen *Salmonella enterica* serovar *Typhimurium*. Differentially expressed genes involved in both immune and inflammatory responses were highly represented. While nF-κB target genes where increased 24h after infection, the nF-κB pathway was suppressed thereafter. The authors proposed that this nF-κB suppression was a mechanism by which *S. Typhimurium* established carrier status in pigs. Chowdhury *et al.* (2007) also investigated gene expression profiles in the small intestinal epithelium of germfree and conventional neonatal piglets. They found that the intestinal microbiota triggered upregulation of genes involved in biological processes such as epithelial cell turnover, nutrient transport and metabolism, xenobiotic metabolism, JAK-STAT signaling pathway, and immune response.

Dvorak *et al.* (2005) created a cDNA microarray from libraries enriched for genes expressed in the Peyer's patch to examine the biological function of Peyer's patch tissue. They uncovered 11 genes having immune functions relevant to Peyer's patch tissue and the small intestine.

These studies illustrate that the development and composition of the intestinal commensal microbiota has major effects on the host mucosal immune system. Studying these interactions using novel molecular techniques could lead to effective ways of improving the nutritional and immunological status of the host gut. Such findings have obvious commercial relevance not only to animal health but also to the human health sector; firstly, by identifying potentially novel bacterial strains for development as new generation probiotics and secondly, by providing clearer evidence of their mode of action and therapeutic/prophylactic efficacy.

Host-microbe interaction: practical applications

Mortality resulting from infections during the immediate post-weaning period represents a major financial penalty to the pig industry. It is estimated that weaning mortality levels in the EU amount to approximately 17% of the pig population, and a substantial part of these losses are associated with mucosal infections (Lalles *et al.*, 2007). Removal from the sow and littermates at weaning is stressful and accompanied by a multitude of factors (reduced feed intake, introduction of new dietary antigens from the weaning diet, removal of maternal immune protection via milk, and disruption of the microbiota) that make the piglet susceptible to infection. Intensive farming practice in Europe dictates weaning at an early age (21–35 d), which probably exacerbates susceptibility to infection in these immature animals (Lalles *et al.*, 2007).

Post-weaning diarrhoea is mainly caused by enterotoxigenic *Escherichia coli* K88 (Moon and Bunn, 1993; Osek, 1999). Porcine circovirus 2 is the causative pathogen associated with post-weaning multisystemic wasting syndrome (PMWS). Other diseases that have a major impact on pig health during this time include Rotavirus, Salmonella, Swine Dysentery and Haemophilus. Non-specific colitis is also a serious problem in growing and finishing pigs, and significantly impairs animal performance and has striking similarities to human inflammatory bowel disease.

Until recently, methods of disease control at weaning relied on the subtherapeutic use of antibiotic growth promoters (Dritz *et al.*, 2002; Gaskins *et al.*, 2002). Inclusion of these substances in animal feeds improves growth rates and feed conversion efficiency, as well as protecting against pathogenic bacteria. But a European ban on antibiotic growth promoters, partly due to the increased prevalence of antibiotic-resistant bacteria, necessitates the need for alternative methods of immuno-competence and disease control (Anadon, 2006).

One possible avenue to pursue is the application of dietary ingredients to manipulate the gut microbiota, in order to improve intestinal function and a healthy gastrointestinal tract. An approach that has received much attention recently is the

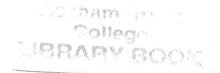

use of pro- and prebiotics. Probiotics are defined as "Live micro-organisms which when administered in adequate amounts confer a health benefit on the host" (FAO 2001). Prebiotics are food additives that skew the intestinal microbial community towards the colonisation of so-called 'good' bacteria, which have health benefits for the host (Tako *et al.*, 2008).

Oral ingestion of pro- and prebiotics could be beneficial to the host and influence succession at different stages because microbial succession is an ongoing process. This is especially useful during stressful periods such as weaning, when the animal is susceptible to colonisation by pathogens. One way in which pre- and probiotics are thought to prevent gut colonisation of exogenous pathogens is through competition for biological niches according to for instance oxygen, pH or nutrient requirements. Probiotic bacteria can also produce antibacterial compounds including hydrogen peroxide, organic acids and bacteriocins. For instance, the Abp 118 bacteriocin produced by *Lactobacillus salivarius* has antilisterial effects in mice (Corr *et al.*, 2007). Finally, as mentioned before, these bacteria potentially modulate the systemic immune response through the mucosal immune system (Corth *et al.*, 2007).

Commonly investigated prebiotics include inulin and inulin-type fructans (Tako *et al.*, 2008). Inulin improves iron and calcium absorption, and is fermented in the colon to produce short chain fatty acids (SCFA) such as butyrate, thereby stimulating the growth of health-promoting bacteria such as bifidobacteria and lactobacilli (Tako *et al.*, 2008). Butyrate also has direct effects on colonic health, by regulating processes associated with proliferation, differentiation and apoptosis of epithelial cells (Tako *et al.*, 2008).

Probiotics have been used in diets for pigs to improve growth performance and decrease the incidence of diarrhoea and subsequent mortality rates (Lalles *et al.*, 2007). The probiotic species mostly investigated in pigs are lactobacilli, enterococci and yeast with *Lactobacillus* species currently being in practical use as probiotics (Takahashi *et al.*, 2007). The lactic-acid producer *Pediococcus acidilactici* increases weight gain in piglets post-weaning, and has a positive effect on the morphology of the ileum by increasing villus height and crypt depth (Di Giancamillo *et al.*, 2008). The live yeast *Saccharomyces cerevisiae* spp *boulardii* has potential beneficial effects on the structure of the gut (Baum *et al.*, 2002; Bontempo *et al.*, 2006).

Summary

The mammalian gastrointestinal tract contains a huge number of micro-organisms, collectively known as the microbiota. Microbial colonisation of the intestine drives the development of the immune system. Cross-talk between the microbiota and the mucosal immune system is carefuly regulated as the immune system must be able to mount active responses against pathogens but maintain tolerance against harmless food and commensal bacterial antigens. The pig is especially susceptible to mortality in the critical post-weaning period. The ban on antibiotic growth promoters means that alternative methods of disease control are necessary. Pro- and prebiotics could be useful therapeutics in this respect, and their potential beneficial effects are currently being investigated.

Acknowledgements

The authors acknowledge the support of the Scottish Government Rural and Environment Research and Analysis Directorate (RERAD).

References

Alam M., Midtvedt T., and Uribe A. (1994). Differential cell kinetics in the ileum and colon of germfree rats. *Scandinavian Journal of Gastroenterology* **29**: 445-451.

Anadon A. (2006). WS14 The EU ban of antibiotics as feed additives (2006): alternatives and consumer safety. *Journal of Veterinary Pharmacology and Therapeutics* **29**: 41-44.

Bach J.F. (2005). Six questions about the hygiene hypothesis. *Cellular Immunology* **233**: 158-161.

Backhed F., Ding H., Wang T., Hooper L.V., Koh G.Y., Nagy A., Semenkovich C.F., and Gordon J.I. (2004). The gut microbiota as an environmental factor that regulates fat storage. *Proceedings of the National Academy of Sciences* **101**: 15718-15723.

Bailey M., Haverson K., Inman C., Harris C., Jones P., Corfield G., Miller B., and Stokes C. (2005). The influence of environment on development of the mucosal immune system. *Veterinary Immunology and Immunopathology* **108**: 189-198.

Baum B., Liebler-Tenorio E.M., Enss M.L., Pohlenz J.F., and Breves G. (2002). *Saccharomyces boulardii* and *Bacillus cereus* var. Toyoi influence the morphology and the mucins of the intestine of pigs. *Zeitschrift fur Gastroenterologie* **40**: 277-284.

Bontempo V., Di Giancamillo A., Savoini G., Dell'Orto V., and Domeneghini C. (2006). Live yeast dietary supplementation acts upon intestinal morpho-functional aspects and growth in weanling piglets. *Animal Feed Science and Technology* **129**: 224-236.

Butler J.E., Sun J., Weber P., Navarro P., and Francis D. (2000). Antibody repertoire development in fetal and newborn piglets, III. Colonization of the gastrointestinal tract selectively diversifies the preimmune repertoire in mucosal lymphoid tissues. *Immunology* **100**: 119-130.

Chowdhury S., King D., Willing B., Band M., Beever J., Lane A., Loor J.J., Marini J.C., Rund L.A., Schook L.B., Van Kessel A.G., and Gaskins H.R. (2007). Transcriptome profiling of the small intestinal epithelium in germfree versus conventional piglets. *BMC Genomics* **8**: 215.

Corr S.C., Li Y., Riedel C.U., O'Toole P.W., Hill C., and Gahan C.G. (2007). Bacteriocin production as a mechanism for the antiinfective activity of *Lactobacillus salivarius* UCC118. *Proceedings of the National Academy of Sciences* **104**: 7617-7621.

Corthesy B., Gaskins H.R., and Mercenier A. (2007). Cross-Talk between probiotic bacteria and the host immune system. *Journal of Nutrition* **137**: 781S-790.

Di Giancamillo A., Vitari F., Savoini G., Bontempo V., Bersani C., Dell'Orto V., and Domeneghini C. (2008). Effects of orally administered probiotic *Pediococcus acidilactici* on the small and large intestine of weaning piglets. A qualitative and quantitative micro-anatomical study. *Histology and Histopathology* **23**: 651-664.

Dritz S.S., Tokach M.D., Goodband R.D., and Nelssen J.L. (2002). Effects of administration of antimicrobials in feed on growth rate and feed efficiency of pigs in multisite production systems. *Journal of the American Veterinary Medical Association* **220**: 1690-1695.

Dvorak C.M.T., Hyland K.A., Machado J.G., Zhang Y., Fahrenkrug S.C., and Murtaugh M.P. (2005). Gene discovery and expression profiling in porcine peyer's patch. *Veterinary Immunology and Immunopathology* **105**: 301-315.

Dvorak C.M., Hirsch G.N., Hyland K.A., Hendrickson J.A., Thompson B.S., Rutherford M.S., and Murtaugh M.P. (2006). Genomic dissection of mucosal immunobiology in the porcine small intestine. *Physiological Genomics* **28**: 5-14.

Eckburg P.B., Bik E.M., Bernstein C.N., Purdom E., Dethlefsen L., Sargent M., Gill S.R., Nelson K.E., and Relman D.A. (2005). Diversity of the human intestinal microbial flora. *Science* **308**: 1635-1638.

Falk P.G., Hooper L.V., Midtvedt T., and Gordon J.I. (1998). Creating and maintaining the gastrointestinal ecosystem: What we know and need to know from gnotobiology. *Microbiology and Molecular Biology Review* **62**: 1157-1170.

Fanaro S., Chierici R., Guerrini P., and Vigi V. (2003). Intestinal microflora in early infancy: composition and development. *Acta Paediatrica* **92**: 48-55.

Gaskins H.R., Collier C.T., and Anderson D.B. (2002). Antibiotics as growth promotants: mode of action. *Animal Biotechnology* **13**: 29-42.

Green G.L., Brostoff J., Hudspith B., Michael M., Mylonaki M., Rayment N., Staines N., Sanderson J., Rampton D.S., and Bruce K.D. (2006). Molecular characterization of the bacteria adherent to human colorectal mucosa. *Journal of Applied Microbiology* **100**: 460-469.

Haverson K., Singha S., Stokes C.R., and Bailey M. (2000). Professional and non-professional antigen-presenting cells in the porcine small intestine. *Immunology* **101**: 492-500.

Hayashi H., Takahashi R., Nishi T., Sakamoto M., and Benno Y. (2005). Molecular analysis of jejunal, ileal, caecal and recto-sigmoidal human colonic microbiota using 16S rRNA gene libraries and terminal restriction fragment length polymorphism. *Journal of Medical Microbiology* **54**: 1093-1101.

Huang F.P., Platt N., Wykes M., Major J.R., Powell T.J., Jenkins C.D., and MacPherson G.G. (2000). A discrete subpopulation of dendritic cells transports apoptotic intestinal epithelial cells to T cell areas of mesenteric lymph nodes. *Journal of Experimental Medicine* **191**: 435-444.

Kelly D. and King T.P. (2001). Digestive physiology and development in pigs. In The Weaner Pig. Nutrition and Management. M.A. Varley and J. Wiseman, eds. CABI Publishing, U.K.

Kelly D., Campbell J.I., King T.P., Grant G., Jansson E.A., Coutts A.G.P., Pettersson S., and Conway S. (2004). Commensal anaerobic gut bacteria attenuate inflammation by regulating nuclear-cytoplasmic shuttling of PPAR-[gamma] and RelA. *Nature Immunology* **5**: 104-112.

Klaasen H.L., Van der Heijden P.J., Stok W., Poelma F.G., Koopman J.P., Van den Brink M.E., Bakker M.H., Eling W.M., and Beynen A.C. (1993). Apathogenic, intestinal, segmented, filamentous bacteria stimulate the mucosal immune system of mice. *Infection and Immunity* **61**: 303-306.

Lallès J.P., Bosi P., Smidt H., and Stokes C.R. (2007). Nutritional management of gut health in pigs around weaning. *Proceedings of the Nutrition Society* **66**: 260-268.

Leser T.D., Amenuvor J.Z., Jensen T.K., Lindecrona R.H., Boye M., and Moller K. (2002). Culture-independent analysis of gut bacteria: the pig gastrointestinal tract microbiota revisited. *Applied and Environmental Microbiology* **68**: 673-690.

Ley R.E., Turnbaugh P.J., Klein S., and Gordon J.I. (2006). Microbial ecology: Human gut microbes associated with obesity. *Nature* **444**: 1022-1023.

Ley R.E., Hamady M., Lozupone C., Turnbaugh P.J., Ramey R.R., Bircher J.S., Schlegel M.L., Tucker T.A., Schrenzel M.D., Knight R., and Gordon J.I. (2008). Evolution of mammals and their gut microbes. *Science* **320**: 1647-1651.

Mackie R.I., Sghir A., and Gaskins H.R. (1999). Developmental microbial ecology of the neonatal gastrointestinal tract. *American Journal of Clinical Nutrition* **69**: 1035S-11045.

Macpherson A.J. and Uhr T. (2004). Induction of protective IgA by intestinal dendritic cells carrying commensal bacteria. *Science* **303**: 1662-1665.

Matsumoto S., Setoyama H., and Umesaki Y. (1992). Differential induction of major histocompatibility complex molecules on mouse intestine by bacterial colonisation. *Gastroenterology* **103**: 1777-1782.

Mazmanian S.K., Liu C.H., Tzianabos A.O., and Kasper D.L. (2005). An immunomodulatory molecule of symbiotic bacteria directs maturation of the host immune system. *Cell* **122**: 107-118.

Medzhitov R. and Janeway C.A. (1997). Innate immunity: impact on the adaptive immune response. *Current Opinion in Immunology* **9**: 4-9.

Meyerholz D.K., Stabel T.J., and Cheville N.F. (2002). Segmented filamentous bacteria interact with intraepithelial mononuclear cells. *Infection and Immunity* **70**: 3277-3280.

Moon H.W. and Bunn T.O. (1993). Vaccines for preventing enterotoxigenic Escherichia coli infections in farm animals. *Vaccine* **11**: 213-220.

Okada Y., Setoyama H., Matsumoto S., Imaoka A., Nanno M., Kawaguchi M., and Umesaki Y. (1994). Effects of fecal microorganisms and their chloroform-resistant variants derived from mice, rats, and humans on immunological and physiological characteristics of the intestines of ex-germfree mice. *Infection and Immunity* **62**: 5442-5446.

Osek J. (1999). Prevalence of virulence factors of *Escherichia coli* strains isolated from diarrheic and healthy piglets after weaning. *Veterinary Microbiology* **68**: 209-217.

Pluske J.R., Durmic Z., Payne H.G., Mansfield J., Mullan B.P., Hampson D.J., and Vercoe P.E. (2007). Microbial diversity in the large intestine of pigs born and reared in different environments. *Livestock Science* **108**: 113-116

Pryde S.E., Richardson A.J., Stewart C.S., and Flint H.J. (1999). Molecular analysis of the microbial diversity present in the colonic wall, colonic lumen, and cecal lumen of a pig. *Applied and Environmental Microbiology* **65**: 5372-5377.

Rakoff-Nahoum S., Paglino J., Eslami-Varzaneh F., Edberg S., and Medzhitov R. (2004). Recognition of commensal microflora by Toll-like receptors is required for intestinal homeostasis. *Cell* **118**: 229-241.

Rescigno M. (2001). Dendritic cells express tight junction proteins and penetrate gut epithelial monolayers to sample bacteria. *Nature Immunology* **2**: 361-367.

Rothkotter H.-J., Mollhoff S., and Pabst R. (1999). The influence of age and breeding conditions on the number and proliferation of intraepithelial lymphocytes in pigs. *Scandinavian Journal of Immunology* **50**: 31-38.

Russell E.G. (1979). Types and distribution of anaerobic bacteria in the large intestine of pigs. *Applied and Environmental Microbiology* **37**: 187-193.

Salminen S., Bouley C., Boutron-Ruault M.C., Cummings J.H., Franck A., Gibson G.R., Isolauri E., Moreau M.C., Roberfroid M., and Rowland I. (1998). Functional food science and gastrointestinal physiology and function. *British Journal of Nutrition* **80**: S147-S171.

Salzman N.H., de Jong H., Paterson Y., Harmsen H.J.M., Welling G.W., and Bos N.A. (2002). Analysis of 16S libraries of mouse gastrointestinal microflora reveals a large new group of mouse intestinal bacteria. *Microbiology* **148**: 3651-3660.

Sharma R. and Schumacher R. (1995). Morphometric analysis of intestinal mucins under different dietary conditions and gut flora in rats. *Digestive Diseases and Sciences* **40**: 2532-2539.

Stappenbeck T.S., Hooper L.V., and Gordon J.I. (2002). Developmental regulation of intestinal angiogenesis by indigenous microbes via Paneth cells. *Proceedings of the National Academy of Sciences* **99**: 15451-15455.

Strachan D.P. (1989). Hay fever, hygiene, and household size. *British Medical Journal* **18**: 1259-1260.

Suau A., Bonnet R., Sutren M., Godon J.J., Gibson G.R., Collins M.D., and Dore J. (1999). Direct analysis of genes encoding 16S rRNA from complex communities reveals many novel molecular species within the human gut. *Applied and Environmental Microbiology* **65**: 4799-4807.

Swords W.E., Wu C.C., Champlin F.R., and Buddington R.K. (1993). Postnatal changes in selected bacterial groups of the pig colonic microflora. *Biology of the neonate* **63**: 191-200.

Takahashi S., Egawa Y., Simojo N., Tsukahara T., and Ushida K. (2007). Oral administration of *Lactobacillus plantarum* strain Lq80 to weaning piglets stimulates the growth of indigenous lactobacilli to modify the lactobacillal population. *Journal of General and Applied Microbiology* **53**: 325-332.

Tako E., Glahn R.P., Welch R.M., Lei X., Yasuda K., and Miller D.D. (2008). Dietary inulin affects the expression of intestinal enterocyte iron transporters, receptors and storage protein and alters the microbiota in the pig intestine. *British Journal of Nutrition* **99**: 472-480.

Talham G.L., Jiang H.Q., Bos N.A., and Cebra J.J. (1999). Segmented filamentous bacteria are potent stimuli of a physiologically normal state of the murine gut mucosal immune system. *Infection and Immunity* **67**: 1992-2000.

Tuggle C.K., Wang Y., and Couture O. (2007). Advances in swine transcriptomics. *International Journal of Biological Sciences* **3**: 132-152.

Umesaki Y., Setoyama S., Matsumoto S., and Okada Y. (1993). Expansion of T-cell receptor-bearing intestinal intraepithelial lymphocytes after microbial colonisation in germ-free mice and its independence from thymus.

Immunology **79**: 32-37.

Umesaki Y., Okada Y., Matsumoto S., Imaoka A., and Setoyama H. (1995). Segmented filamentous bacteria are indigenous intestinal bacteria that activate intraepithelial lymphocytes and induce MHC class II molecules and fucosyl asialo GM1 glycopolipids on the small intestinal epithelial cells in the ex-germ-free mouse. *Microbiology and Immunology* **39**: 555-562.

Umesaki Y., Setoyama H., Matsumoto S., Imaoka A., and Itoh K. (1999). Differential roles of segmented filamentous bacteria and clostridia in development of the intestinal immune system. *Infection and Immunity* **67**: 3504-3511.

Wang Y., Qu L., Uthe J.J., Bearson S.M.D., Kuhar D., Lunney J.K., Couture O.P., Nettleton D., Dekkers J.C., and Tuggle C.K. (2007). Global transcriptional response of porcine mesenteric lymph nodes to *Salmonella enterica* serovar Typhimurium. *Genomics* **90**: 72-84.

Wills-Karp M., Santeliz J., and Karp C.L. (2001). The germless theory of allergic disease: revisiting the hygiene hypothesis. *Nature Reviews Immunology* **1**: 69-75.

Wilson A.D., Haverson K., Southgate K., Bland P.W., Stokes C.R., and Bailey M. (1996). Expression of major histocompatibility complex class II antigens on normal porcine intestinal endothelium. *Immunology* **88**: 98-103.

Wostmann B.S. (1996). Germfree and gnotobiotic animal models: background and applications. Boca Raton, FL: CRC Press.

Zoetendal E.G., Akkermans A.D., and de Vos W.M. (1998). Temperature gradient gel electrophoresis analysis of 16S rRNA from human fecal samples reveals stable and host-specific communities of active bacteria. *Applied and Environmental Microbiology* **64**: 3854-3859.

Zoetendal E.G., von Wright A., Vilpponen-Salmela T., Ben-Amor K., Akkermans A.D.L., and de Vos W.M. (2002). Mucosa-associated bacteria in the human gastrointestinal tract are uniformly distributed along the colon and differ from the community recovered from feces. *Applied and Environmental Microbiology* **68**: 3401-3407.

12

THE ROLE OF FIBRE IN GUT HEALTH

KNUD ERIK BACH KNUDSEN, METTE SKOU HEDEMANN AND HELLE NYGAARD LÆRKE
Department of Animal Health, Welfare and Nutrition, Faculty of Agricultural Sciences, Aarhus University, Denmark

Introduction

Fibres are important components of all but a few feedstuffs used in the feeding of pigs (Bach Knudsen, 1997). They are resistant to digestion by endogenous enzymes in the small intestine thereby becoming the main substrate for bacterial fermentation, particularly in the large intestine (Bach Knudsen *et al.*, 2001). Because of the physical properties of fibres they interact both with the microflora and the mucosa of all sites of the gastrointestinal tract. In this way fibres have an important role in the complex interaction between the diet, the mucosa and the commensal microflora – all of which are considered important in "gut health" (Montagne *et al.*, 2003). However, in the literature there is conflicting evidence as to whether fibres exert a beneficial or detrimental influence of gut health. For example, an almost fibre-free rice-based diet supplemented with animal protein has been shown to reduce the susceptibility to enteric disorders including post weaning enteric disorders (PWED) (McDonald *et al.*, 1999; McDonald *et al.*, 2001; Hopwood *et al.*, 2004), and swine dysentery (Durmic *et al.*, 1998). The same was the case with fibre from the outer hull of barley (Bertschinger *et al.*, 1978), rich in insoluble fibre, whereas feeding barley meal and guar gum has been associated with increased susceptibility to PWED (McDonald *et al.*, 1999; McDonald *et al.*, 2001; Hopwood *et al.*, 2004), swine dysentery (Durmic *et al.*, 1998) or porcine intestinal spirochaetosis (Hampson *et al.*, 2000). In a recent study where growing pigs were fed a highly fermentable fibre-rich diet based on dried chicory roots and sweet lupins the animals were completely protected against the infection with *Brachyspira hyodysenteria* after experimental challenge (Thomsen *et al.*, 2007). Accordingly, the results on the impact of fibre on gut health are conflicting. This chapter will address different aspects of the chemical and physicochemical characteristics of

211

fibre, how fibre influences the gut lumen, the commensal microbiota, and interacts with the intestinal mucosa thereby influencing gut health.

The concept of gut health

The concept of "gut health" is complex and, at present, an ill-defined notion (Montagne *et al.*, 2003). Conway (1994) proposed that there are three major components of "gut health", namely the diet, the mucosa and the commensal flora (Figure 1). The mucosa is composed of the digestive epithelium, the gut-associated lymphoid tissue (GALT) and the mucus overlying the epithelium. The GALT, commensal bacteria, mucus and host epithelial cells interact with each other forming a fragile and dynamic equilibrium within the alimentary tract that ensures efficient functioning and absorption capacity of the digestive system. The feed should be selected to favour conditions in the gut that create and stabilize this balance between the host, the microflora and environment, and to prevent disturbance of the structure and function of the gut. In this respect, the relative "gut health" value of a dietary component or diets should rest with their capacity either to stabilize or to perturb this equilibrium. It is, however, also clear that such a relative evaluation inevitably will result in different outcomes with the same feedstuff/feed ingredients depending on the experimental setting.

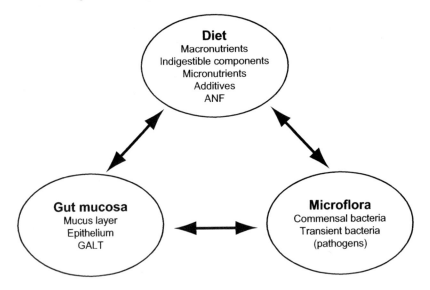

Figure 1. Schematic representation of the different elements in the gut ecosystem making up the concept of gut health. Modified from Conway (1994) as discussed by Montagne *et al.* (2003).

Fibre

TERMINOLOGY

Fibre is not a well-defined chemical entity, but a term that in both human and animal nutrition literature has been defined by the methods applied for its analysis. In this chapter the term fibre will be restricted to the sum of non-starch polysaccharides (NSP) and lignin, while non-digestible carbohydrates (NDC) are defined as the sum of non-digestible oligosaccharides (NDO), resistant starch (RS) and NSP. Prebiotic carbohydrates will be used for carbohydrates that are: "a non-digestible food ingredient which beneficially affects the host by selectively stimulating the growth and/or activating the metabolism of one or a limited number of health-promoting bacteria in the intestinal tract thus improving the host's intestinal physiology" (Gibson & Roberfroid, 1995). An overview of NDC and lignin is given in Table 1.

THE CHEMISTRY OF FIBRE

Fibre is primarily found in the plant cell wall (McDougall *et al.*, 1996) that consists of a series of polysaccharides often associated and/or substituted with proteins and phenolic compounds, and in some cells together with the phenolic polymer lignin (Theander *et al.*, 1989). The building blocks of the cell wall polysaccharides are the pentoses arabinose and xylose, the hexoses glucose, galactose and mannose, the 6-deoxyhexoses rhamnose and fucose, and the uronic acids glucuronic and galacturonic acids (or their 4-O-methyl ethers). Although the cell wall polysaccharides are built from only 10 common monosaccharides, each monosaccharide can exist in two ring (pyranose and furanose) forms, and these residues can be linked through glycosidic bonds at any one of their three, four or five available hydroxyl groups and in two (α or β) orientations. As a result, cell wall polysaccharides can adopt a huge number of three-dimensional shapes and thereby offer a vast range of functional surfaces (McDougall *et al.*, 1996). The NSP can also be linked to lignin and suberin, which provide hydrophobic surfaces and which stiffen the walls thus preventing biochemical degradation of the walls. In addition, charged groups on polysaccharides, i.e. the acid group on galacturonic and glucuronic acids, can affect the ionic properties.

NON-CELL WALL POLYSACCHARIDES

Some plant materials also contain intracellular NSP as storage carbohydrates such as fructans in Jerusalem artichoke and chicory roots, and mannans in palm

Table 1. Overview of non-digestible carbohydrates and lignin in feedstuffs and feed additives

Category	Monomeric residues	Examples of source
Non-digestible oligosaccharides (DP 3-9)		
α-galactosides		
(Raffinose, stachyose, verbascose)	Galactose, glucose, fructose	Soybean meal, peas, rape seed meals etc.
Fructo-oligosaccharides	Fructose	Cereals, feed additives
Trans-galacto-oligosaccharides	Galactose, glucose	Feed additives
Xylo-oligosaccharides	Xylose, arabinose	Feed additives
Polysaccharides (DP≥10)		
A. Resistant starch (RS)		
Physical inaccessible - RS1	Glucose	Peas, faba beans
Native - RS2	Glucose	Potato
Retrograded - RS3	Glucose	Heat treated starch rich products
Chemically modified – RS4	Glucose	Chemically modified starch
B. Non-starch (NSP)		
Cell Wall NSP		
Cellulose	Glucose	Most feedstuffs
Mixed linked ß-glucans	Glucose	Barley, oats, rye
Arabinoxylans	Xylose, arabinose	Rye, wheat, barley, cereals by-products
Arabinogalactans	Galactose, arabinose	Cereal flours
Xyloglucans	Glucose, xylose	Pea hulls
Rhamnogalacturans	Uronic acids, rhamnose	Soybean meal, sugar beet fibre/pulp
Galactans	Galactose	Lupins
Non-cell Wall NSP		
Fructans	Fructose	Jerusalem artichoke, chicory roots, rye
Mannans	Mannose	Coconut cake, palm cake
Pectins	Uronic acids, rhamnose	Feed additives
Guar gum	Galactose, mannose	Feed additives
Lignin	Phenylpropanoid	Barley hulls, oat hulls

DP, degree of polymerisation; RS, resistant starch; NSP, non-starch polysaccharides.

and coconut cake. In contrast to the plant cell wall, lignin is not associated with storage NSP.

FIBRE FEED ADDITIVES

A number of purified soluble and viscous, and non-viscous polysaccharides such as pectins of different origin, inulin, alginates, carrageenans, gum xanthan, guar gum or gum arabic (acacia) as well as carboxymethylcellulose and insoluble polysaccharides as cellulose are frequently used as feed additives in studies with pigs. The practical use of these polysaccharides, however, is limited.

RESISTANT STARCH

Native starch is a semi-crystalline material synthesised roughly as spherical granules in many plant tissues of which cereals and pulses (peas and beans) are the most important feedstuffs in pig nutrition (Bach Knudsen, 1997). Pure starch consists predominantly of α-glucan in the form of amylose and amylopectin. Amylose is a linear $\alpha(1\text{-}4)$- linked molecule, while amylopectin is a much larger, heavily branched by $\alpha(1\text{-}6)$- linkages. The two α-glucans are present in various proportions in the starch granules; amylopectin forms a branched helical crystalline system interspersed with amorphous lamella. Although all starch potentially can be digested by α-amylase and the brush-border enzymes in the small intestine (Gray, 1992), a certain fraction of starch will resist enzymatic digestion in the small intestine (resistant starch) either because it is trapped within whole plant cells matrices (RS_1), the starch granules are resistant (RS_2), the starch is retrograded (RS_3), or the starch is chemically modified (RS_4) (Englyst *et al.*, 1992).

NON-DIGESTIBLE OLIGOSACCHARIDES

Non-digestible oligosaccharides are present in a number of predominantly protein-rich feedstuffs as α-galactosides - raffinose, stachyose, verbascose and ajugose or as fructooligosaccharides, as in the fructan fraction in Jerusalem artichoke and chicory roots. NDO may also be incorporated into the pig's diet as isolates of fructo-oligosaccharides from partly hydrolysed inulin or enzymatically synthesised, as trans-galacto-oligosaccharides or as xylo-oligosaccharides (Flickinger *et al.*, 2003).

Physico-chemical properties of fibre

The physicochemical properties – hydration properties and viscosity – of fibre are linked to the type of polymers that make up the cell wall and their intermolecular association (McDougall *et al.*, 1996). The hydration properties are characterised by the swelling capacity, solubility, water holding capacity, and water binding capacity. The latter two have been used interchangeably in the literature since both reflect the ability of a fibre source to immobilise water within its matrix. The first part of the solubilisation process of polymers is swelling in which incoming water spreads the macromolecules until they are fully extended and dispersed - the cell wall in Figure 2 expands in the three dimensional space (Thibault *et al.*, 1992). Solubilisation is not possible in the case of polysaccharides that adopt regular, ordered structures (e.g. cellulose or linear arabinoxylans) because the linear structure increases the strength of the non-covalent bonds, which stabilise the ordered conformation. Under these conditions only swelling can occur (Thibault *et al.*, 1992). The majority of polysaccharides give viscous solutions if dissolved in water (Morris, 1992). The viscosity is dependent on the primary structure, molecular weight of the polymer, and concentration. Large molecules increase the viscosity of diluted solutions and their ability to do so depends primarily on the volume they occupy. Although a range of polysaccharides by analytical definitions are soluble, their in vivo solubility may be restricted in the feed matrix thus limiting their viscosity elevating properties.

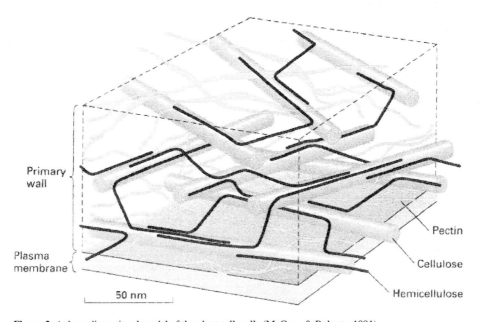

Figure 2. A three-dimensional model of the plant cell walls (McCann & Roberts, 1991).

The gut – the reaction tube for nutrient degradation and absorption

The gastrointestinal tract of pigs can be considered as a tube with regions that have different structure and functional elements, which provide optimal conditions for the digestion and absorption processes. Gastric emptying regulates the flow of digesta from the stomach to the small intestine (Low, 1990) and the digesta moves at a higher velocity in the proximal small intestine compared to the more distal segments (Wilfart *et al.*, 2007). The main determinants of the composition of digesta in the stomach and the upper part of the small intestine are the dietary composition and particularly the amount of non-digestible components, and the endogenous secretion from the stomach, intestine, pancreas and gall bladder (Johansen & Bach Knudsen, 1994; Johansen *et al.*, 1996). In these regions, the main contributor to the hydrolytic capacity comes from the endogenous enzymes secreted to the stomach and small intestine and the enzymes located on the brush border of the small intestine (Kidder & Manners, 1980). As the digesta moves distally, flow rate and oxygen content decline, and the composition changes as a result of digestive, secretory and microbial processes. In the large intestine, the microflora is the main contributor to the hydrolytic capacity (Louis *et al.*, 2007).

THE GUT MUCOSA

The mucosa of the small intestine "traps" the compounds released by the hydrolytic processes (glucose from starch; amino acids and peptides from proteins and fatty acids and monoacylglycerols from lipids) and absorbs them into the body (Gray, 1992). The epithelial layer is a semipermeable membrane that efficiently regulates the exchange of materials between the body and the lumenal contents, and is metabolically very active. Furthermore, the secretions and the glycoproteins of the brush border membrane influence the adherence and the metabolic activity of bacteria (Kelly *et al.*, 1994). There are also regional differences in the mucosal architecture. The height of the villi is reduced from the proximal (e.g. the regions with high nutrient influx) to distal small intestine and with barely any present in the colon (Jin *et al.*, 1994; Brunsgaard, 1997).

The size, volume and morphological structure of the tract adapt to the composition of the diets provided in the different periods of the pig's life and to the age of the animals. The strongest and most significant change in morphological structure occurs during the transition from mother's milk before weaning to the solid plant-based feed after weaning. In this period the effect of diet composition on mucosal integrity in the small intestine is overridden by diminished feed intake (van Beers-Schreurs *et al.*, 1998; Spreeuwenberg *et al.*, 2001) (Figure 3). The voluntary feed intake in the immediate post-weaning period is low and extremely variable and it is not until the end of the second week after weaning that the intake of energy reaches the same level as in the pre-weaning period (Le Dividich & Herpin, 1994). This is presumably also responsible for the lower villus height and lower crypt depth in middle small intestine in the immediate post-weaning period compared with growing pigs and sows. For the distal part of the small intestine and the middle colon, however, the difference in morphological structure is somewhat smaller (Table 2).

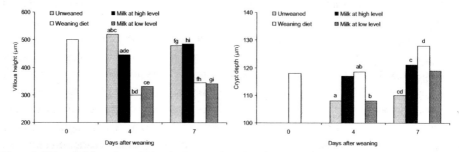

Figure 3. Villous height and crypth dept in the small intestine of unweaned pigs, weaned pigs offered a high sow milk diet, a weaning diet or a low sow milk diet at weaning at d 4 and 7 after weaning. Values are means ±SEM, n = 6. Bars with the same letter differ, p < 0.05. Data from: van Beers-Schreurs *et al.* (1998).

Table 2. Villus height and crypt depth at 0.50 and 0.90 of the pyloro-ileal intestinal length (SI50 and SI90) and at 0.50 of caecal-rectal colonic length (Co50) in piglets 9 days post weaning, in growing pigs and sows

Intestinal segment	Piglets[1]	Growing pigs[2]	Sows[3]
		Villus height, mm	
SI50	358	486	443
SI90	354	389	-
		Crypt depth, mm	
SI50	381	297	213
SI90	300	301	-
Co50	365	431	330

Data from: [1]Hedemann *et al.* (2006), [2]Hedemann *et al.*, unpublished, and [3]Serena *et al.* (2008a)

The addition of soluble fibre to the diet of piglets generally causes an increase in the viscosity of the intestinal contents, which may increase the rate of villus cell loss leading to villus atrophy. This has been seen in studies using pectin (Hedemann *et al.*, 2006) and carboxymethylcellulose (CMC, a water soluble synthetic viscous polysaccharide which is resistant to microbial fermentation; McDonald *et al.*, 2001). However, in the study of McDonald *et al.* (2001) pigs fed a low-viscosity

CMC had increased villus height suggesting that viscosity may be beneficial up to a threshold. Using CMC in piglet feed increased the crypt depth (McDonald *et al.*, 2001) whereas pectin-fed piglets had lower crypts than piglets fed a low fibre diet (Hedemann *et al.*, 2006) suggesting that the type of soluble fibre influences the response. The villus height/crypt depth ratio is a useful criterion for estimating the likely digestive capacity of the small intestine. Feeding high-viscosity CMC the ratio decreased (McDonald *et al.*, 2001) whereas it was maintained when feeding pectin (Hedemann *et al.*, 2006).

Inclusion of 100 g wheat straw (insoluble fibre)/kg low fibre diet resulted in deeper crypts in the jejunum and ileum and augmented cell division in growing pigs (Jin *et al.*, 1994). Similar results were not found in newly weaned piglets where fibre concentration (73 vs. 145 g/kg dry matter) did not affect the intestinal morphology (Hedemann *et al.*, 2006). The increased crypt-cell proliferation induced by fibre may be explained by the trophic effect of short-chain fatty acids (SCFA) and especially butyrate. The effect of SCFA is not restricted to the colon, and SCFA also stimulate cell proliferation and growth of the small intestine. In piglets the microflora may, however, not be fully adapted to fibre (Jensen, 1998). In growing pigs the effect of fibre on colonic morphology is conflicting. It depends on the botanic origin and fermentation properties of the fibre and the composition of the microflora in the colon of pigs (Williams *et al.*, 2001).

DIGESTION AND ABSORPTION

Immediately after weaning at 3 weeks of age, there is insufficient production of pancreatic enzymes required for starch digestion (Efird *et al.*, 1982) but of the brush-border enzymes it is only the activity of maltase and glycoamylase which is directly affected by feed intake in the post-weaning period (Kelly *et al.*, 1991). This is the likely cause for the compromised digestive capacity of the small intestine up to 10 days post weaning as compared to piglets 14-28 days post weaning, growing pigs and sows (Table 3). Gelatinising the starch, which increases the surface area and thereby the interactions between the starch and the digestive enzymes may, however, increase the digestibility of starch in piglets (10 days post-weaning; Hopwood *et al.*, 2004) to a level only slightly lower than in growing pigs where gelatinised starch is almost completely digested (Bach Knudsen *et al.*, 2005). These conditions have a profound influence on the type of substrate available for the microbial fermentation in the large intestine; in the critical post-weaning period up to 10 days post weaning, starch is the main substrate for microbial fermentation irrespective the fibre concentrations in the diet. This is in contrast to the situation in growing pigs and sows where fibre is by far the most important dietary factor influencing the flow of nutrients from the small to the large intestine

(Bach Knudsen *et al.*, 2008). In the large intestine, the rate and overall degree of degradation of fibre polysaccharides is influenced by the chemical nature of the plant fibre, the solubility, and the degree of lignification. Thus, β-glucan, soluble AX, and pectins are all rapidly degraded in the caecum and proximal colon (Bach Knudsen *et al.*, 1993; Canibe & Bach Knudsen, 1997; Glitsø *et al.*, 1998) while the more insoluble plant fibre, e.g. cellulose and insoluble arabinoxylans, is degraded more slowly at more distal locations of the colon (Bach Knudsen *et al.*, 1993; Glitsø *et al.*, 1998).

Table 3. The digestibility (proportion of intake) of starch and non-starch polysaccharides in the small intestine and total tract of piglets, growing pigs and sows

	N	Small intestine		Total tract	
		Starch	NSP	Starch	NSP
Piglets, 0-10 days post-weaning[1]	9	0.75	0.03	0.99	0.57
Piglets, 14-28 days post-weaning[2]	8	0.95	0.14	1.00	0.67
Growing pigs[3]	78	0.96	0.21	1.00	0.70
Sows[4]	3	0.93	0.30	0.99	0.64

N = number of diets.
Data from: [1]Lærke *et al.* (2003); Hopwood *et al.* (2004), [2]Gdala *et al.* (1997); Jensen *et al.* (1998); Pluske *et al.* (2007), [3]Bach Knudsen *et al.* (2008), and [4]Serena *et al.* (2008b).

The substantial malabsorption of starch in the first 10 days post weaning could potentially overload the large intestine with readily fermentable nutrients thereby reducing the degradation of NSP. As shown in Table 3, the digestibility of NSP in the immediate post-weaning period is also slightly lower than in older pigs. Moreover, the gut as a whole is also less efficient in handling diets enriched in soluble and insoluble fibre than growing pigs and sows presumably because of the lower enzymatic digestion capacity for all compounds in the small intestine in that time frame (Figure 4).

MICROBIAL COMMUNITY

Already at weaning the gastrointestinal tract of pigs is densely populated with bacteria but the community is very unstable (Janczyk *et al.*, 2007; Pieper *et al.*, 2008). It takes at least 5-10 days for the intestinal bacterial community to be re-established and to adapt its activity to the new feeding situation with complex plant materials at the expense of the liquid compounds from milk (Janczyk *et al.*, 2007;

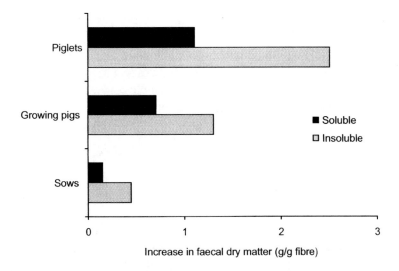

Figure 4. Effect of soluble and insoluble fibre on the faecal bulking in piglets, growing pigs and sows. Data from: Bach Knudsen and Hansen, (1991); Pedersen *et al.* (2003); Serena *et al.* (2008b).

Pieper *et al.*, 2008). As long as the microbial community is stable and not disturbed by enterobacteria, members of the lactobacilli family are the dominating bacterial groups and lactic acid by far the most important metabolic end-product. The concentration of lactic acid increases several-fold within the first 11 days after weaning and with a concomitant drop in pH (Janczyk *et al.*, 2007; Pieper *et al.*, 2008). In growing pigs, gram-positive strict anaerobic streptococci, lactobacilli, eubacteria, clostridia and peptostreptococci, comprise the major part of the total culturable flora (Jensen, 2001). While it is difficult to change the flora composition in the immediate post-weaning period, prebiotic carbohydrates in the form of fructose containing oligo- and polysaccharides can be used specifically to stimulate lactic acid producing bacteria (*Lactobacillus* spp. together with *Bifidobacterium* spp.; Mikkelsen *et al.*, 2004; Mølbak *et al.*, 2007; Wellock *et al.*, 2007). Stimulation of these groups of microorganisms is generally considered beneficial as attachment of these harmless bacteria to the mucosa may protect the animals from gut infection. Since fructose containing oligo- and polysaccharides are readily fermentable they further reduce luminal pH (Houdijk *et al.*, 2002; Bach Knudsen *et al.*, 2003) and potentially reduce the proliferation and establishment of pH sensitive enteropathogenic strains of *Escherichia coli, Salmonella, Shingella* or some clostridia (Gibson & Wang, 1994; Macfarlane *et al.*, 2006). Feeding a diet containing dried chicory roots and sweet lupins to growing pigs were found to stimulate *Bifidobacterium thermoacidophilum* and *Megasphaera elsdenii*, which inhibited *B. hyodysenteriae* to be established (Mølbak *et al.*, 2007). An improved ratio between lactobacilli and coliform and reduced luminal pH in digesta have also been found in a study with piglets fed diets containing inulin (Wellock *et al.*, 2008). In addition to the horizontal variation in bacterial composition, there is also a vertical gradient of species distribution (Kelly *et al.*, 1994; Macfarlane *et al.*, 2006). The mucosa provides an environment that differs physically and chemically from those of the digesta. It is also recognised that the bacteria associated with the mucosa are likely to have a greater potential to influence the host than those present in the lumen (Kelly *et al.*, 1994; Macfarlane *et al.*, 2006). However, much more is known about the bacteria of the lumen than those attached to the mucosa.

END-PRODUCT FORMATION

The concentration of SCFA in the colon content increases post-weaning (van Beers-Schreurs *et al.*, 1998; Bruininx *et al.*, 2004) and, although the concentration of SCFA in the lumen of the large intestine in piglets (Wellock *et al.*, 2008) is comparable to what is found with older animals (growing pigs and sows; Bach Knudsen & Hansen, 1991; Serena *et al.*, 2008a), the type of substrate may have a profound influence on the composition of fermentation end-products. The range of carbohydrates that arrive in the large intestine from the diet is enormous. While starch will dominate in the immediate post-weaning period (Table 3), fibres in various forms will later on be the major contributor (Bach Knudsen *et al.*, 2008). The high load of starch in the immediate post-weaning period is responsible for the relatively high butyrate concentration at that stage (Pluske *et al.*, 2007), which further can be stimulated by the inclusion of RS_2 from raw potato in the diets of piglets (Hedemann & Bach Knudsen, 2007) but also for growing pigs (van der Meulen *et al.*, 1997). In older pigs and sows, where fibre polysaccharides are the main substrate for microbial fermentation, overall degree of degradation of these polymers is influenced by the chemical nature of the plant fibre, the solubility, and the degree of lignification. In the caecum and proximal colon the carbohydrate supply is usually plenty to support a high activity of the microbial community, while carbohydrates become a limiting factor for high SCFA generation in the more distal locations of the colon (Bach Knudsen *et al.*, 1993; Glitsø *et al.*, 1998). In these regions other substances like protein and endogenous materials are of greater importance. These conditions influence the concentrations and molar proportions of organic acids; the concentrations of SCFA and the ratio between saccharolytic derived SCFA (acetate, propionate, and butyrate) and proteolytic derived acids (iso-butyrate, and isovalerate) decline from the proximal to the distal large intestine (Bach Knudsen *et al.*, 1993). The concentration of potential toxic components like NH_3, indoles, phenols, secondary bile acids are also higher in the distal compared to the proximal colon (Glitsø *et al.*, 1998).

Impact of fibre on gut health and resistance to infection

As discussed above, fibres and other NDCs play an important role for the function of the gastrointestinal tract of pigs at all ages. However, to what extent the fibres and the other NDCs can be used proactively to modulate digestion events in all regions of the intestinal tract thereby reducing the susceptibility to enteric disorders is still open for discussion.

FIBRE AND POST WEANING ENTERIC DISORDERS

It is well established that post-weaning diarrhoea caused by enterotoxigenic strains of *Eschericia coli*, which colonise the small intestine, is a multifactorial condition that is influenced by diet (Hampson, 1997). High level of dietary protein has been shown to predispose to the condition (Prohaszka & Baron, 1980), whereas fibre present naturally in the feedstuffs or provided as isolates has demonstrated both beneficial and detrimental effects on the development of PWED. For example, fibre from the outer hull of barley, rich in insoluble fibre, reduces severity of PWED (Smith & Halls, 1968), whereas barley meal, high in soluble β-glucan, has been associated with increased susceptibility (Smith & Halls, 1968; Hopwood *et al.*, 2004). Studies with soluble and viscous NSP in the form of guar gum and CMC have further been shown to exacerbate experimental PWED whereas an almost fibre free cooked rice based diet was more protective (McDonald *et al.*, 1999; McDonald *et al.*, 2001; Montagne *et al.*, 2004). Peroral administration of pectin to pigs was found to reduce the fluid accumulation in intestinal loops challenged to different dilutions of enteropatogenic *E. coli* strains (Larsen, 1981) but when pectins were included in either a diets based on wheat and barley flour or wholegrain wheat and barley there was no difference in the frequency of spontaneous PWED (Bach Knudsen *et al.*, unpublished). However, in a recent study where NDC in form of inulin was provided to piglets there were fewer cases of diarrhoea and an improved gut health, as indicated by a lower colonic digeta pH and increased *Lactobacillus*:coliform ratio when compared to piglets on a diet with insoluble fibre from cellulose (Wellock *et al.*, 2008). Taken as a whole, soluble and viscous fibre seems be an important characteristic that predisposes to PWED, possibly because the solubilised polysaccharides provide favourable microenvironment for the enterotoxigenic *E. coli*. In this respect, the structural organisation of the solubilised polysaccharide (type of linkages, degree of branching etc.) can be expected to play a major role for the susceptibility of soluble polysaccharide to predispose to PWED.

FIBRE AND SWINE DYSENTERY

Swine dysentery is a major problem in many parts of the world. The disease is caused by the anaerobic intestinal spirochaete *Brachyspira hyodysenteriae*, which colonise the crypts of the large intestine and induce severe mucohaemorrhagic colitis and dysentery (Hampson *et al.*, 1997). Studies with gnotobiotics pigs have shown that colonisation by the spirochaete and lesion formation is enhanced by the presence of other species of anaerobic bacteria (Whipp *et al.*, 1979). Earlier field studies have indicated that a protective effect was obtained when pigs with swine dysentery were changed from a maize-based diet to a diet based on maize silage (Prohaszka & Lukacs, 1984). The interpretation was that the maize silage lowered the pH in the digesta in the large intestine, thereby inhibiting the growth of *B. hyodysenteriae*. A series of studies performed by an Australian group, however, could not confirm this. Rather, the Australian studies identify a very digestible diet based on cooked white rice and animal protein to be protective against colonisation by the spirochaete or development of swine dysentery after experimental challenge (Pluske *et al.*, 1996; Siba *et al.*, 1996). When the cooked rice or the animal protein were mixed with either *lupinus* spp. or wheat, disease occurred after challenge. The authors identified the protective effect to be the low level of fibre and RS in cooked rice that limited the fermentation in the large intestine and in this way suppressed the commensal microflora, which normally facilitate colonisation with the spirochaete (Pluske *et al.*, 1998). A direct physical effect of the limited amount of residues that is passed to the large intestine could also play a role. In follow up studies, maize and sorghum, when steam-flaked, and oat chaff also reduced the incidence of disease after experimental challenge, whereas soluble fibre and RS were two important dietary components that promote fermentation in the large intestine and were associated with high incidence of swine dysentery (Durmic *et al.*, 1997; Durmic *et al.*, 1998; Pluske *et al.*, 1998). The potential of using exogenous enzymes to improve the digestibility of wheat and sorghum-based diets and thereby to obtain a similar protective effect as of the cooked white rice diet has also been tested with variable results (Durmic *et al.*, 1997). While the Australian works consistently have shown cooked white rice supplemented with animal protein to have a protective effect on the expression of swine dysentery after experimental challenge it has been difficult to reproduce these findings outside Australia. In a Danish study it was not possible by the rice diet to prevent the development of swine dysentery upon experimental infection (Lindecrona *et al.*, 2000), and increasing the level of fibre or RS did not result in any higher incidence of disease. However, clinical symptoms and pathological lesions were more severe when the level of fibre was increased. The reason for the failure to confirm the Australian work in Denmark is not easy to explain but, since the colonisation with *B. hyodysenteria* requires a component of the anaerobic microflora to be expressed, differences in the intestinal microflora at the study site can influence the outcome.

An alternative to the use of cooked rice, which is difficult to implement commercially under practical conditions, is to stimulate the beneficial microorganisms, i.e. lactic acid bacteria by specific prebiotic carbohydrates. This was done in a recent study when growing pigs were fed either a conventional pig diets or a diet containing NDC from chicory roots and sweet lupins and experimentally infected with *Brachyspira hyodysenteriae* alone or in combination with the whip worm *Tricuris suis*. The outcome was that the pigs that were fed the diet containing the dried chicory roots and lupins were completely protected against the development of swine dysentery (Thomsen *et al.*, 2007) (Figure 5). Terminal restriction fragment length polymorphism analysis of colonic contents showed that pigs fed the fructan-rich chicory root diet had a higher proportion of *Bifidobacterium thermoacidophilum* and *Megasphaera elsdenii*, which were thought to inhibit the establishment of *B. hyodysenteriae* (Mølbak *et al.*, 2007). Studies with inulin, the main component of the fructans in chicory roots, have shown that inulin lowers pH of colonic digesta, and at a high dose stimulated lactic acid formation in the caecum (Bach Knudsen *et al.*, 2003) and increased *Lactobacillus*:coliform ratio (Wellock *et al.*, 2008).

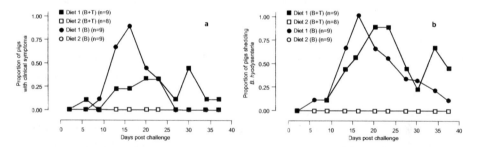

Figure 5. Proportion of pigs with clinical symptoms of swine dysentery (a) and faecal re-isolation of *B. hyodysenteria* (b) after experimental *B. hyodysenteria* challenge of pigs fed a control diet (Diet 1) and a diet containing fructans and lupins (Diet 2). Values are the mean of the means of three subgroups. Data from: Thomsen *et al.* (2007).

Conclusion

The fibre fraction represents a diverse group of polymers present as cell wall and storage components in all but a few feedstuffs. When ingested, the fibre components interact with the digestive processes along the entire gastrointestinal tract, with the microbial community, and influence the structure and function of the gut. The direct effect of fibre the first two weeks after weaning (weaning age 3-4 weeks), however, is blurred by an extremely variable feed intake and low digestibility of starch in the small intestine, that makes it difficult to assess the specific effects of soluble and insoluble fibre on gut health. With current knowledge, recommendations are to feed a diet containing a mixture of soluble and insoluble fibre and supplement with prebiotic carbohydrates other than fibre in the first week after weaning to specifically stimulate lactobacilli bacteria over enteropathogenic bacteria. The same strategy can be recommended used in herds with disease problems caused by enteropathogenic bacteria.

Literature cited

Bach Knudsen, K.E. (1997) Carbohydrate and lignin contents of plant materials used in animal feeding. *Animal Feed Science and Technology* 67, 319-338.

Bach Knudsen, K.E. and Hansen, I. (1991) Gastrointestinal implications in pigs of wheat and oat fractions 1. Digestibility and bulking properties of polysaccharides and other major constituents. *British Journal of Nutrition* 65, 217-232.

Bach Knudsen, K.E., Jensen, B.B. and Hansen, I. (1993) Digestion of polysaccharides and other major components in the small and large intestine of pigs fed on diets consisting of oat fractions rich in ß-D-glucan. *British Journal of Nutrition* 70, 537-556.

Bach Knudsen, K.E., Jørgensen, H., Lindberg, J.E. and Ogle, B. (2001) Intestinal degradation of dietary carbohydrates - from birth to maturity. In *Digestive physiology in pigs. Proceedings of the 8th Symposium, Sweden 20-22 June 2000; 90 ref.*, pp. 109-120. Wallingford: CABI Publishing.

Bach Knudsen, K.E., Lærke, H.N. and Jørgensen, H. (2008) The role of fibre in nutrient utilization and animal health. In *Proceedings of the 29th Western Nutrition Conference*, pp. 93-107: Edmonton, Canada: University of Alberta.

Bach Knudsen, K.E., Petkevicius, S., Jørgensen, H. and Murrel, K.D. (2003) A high load of rapidly fermentable carbohydrates reduces worm burden in infected pigs. In *Manipulating pig production IX*, pp. 169 [JE Paterson, editor]. Werribee, Australia: Australasian Pig Science Association Inc.

Bach Knudsen, K.E., Serena, A., Kjaer, A.K., Jørgensen, H. and Engberg, R. (2005) Rye bread enhances the production and plasma concentration of butyrate but not the plasma concentrations of glucose and insulin in pigs. *Journal of Nutrition* 135, 1696-1704.

Bertschinger, H.U., Eggenberger, E., Jucker, H. and Pfirter, H.P. (1978) Evaluation of low nutrient, high fibre diets for the prevention of porcine *Escherichia coli* enterotoxaemia. *Veterinary Microbiology* 3, 281-290.

Bruininx, E.M.A.M., Schellingerhout, A.B., Binnendijk, G.P., Peet-Schwering,

C.M.C. van der Schrama, J.W., Hartog, L.A. den, Everts, H. and Beynen, A.C. (2004) Individually assessed creep food consumption by suckled piglets: influence on post-weaning food intake characteristics and indicators of gut structure and hind-gut fermentation. *Animal Science* 78, 67-75.

Brunsgaard, G. (1997) Morphological characteristics, epithelial cell proliferation, and crypt fission in cecum and colon of growing pigs. *Digestive Diseases and Science* 42, 2384-2393.

Canibe, N. and Bach Knudsen, K.E. (1997) Apparent digestibility of non-starch polysaccharides and short-chain fatty acids production in the large intestine of pigs fed dried or toasted peas. *Acta Agriculturae Scandinavica* 47, 106-116.

Conway, P. (1994) *Function and regulation of the gastrointestinal microbiota of the pig.* Eds. W.B. Souttrant and H. Hagemeister. Dummerstof: EAAP Publication no. 80.

Durmic, Z., Pethick, D.W., Mullan, B.P., Schulze, H. and Hampson, D.J. (1997) The effects of extrusion and enzyme addition in wheat-based diets on fermentation in the large intestine and expression of swine dysentery. In: *Manipulating Pig Production*, p180. Werribee, Australia. Australasian Pig Science Association.

Durmic, Z., Pethick, D.W., Pluske, J.R. and Hampson, D.J. (1998) Changes in bacterial populations in the colon of pigs fed different sources of dietary fibre, and the development of swine dysentery after experimental infection. *Journal of Applied Microbiology* 85, 574-582.

Efird, R.C., Armstrong, W.D. and Herman, D.L. (1982) The development of digestive capacity in young pigs: effects of age and weaning system. *Journal of Animal Science* 55, 1380-1387.

Englyst, H.N., Kingman, S.M. and Cummings, J.H. (1992) Classification and measurement of nutritionally important starch fractions. *European Journal of Clinical Nutrition* 46, S33-50.

Flickinger, E.A., Van Loo, J. and Fahey, G.C., Jr. (2003) Nutritional responses to the presence of inulin and oligofructose in the diets of domesticated animals: a review. *Critical Review Food Science and Nutrion* 43, 19-60.

Gdala, J., Johansen, H.N., Bach Knudsen, K.E., Knap, I.H., Wagner, P. and Jorgensen, O.B. (1997) The digestibility of carbohydrates, protein and fat in the small and large intestine of piglets fed non-supplemented and enzyme supplemented diets. *Animal Feed Science and Technology* 65, 15-33.

Gibson, G.R. and Roberfroid, M.B. (1995) Dietary modulation of the human colonic microbiota: introducing the concept of prebiotics. *Journal of Nutrition* 125, 1401-1412.

Gibson, G.R. and Wang, X. (1994) Regulatory effects of bifidobacteria on the growth of other colonic bacteria. *Journal of Applied Bacteriology* 77, 412-420.

Glitsø, L.V., Brunsgaard, G., Højsgaard, S., Sandström, B. and Bach Knudsen, K.E. (1998) Intestinal degradation in pigs of rye dietary fibre with different structural characteristics. *British Journal of Nutrition* 80, 457-468.

Gray, G.M. (1992) Starch digestion and absorption in nonruminants. *Journal of Nutrition* 122, 172-177.

Hampson, D.J. (1997) Dietary influence on porcine postweaning diarrhoea. In: *Manipulating Pig Production*, pp 202-215 (Eds. J.L. Barnes, E.S. Batterham, G.M. Cronin, C. Hansen, P.H. Hemsworth, D.P. Hennesey, P.E. Huges, N.E. Johnston and T.B. King) Werribee, Australia. Australasian Pig Science Association.

Hampson, D.J., Atyeo, R.F. and Combs, B.G. (1997) Swine dysentery. In *Intestinal Spirochaetes in Domestic Animals and Humans*, pp. 175-209 [D.J. Hampson and T.B. Stanton, editors]. Wallingford, England: CAB International.

Hampson, D.J., Robertson, I.D., La, T., Oxberry, S.L. and Pethick, D.W. (2000) Influences of diet and vaccination on colonisation of pigs by the intestinal spirochaete Brachyspira (Serpulina) pilosicoli. *Veterinary Microbiology* 73, 75-84.

Hedemann, M.S. and Bach Knudsen, K.E. (2007) Resistant starch for weaning pigs – Effect on concentration of short chain fatty acids in digesta and intestinal morphology. *Livestock Science* 108, 175-177.

Hedemann, M.S., Eskildsen, M., Laerke, H.N., Pedersen, C., Lindberg, J.E., Laurinen, P. and Bach Knudsen, K.E. (2006) Intestinal morphology and enzymatic activity in newly weaned pigs fed contrasting fiber concentrations and fiber properties. *Journal of Animal Science* 84, 1375.

Hopwood, D.E., Pethick, D.W., Pluske, J.R. and Hampson, D.J. (2004) Addition of pearl barley to a rice-based diet for newly weaned piglets increases the viscosity of the intestinal contents, reduces starch digestibility and exacerbates post-weaning colibacillosis. *British Journal of Nutrition* 92, 419-427.

Houdijk, J.G., Hartemink, R., Verstegen, M.W. and Bosch, M.W. (2002) Effects of dietary non-digestible oligosaccharides on microbial characteristics of ileal chyme and faeces in weaner pigs. *Archives of Animal Nutrition* 56, 297-307.

Janczyk, P., Pieper, R., Smidt, H. and Souffrant, W.B. (2007) Changes in the diversity of pig ileal lactobacilli around weaning determined by means of 16S rRNA gene amplification and denaturing gradient gel electrophoresis. *FEMS Microbiology and Endocrinology* 61, 132-140.

Jensen, B.B. (1998) The impact of feed additives on the microbial ecology of the gut in young pigs. *Journal of Animal and feed Sciences* 7, 45-64.

Jensen, B.B. (2001) Possible ways of modifying type and amount of products from microbial fermentation in the gut. In *Gut Environment of pigs*, pp.

181-200 [A Piva, KE Bach Knudsen and JE Lindberg, editors]. Nottingham: Nottingham University Press.

Jensen, M.S., Bach Knudsen, K.E., Inborr, J. and Jakobsen, K. (1998) Effect of [beta]-glucanase supplementation on pancreatic enzyme activity and nutrient digestibility in piglets fed diets based on hulled and hulless barley varieties. *Animal Feed Science and Technology* 72, 329-345.

Jin, L., Reynolds, L.P., Redmer, D.A., Caton, J.S. and Crenshaw, J.D. (1994) Effects of dietary fiber on intestinal growth, cell proliferation, and morphology in growing pigs. *Journal of Animal Science* 72, 2270-2278.

Johansen, H.N. and Bach Knudsen, K.E. (1994) Effects of wheat-flour and oat mill fractions on jejunal flow, starch degradation and absorption of glucose over an isolated loop of jejunum in pigs. *British Journal of Nutrition* 72, 299-313.

Johansen, H.N., Bach Knudsen, K.E. and Sandström, B. (1996) Effect of varying content of soluble dietary fibre from wheat flour and oat milling fractions on gastric emptying in pigs. *British Journal of Nutrition* 75, 339-351.

Kelly, D., Begbie, R. and King, T.P. (1994) Nutritional influences on interactions between bacteria and the small intestinal mucosa. *Nutrition Research Reviews* 7, 233-257.

Kelly, D., Smyth, J.A. and McCracken, K.J. (1991) Digestive development of the early-weaned pig. 2. Effect of level of food intake on digestive enzyme activity during the immediate post-weaning period. *British Journal of Nutrition* 65, 181-188.

Kidder, D.E. and Manners, M.J. (1980) The level and distribution of carbohydrases in the small intestine mucosa of pigs from three weeks of age to maturity. *British Journal of Nutrition* 43, 141-153.

Larsen, J.L. (1981) Effect of pectin on secretion in pig jejunal loops to enetropathogenic E. coli or enterrotoxin (LT). A preliminary report. *Nordisk Veterinærmedicin* 33, 218-213.

Le Dividich, J. and Herpin, P. (1994) Effects of climatic conditions on the performance, metabolism and health status of weaned piglets: a review. *Livestock Production Science* 38, 79-90.

Lindecrona, R.H., Jensen, B.B., Jensen, T.K. and Møller, K. (2000) *The influence of diet on the development of swine dysentery.* Proc. 16th International Pig Veterinary Society Congress (Eds. C. Cargill and S. McOrist) Adelaide, Australia.

Louis, P., Scott, K.P., Duncan, S.H. and Flint, H.J. (2007) Understanding the effects of diet on bacterial metabolism in the large intestine. *Journal of Applied Microbiology* 102, 1197-1208.

Low, A.G. (1990) Nutritional regulation of gastric secretion, digestion and emptying. *Nutrition Research Reviews* 3, 229-252.

Lærke, H.N., Hedemann, M.S., Pedersen, C., Laurinen, P., Lindberg, J.E. and Bach Knudsen, K.E. (2003) Limitation in starch digestion in the newly weaned pig. Does it relate to physico-chemical properties or enzyme activity in the gut? In *Proceedings of the 9th Symposium of Digestive Physiology of Pigs Vol 2*, pp. 149-151 [RO Ball, editor]. Banff, Alberta, Canada: University of Alberta Department of Agriculture, Food and Nutritional Science.

Macfarlane, S., Macfarlane, G.T. and Cummings, J.H. (2006) Review article: prebiotics in the gastrointestinal tract. *Alimentary Pharmacology Therapeutics* 24, 701-714.

McCann, M.C. and Roberts, K. (1991) Architecture of the primary cell wall. In *The Cytoskeletal Basis of Plant Growth and Form*, pp. 109-129 [CW Lloyd, editor]. London: Academic Press.

McDonald, D.E., Pethick, D.W., Mullan, B.P. and Hampson, D.J. (2001) Increasing viscosity of the intestinal contents alters small intestinal structure and intestinal growth, and stimulates proliferation of enterotoxigenic Escherichia coli in newly-weaned pigs. *British Journal of Nutrition* 86, 487-498.

McDonald, D.E., Pethick, D.W., Pluske, J.R. and Hampson, D.J. (1999) Adverse effects of soluble non-starch polysaccharide (guar gum) on piglet growth and experimental colibacillosis immediately after weaning. *Research in Veterinary Science* 67, 245-250.

McDougall, G.J., Morrison, I.M., Stewart, D. and Hillman, J.R. (1996) Plant cell walls as dietary fibre: Range, structure, processing and function. *Journal of the Science of Food and Agriculture* 70, 133-150.

Mikkelsen, L.L., Knudsen, K.E.B. and Jensen, B.B. (2004) In vitro fermentation of fructo-oligosaccharides and transgalacto-oligosaccharides by adapted and unadapted bacterial populations from the gastrointestinal tract of piglets. *Animal Feed Science and Technology* 116, 225-238.

Montagne, L., Cavaney, F.S., Hampson, D.J., Lalles, J.P. and Pluske, J.R. (2004) Effect of diet composition on postweaning colibacillosis in piglets. *Journal of Animal Science* 82, 2364-2374.

Montagne, L., Pluske, J.R. and Hampson, D.J. (2003) A review of interactions between dietary fibre and the intestinal mucosa, and their consequences on digestive health in young non-ruminant animals. *Animal Feed Science and Technology* 108, 95-117.

Morris, E.R. (1992) Physico-chemical properties of food polysaccharides. In *Dietary fibre: A component of food: Nutritional function in health and disease*, pp. 41-55 [TF Schweizer and CA Edwards, editors]. London: Springer-Verlag.

Mølbak, L., Thomsen, L., Jensen, T., Bach Knudsen, K.E. and Boye, M. (2007) Increased amount of Bifidobacterium thermoacidophilum and Megashpaera elsdenii in the colonic microbiota of pigs fed a swine dysentery preventive diet containing chicory roots and sweet lupine. *Journal of Applied Microbiology* (Accepted).

Pedersen, C., Lærke, H.N., Lindberg, J.E., Hedemann, M.S., Laurinen, P. and Bach Knudsen, K.E. (2003) Digestibility and performance in newly weaned piglets fed diets with contrasting fibre levels and fibre properties. In *Proceedings of the 9th Symposium of Digestive Physiology of Pigs Vol 2*, pp. 128-130 [RO Ball, editor]. Banff, Alberta, Canada: University of Alberta Department of Agriculture, Food and Nutritional Science.

Pieper, R., Janczyk, P., Zeyner, A., Smidt, H., Guiard, V. and Souffrant, W.B. (2008) Ecophysiology of the developing total bacterial and Lactobacillus communities in the terminal small intestine of weaning piglets. *Microb Ecol*, DOI 10.1007/s00248-00008-09366-y.

Pluske, J.R., Durmic, Z., Pethick, D.W., Mullan, B.P. and Hampson, D.J. (1998) Confirmation of the role of rapidly fermentable carbohydrates in the expression of swine dysentery in pigs after experimental infection. *Journal of Nutrition* 128, 1737-1744.

Pluske, J.R., Montagne, L., Cavaney, F.S., Mullan, B.P., Pethick, D.W. and Hampson, D.J. (2007) Feeding different types of cooked white rice to piglets after weaning influences starch digestion, digesta and fermentation characteristics and the faecal shedding of beta-haemolytic Escherichia coli. *British Journal of Nutrition* 97, 298-306.

Pluske, J.R., Siba, P.M., Pethick, D.W., Durmic, Z., Mullan, B.P. and Hampson, D.J. (1996) The incidence of swine dysentery in pigs can be reduced by feeding diets that limit the amount of fermentable substrate entering the large intestine. *Journal of Nutrition* 126, 2920-2933.

Prohaszka, L. and Baron, F. (1980) The predisposing role of high protein supplies in enteropathogenic *Escherichia coli* infections of weaned pigs. *Zentralblatt für Veterinärmedizin B* 27, 222-232.

Prohaszka, L. and Lukacs, K. (1984) Influence of the diet on the antibacterial effect of volatile fatty acids on the development of swine dysentery. *Zentralblatt für Veterinärmedizin B* 31, 779-785.

Serena, A., Hedemann, M.S. and Bach Knudsen, K.E. (2008a) Influence of dietary fiber on luminal environment and morphology in the small and large intestine of sows. *Journal of Animal Science* 86, 2217-2227.

Serena, A., Jørgensen, H. and Bach Knudsen, K.E. (2008b) Digestion of carbohydrates and utilization of energy in sows fed diets with contrasting levels and physicochemical properties of dietary fiber. *Journal of Animal Science* 86, 2208-2216.

Siba, P.M., Pethick, D.W. and Hampson, D.J. (1996) Pigs experimentally infected with Serpulina hyodysenteriae can be protected from developing swine dysentery by feeding them a highly digestible diet. *Epidemiology and*

Infection 116, 207-216.

Smith, H.W. and Halls, S. (1968) The production of oedema disease and diarrhoea in weaned pigs by the oral administration of *Escherichia coli*:factors that influence the course of the experimental disease. *Journal of Medical Microbiology* 1, 45-59.

Spreeuwenberg, M.A.M., Verdonk, J.M.A.J., Gaskins, H.R. and Verstegen, M.W.A. (2001) Small intestine epithelial barrier function is compromised in pigs with low feed intake at weaning. *Journal of Nutrition* 131, 1520-1527.

Theander, O., Westerlund, E., Åman, P. and Graham, H. (1989) Plant cell walls and monogastric diets. *Animal Feed Science and Technology* 23, 205-225.

Thibault, J.-F., Lahaye, M. and Guillon, F. (1992) Physico-chemical properties of food plant cell walls. In *Dietary fibre: A component of food: Nutritional function in health and disease*, pp. 21-39 [TF Schweizer and CA Edwards, editors]. London: Springer-Verlag.

Thomsen, L.E., Knudsen, K.E.B., Jensen, T.K., Christensen, A.S., Moller, K. and Roepstorff, A. (2007) The effect of fermentable carbohydrates on experimental swine dysentery and whip worm infections in pigs. *Veterinary Microbiology* 119, 152-163.

van Beers-Schreurs, H.M.G., Nabuurs, M.J.A., Vellenga, L., Kalsbeek-van der Valk, H.J., Wensing, T. and Breukink, H.J. (1998) Weaning and the weanling diet influence the villous height and crypt depth in the small intestine of pigs and alter the concentrations of short-chain fatty acids in the large intestine and blood. *Journal of Nutrition* 128, 947-953.

van der Meulen, J., Bakker, G.C.M., Bakker, J.G.M., de Visser, H., Jongbloed, A.W. and Everts, H. (1997) Effect of resistant starch on net portal-drain viscera flux of glucose, volatile fatty acids, urea and ammonia in growing pigs. *Journal of Animal Science* 75, 2697-2704.

Wellock, I.J., Houdijk, J.G.M. and Kyriazakis, I. (2007) Effect of dietary non-starch polysaccharide solubility and inclusion level on gut health and the risk of post weaning enteric disorders in newly weaned piglets. *Livestock Science* 108, 186-189.

Wellock, I.J., Fortomaris, P.D., Houdijk, J.G., Wiseman, J. and Kyriazakis, I. (2008) The consequences of non-starch polysaccharide solubility and inclusion level on the health and performance of weaned pigs challenged with enterotoxigenic Escherichia coli. *British Journal of Nutrition* 99, 520-530.

Whipp, S.C., Robinson, I.M., Harris, D.L., Glock, R.D., Mathews, P.J. and Alexander, T.J.L. (1979) Pathogenic synergism between *Treponema hyodysenteria* and other selected anaerobes in gnotobiotic pigs. *Infection and Immunity* 26, 1042-1047.

Wilfart, A., Montagne, L., Simmins, H., Noblet, J. and Milgen, J. (2007) Digesta transit in different segments of the gastrointestinal tract of pigs as affected by insoluble fibre supplied by wheat bran. *British Journal of Nutrition* 98, 54-62.

Williams, B.A., Verstegen, M.W.A. and Tamminga, S. (2001) Fermentation in the large intestine of single-stomached animals and its relationship to animal health. *Nutrition Research Reviews* 14, 207-227.

13

BIOFUELS AND THE ANIMAL FEED SECTOR: HOW BIO-REFINING CROPS CAN MAKE BETTER USE OF LAND TO MEET OUR NEEDS FOR FEED AND LOW CARBON BIOFUELS

JOHN PINKNEY
Ensus Biofuels, UK

Introduction

As the manufacture of biofuels grows, questions are being asked as to whether such a strategy can be supported without putting unacceptable pressure on the food supply chain. This chapter critically assesses the arguments and looks in particular at the impact of biorefining wheat in Europe to both provide a new source of protein concentrate for the animal feed sector, and to support the growth of Bioethanol as a substitute for gasoline/petrol.

In order to respond to the challenge of global warming, transport fuels are a priority for action; they are the source of over 18% of Greenhouse Gas (GHG) emissions in the EU and are notable as the only significant source of GHGs that is increasing. Although more efficient cars and new technologies will inevitably contribute to meeting this challenge, the use of biofuels is an essential element of the strategy to decarbonise transport fuels. Biofuels vary in their contribution to saving carbon. Manufactured in the right way, and using the right feedstock, biofuels can reduce GHGs by at least 50% compared to fossil fuels (2, 3).

Conventionally, land has been used to meet the world's food requirements, while other sources such as oil, coal and gas have been used to meet energy and transport fuel requirements. In other words, today's sun has been used to feed the world and yesterday's sun (over millions of years) has been used to meet the world's energy and fuel needs. The challenge now is to use land and today's sun to meet not only the world's food needs but also its requirements for energy and transport fuel requirements. The critical question is whether this can be done without putting undue pressure on the planet's food supply chain and land use.

Bioethanol is manufactured through the fermentation of sugars. Today this is done by accessing sugars directly (sugar cane and beet) or by breaking down the starch in grains such as wheat to sugar. Biorefineries for the manufacture of bioethanol from cereals also produce a co-product of protein rich animal feed (DDGS) as well as carbon dioxide. Previous studies that have compared the biofuel yields from alternative crops have almost entirely ignored the credit for high protein co-products, such as DDGS from grain crops.

In meeting our food requirements, growing protein in sufficient quantities and concentrations is critical. Although cereal crops such as wheat and maize are efficient at converting the sun's energy, the concentration of protein is too low for animal feed. Soya meal is widely used as a supplement to raise protein levels and Europe today imports about 35 million tonnes of soya meal to use as an animal feed supplement. However soya makes inefficient use of land and of the sun's energy producing only 2.5 t/ha, compared to a yield of 7.7 t/ha for wheat in NW Europe. When cereals are biorefined to make bioethanol, the protein in the co-product DDGS is at a much higher concentration than in the original cereal and can replace soya meal. This means that cereals produce high protein feedstocks as well as low carbon biofuel, thus creating the opportunity for much more effective use of land.

Thus at current yields, the use of cereals to produce bioethanol could enable more effective use of land by growing a greater proportion of crops which are more efficient at converting the sun's energy to food and biofuel products. The use of bioethanol DDGS to replace soya meal could therefore enable large scale EU production of biofuel from wheat and maize of 35 Mt/yr with only a small net increase in the global arable land area. With continued increases in cereal yields, the bioethanol can be obtained with no increase or even a decrease in global cropland area.

For example, with sustainable higher cereals yields and an increased land use of 4 million ha, the supply of biofuel cereals in the EU could be increased by about 110 Mt/yr by 2020. This would enable production of about 44 Mt/yr of bioethanol in the EU, which could replace more than 8% of the EU road transport fuel consumption. The increased protein production from DDGS would reduce EU import of soya meal by 18 Mt/yr and would reduce the area required for growing soya in South America by 6 million ha. This would result in a net decrease in land area of 1.5 million ha.

This is not the whole story. The above analysis considers only wheat grain. When growing wheat, a similar amount of straw and stalks are also produced, ca 8 t/ha, of which half is harvested and is available for use to generate energy, either for power generation, or biofuel. In fact, when this is taken into account wheat has the potential to be an effective way of meeting the world's food, fuel and energy requirements and is more effective than ligno-cellulosic energy crops on arable land.

In summary therefore, this chapter shows that biorefining wheat to biofuels is a much more efficient process than has been generally recognised, which uses little if any net new land, and which, far from competing with food, actually makes a valuable contribution to the food industry by virtue of providing an alternative source of feed protein concentrate. Not only will this substantially help the food industry to cope with future growth, it will also make a massive environmental contribution by reducing the pressure on tropical land, some of which is heavily associated with continued deforestation. The chapter also shows that Europe's capacity to source biofuels from its indigenous cereal production is substantial, with the ability to meet the targets currently being proposed in the European Renewable Energy Directive draft legislation, with minimal if any need for imports or development of costly so called second generation ligno-cellulosic technology.

Summary of key arguments/considerations

CLIMATE CHANGE

A major element in the reduction of global warming is the de-carbonisation of power generation and transport fuels. Many options are available for decarbonisation of power generation, but options for decarbonisation of transport fuels are much more limited. Whilst efforts will continue to be made to use cars less and work will continue on making more efficient cars, a critical part of the strategy to decarbonise transport fuels must be biofuels. The only available technology in the foreseeable future is to produce these from agricultural crops. Therefore as we move to address global warming, we need to use global land area not only for food, but also for low carbon transport fuels and possibly for power generation.

PRESSURE ON LAND

Although the need for fuels as well as food will place substantial additional demands on land, there are several ways in which this increased demand can be, at least partially, accommodated.

- Land can be more fully utilised, by bringing unused land into food and fuel production and by continuing to increase crop yields.
- A market and trade structure which encourages the developing world to develop a vibrant agricultural sector by creating a market for grains in the developed world which takes away the need for distorting subsidies.

- Growth in the production of bioethanol from cereals enables re-optimisation of crops for food and fuel, in order to better utilise existing agricultural land.

FOOD AND FUEL CROP YIELDS

Seed crops vary in their ability to convert sunlight to energy and protein and there is a trade off between the protein concentration and crop yield. High protein concentration crops, such as soya, have a low total yield. Wheat and maize have a low protein concentration, but are very efficient at converting sunlight to energy and protein.

ANIMAL FEED

In order to produce meat and milk efficiently, animals are fed with a range of feeds: mainly seed crops including wheat, maize, rape meal and soya meal. About 70% of the wheat grown in UK and 50% of wheat grown in the EU, is used directly as animal feed, whereas most of the higher protein feeds, such as soya are imported into the EU. The optimum concentration of protein in animal feed e.g. for cattle is around 200 g/kg, whereas cereal grains have a protein content of 80-130 g/kg and oilseed meals such as soya and rape have protein concentrations of 350-500 g/kg. Currently therefore cereals need to be blended with imported oil seed meals to give the optimum protein concentration. However, when biofuels are produced from cereal crops, such as wheat and maize, the non starch part of the grain is concentrated into a co-product – distillers dried grain and solubles (DDGS), with a protein concentration of 250-350 g/kg. Therefore, DDGS can be used to replace some of the soya meal for blending, to lift the protein concentration to that required for animal feed.

EFFECTIVE BIOETHANOL YIELD

The total protein yield per hectare of wheat and maize is comparable with that of soya, and the fermentation process produces additional protein by growing yeast. Therefore little or no additional land is required to produce biofuels from wheat and maize, after taking into account the land saved by not having to grow soya. Few, if any, studies comparing biofuel yields have taken credit for the biofuel co-products. Although the direct bioethanol yield from wheat is about 2.5 t/ha, the effective yield after taking into account the DDGS co-product can be much higher at 12 t/ha or more. The land that is currently used to grow soyabeans could be used at a higher overall efficiency to grow other crops, such as maize. Production of bioethanol from cereal crops is thus a very effective way to minimise the requirement for extra land to meet growing food and fuel needs by enabling a global re-optimisation of cropping for animal feed.

BIOETHANOL PRODUCTION IN EU

As a result of higher cereals yields, increased land use supported by the abandonment of set aside, and higher productivity from land, particularly in Eastern Europe, the supply of wheat and maize in the EU could be substantially increased by 2020. This would enable production of bioethanol in the EU, which could replace more than 8% of the EU road transport fuel consumption. The increased protein production from the DDGS would reduce EU import of soya meal and reduce the pressure on deforestation in South America.

TECHNOLOGY DEVELOPMENT

Further developments will be needed to:

- develop higher yielding wheat varieties
- reduce energy requirements in bioethanol plants
- avoid degradation of protein in the fermentation and DDGS drying processes
- modify fermentation yeasts to produce essential amino acids (EAAs), to improve the EAA profile in DDGS.

LIGNO-CELLULOSIC ENERGY CROPS

There has been widespread promotion of the production of bioethanol from ligno-cellulosic energy crops, such as miscanthus and short rotation coppice (SRC) willow (where biofuels are the only product), compared to grain crops, which produce both biofuel and food. The potential benefit of energy crops is stated to be that they won't compete with food crops and will give higher biofuel yields. However, energy crops will still compete with food crops, unless they are grown on land that cannot be used for food. In fact, the biomass yield of energy crops is no higher than for wheat and maize and, because the bioethanol conversion from ligno-cellulosic energy crops is lower than from cereal grains, the biofuel yield per hectare from energy crops is significantly lower than that for cereal crops. Also, farmers are reluctant to tie up land to grow perennial energy crops rather than annual crops. Because cereal crops also give a co-product high protein animal feed, there is no case for growing ligno-cellulosic energy crops for biofuel generation on arable land.

GREENHOUSE GAS SAVINGS

Taking into account the use of co-products for animal feed, the effective GHG savings per ha from growing biofuel crops such as cereals and oilseeds are much higher than the direct savings. Although sugar beet and sugar cane have higher direct GHG savings per hectare than grain crops, the co-products are low protein or are not used for animal feed and do little to offset their land use. As a result, the effective biofuel yields from sugar cane and sugar beet are lower than for cereal crops. It is important that when, as proposed in UK and Germany, biofuel incentives are related to GHG savings, the GHG credit for co-products takes proper credit for the protein. This will encourage the most efficient use of land for growing high yield energy plus protein crops, such cereals and rapeseed, rather than sugar cane.

Climate change

The main cause of global warming is GHG emissions. The breakdown of EU GHG emissions by sector (4) is shown in Figure 1.

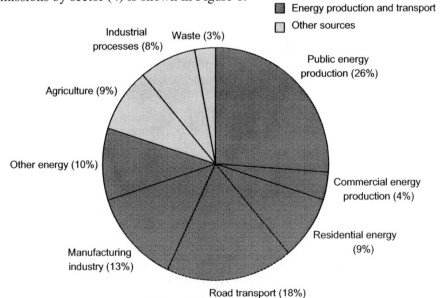

Figure 1. EU27 total GHG emissions by sector 2006

It can be seen that 80% of GHG emissions are related to energy production and transport fuels.

A major step in the reduction of global warming is, therefore, the de-carbonisation of power generation and transport fuels. Many options are available for decarbonisation of power generation, such as nuclear, wind, wave, tidal, solar, burning agricultural crops and residues and carbon sequestration from burning fossil fuels.

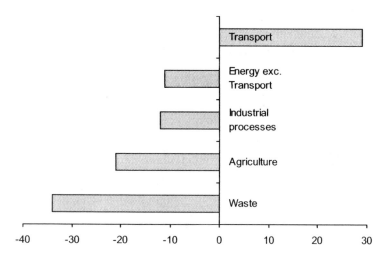

Figure 2. EU27 GHG emissions change 1990-2006

The growth of EU GHG emissions by sector (4) is shown in Figure 2. Since 1990, while all other sectors have seen a significant reduction in GHG emissions, those from transport have increased by more than 25%.

Decarbonisation of transport fuels is just one element in the reduction in the growth of GHG emissions from transport fuels and consumption of transport fuels will need to be reduced by development of more efficient engines and encouraging the use of more efficient means of transport. Options for decarbonisation of transport fuels are much more limited than for power generation and the only technology in the foreseeable future is the production of transport biofuels from agricultural crops. There are other options for non carbon transport, based on hydrogen in fuel cells. However, in order to give GHG savings, the hydrogen would need to be generated from decarbonised electric power. This will therefore give zero GHG savings until the base load power generation sector is completely decarbonised.

It is clear therefore, that as we move to address global warming, we need to use global land area not only for food, but also for transport fuels and possibly also for power generation.

Pressure on land

Although the need for fuels as well as food will place substantial additional demands on land, there are several ways in which this increased demand can be, at least partially, accommodated. These are:

- Vast tracts of land in Africa, South America and Asia can be brought into production if there is an increased demand for food and fuel.

- Continuation of the increase in crop yields, which have been increasing consistently for many years. This is particularly the case in the EU, where the Common Agricultural Policy encouraged higher agricultural output.

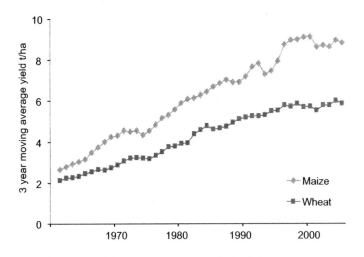

Figure 3. EU 15 cereal yields (Source: FAOStat)

The EU wheat and maize yields have gone up by 2.5% and 2.8% per annum respectively between 1961 and 2006. This has given yield increases over this period of 2.8 times for wheat and 3.4 times for maize (Figure 3).

It is important to note that higher yields have not entailed higher GHG emissions. As shown by Reference 2, GHG emissions from cultivation per tonne of wheat are lower for the high wheat yields obtained in UK and Germany, compared to those for lower yielding countries such as Canada and Ukraine.

The increase in cereals productivity has led to negative real-price inflation. Price trends are shown in Figure 4 for wheat and maize, compared to crude oil.

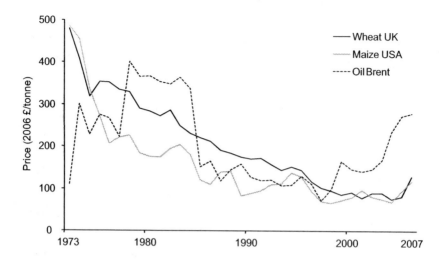

Figure 4. Real price trends in wheat, maize and oil (Source: FAOStat, EIA)

Various factors will enable substantial quantities of biofuel crops to be grown:

- Removal of set-aside mandates will encourage increased food output.

- Import duties and subsidies on particular crops have encouraged non-optimum use of land, for example growing sugar beet in EU and sugar cane in US. Removal of these subsidies will lead to more efficient use of land and resources.

- In developed countries, there is widespread destruction of food, which does not meet supermarket standards.

- The growth in production of bioethanol from cereals enables re-optimisation of crops for food and fuel, in order to better utilise existing agricultural land. This is explained in the following sections.

Eventually, however, the need to use land to grow crops for food as well as fuel will put more pressure on the use of land than historically. Therefore, in considering optimum use of resources, costs and benefits need to be considered in terms of unit land area as well as in terms of per unit of product. For example, alternative options for biofuel production and associated GHG savings need to be considered per unit land area.

Food and fuel crops yields

Food crops produce a range of commercially useful products, including protein, carbohydrate and lipid (oil or fat). The components of plants and their utility using current commercial technology are shown in Table 1.

Table 1. Utilisation of plant components

	Monogastric animals including humans	Ruminant animals	Transport fuels	Heat and power
Sugar	Yes	Yes	Yes	Yes
Starch	Yes	Yes	Yes	Yes
Cellulose	No	Yes	No	Yes
Oil	Yes	Yes	Yes	Yes
Proteins	Yes	Yes	No	Yes
Lignin	No	No	No	Yes

Commercial technology in this case means that the technology is economic, without excessive subsidies. Utilisation of other plant components, using second generation technology to produce transport fuels, will be discussed later.

Three stages need to be considered to determine the relative effectiveness of crops for different applications:

1.   Capturing sunlight to generate primary plant energy in the form of glucose

2.   Efficiency of converting primary energy into crop products

3.   Efficiency of converting plant products into food and fuel.

The rate of sunlight capture to generate primary plant energy has a low efficiency and, as long as water and some other critical resources are available, it is the limiting step in the growth of plants. Total plant yield is, therefore, dependent on the amount of sunlight available, and this varies from region to region. Comparisons of crop yields in this section are therefore average data for a group of countries in NW Europe with reasonably similar climates.

It has been shown (12) that the efficiency of converting primary plant energy into each plant component depends on the component, but is generally the same for all plants. The data from Ref 12 are used in Appendix 1 to give the results shown in Table 2. It can be seen that the conversion efficiencies to carbohydrates are high at 0.96 or more, but for oil, lignin and protein, the conversion efficiencies are somewhat lower.

Table 2. Plant energy conversion for synthesis of individual components

Component	Plant energy conversion efficiency MJ product/MJ substrate
C6 sugar	1.00
Sucrose - beet	1.00
Starch - cereal	0.97
Oil - oilseeds	0.89
Cellulose	0.96
Lignin	0.83
Proteins (available N)	0.82

These efficiencies can be used to determine the amount of the primary energy input that goes into providing useful plant products to give a "primary energy utilisation" for each crop. Crops that are equally effective at using sunlight to make useful products will have a similar "primary energy utilisation". The average yield and composition of various crops in NW European countries have been used to determine the plant primary energy and its utilisation in some alternative crops.

The results for the energy used in the harvested grain crops at average NW Europe yields are shown in Figure 5. The base data and determination of these are shown in Appendix 1.

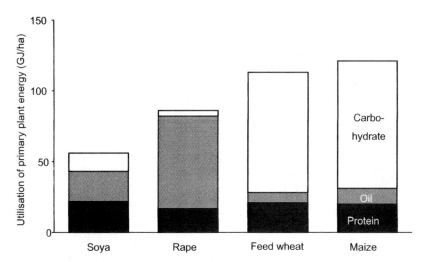

Figure 5. Utilisation of primary plant energy

The amount of energy utilised for plant products by soya beans is substantially lower than for other crops and is half that of wheat and maize. This is mainly due to the primary energy used by soya to fix nitrogen from the air. The inefficiencies of generating the nitrogen to make protein are shown in Appendix 1

The plant energy needed to fix nitrogen from the air in leguminous crops is high, so the efficiency of protein production, when nitrogen is fixed from the air is much lower at 0.34, compared to the efficiency of 0.82 when using available nitrogen in the soil. The overall efficiency for making protein using synthetic nitrogen is 0.64 and includes the mineral energy for the nitrogen. It is clear that whether protein is made by fixing nitrogen, or by the use of synthetic nitrogen, the resource cost per MJ of protein is substantially higher than for other plant components and therefore the 'hard won' protein should be conserved for food, rather than being burnt.

Nitrogen fixation does give a reduction in GHG emissions, compared to using synthetic nitrogen, when considered on the basis of GHG emissions per unit output. However, in an environment where land is a limiting resource, the GHG savings must be considered per unit of land. It is shown in Appendix 7.1 that the GHG savings per unit of nitrogen per unit land area are 1.7 times greater using synthetic nitrogen compared with nitrogen fixation.

The useful primary energy utilisation is calculated in Appendix 1 and shown below for a wider range of harvested crops in NW Europe.

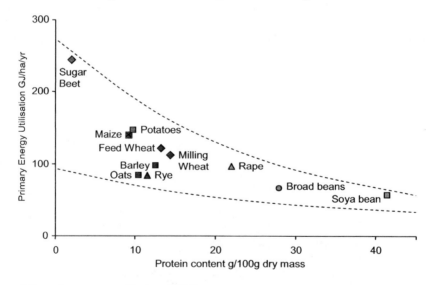

Figure 6. Crop primary energy utilisation - N W Europe

This shows a clear relationship where the higher the concentration of protein per unit dry mass of recovered crop, the less efficient the crop is at capturing energy to produce useful products. This is important in considering the productivity of different crops. Low protein crops can achieve higher energy productivities than low protein crops, but the world needs protein for animal feed as well as energy, so the energy and protein outputs must be considered together.

BIOFUEL PRODUCTION EFFICIENCIES

Different plant products are used to make biofuels, using alternative technologies: Starch and sugar are converted to bioethanol using fermentation, and vegetable oils are converted to biodiesel using transesterification or hydrogenation. In both cases the residual plant components are used as animal feed.

Due to large variations between heat contents of plant products and biofuels, the efficiencies of producing alternative biofuels, are best looked at on an energy basis (rather than mass basis), as shown in Figure 7. These data are explained in Appendix 3.1.

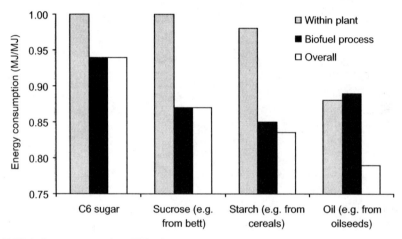

Figure 7. Biofuel energy conversion efficiencies

Taking all the conversion efficiencies into account, the conversion of primary plant energy to biofuel energy is slightly higher for sucrose at 0.86 than starch at 0.83 and oil at 0.80. This means that there is little intrinsic difference in biofuel energy efficiencies using the sun's energy to make sugar, starch or oil in plants.

Animal feed

In order to produce meat and milk efficiently, animals are fed with a range of feeds to provide energy and protein. These animal feeds are mainly seed crops and include wheat, maize, rape meal and soya meal, and are blended to provide an optimum feed for different animals. The blending is operated, primarily to meet the optimum protein and energy levels for animal feed, but also to meet many other factors, such as amino acid requirements. The energy content of different animal feeds is similar, but the protein content varies widely.

Supply of protein sources for animal feed in the EU is tabulated in Appendix 2 and is summarised in Figure 8.

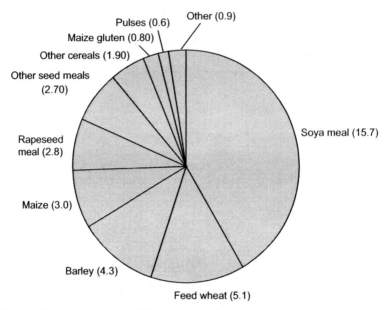

Figure 8. EU Animal feed protein supply (Million tonnes, 2007)

Rapeseed and other seed meals are supplied mainly from within the EU, but nearly all the soya meal is imported. The trend in EU protein imports is shown in Figure 9.

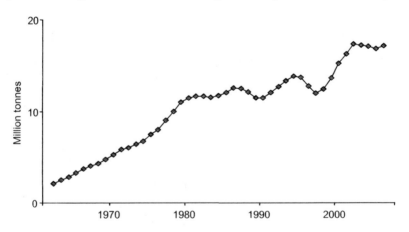

Figure 9. EU 27 Animal feed protein net imports (Source FAOSTAT (Ref 38))

Protein imports are rising steadily and the UK and EU each now import about 50% of their entire animal feed protein requirements. This is a serious problem (11), due to concerns about imported soya and maize products, which come mainly from N and S America, being contaminated with unapproved genetically modified organisms (GMOs).

It can be seen from the data in Appendix 2, that the major animal feed import is of soya meal, which as shown in Figure 7, is the least efficient major crop at utilising sunlight and land to produce plant products.

The protein yield per hectare of different crops, versus their protein concentration, is shown in Appendix 1 and summarised in Figure 10.

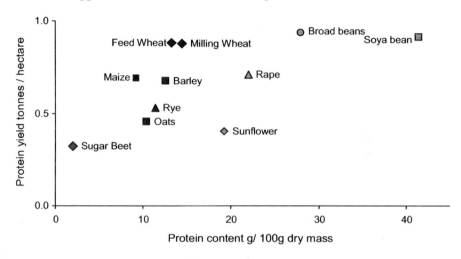

Figure 10. Protein yield and content of crops - NW Europe

It can be seen that many crops have similar protein yields of 0.65 – 0.9 t/ha. Although soya is recognised as being a protein crop, due its high protein content, its protein yield is little higher than wheat and maize.

Protein contents of alternative animal feeds are calculated in Appendix 3 and summarised in Figure 11. Bioethanol will be made from feed wheat.

DDGS is Distillers Dried Grains and Solubles and is the co-product of the production of ethanol from cereals. The optimum level of protein in animal feed e.g. for cattle is around 200 g/kg, whereas cereal grains have a level of protein of 80-130 g/kg and oilseed meals such as soya and rape have protein concentrations of 350-500 g/kg. Low protein concentration cereals are therefore blended with high concentration oil seed meals to give the optimum concentration for animal feed. The reason soya meal is so widely used, despite its inefficiency, is because the high protein concentration enables it to be blended with widely available low protein animal feeds, in order to obtain the optimum protein concentration for compound animal feeds.

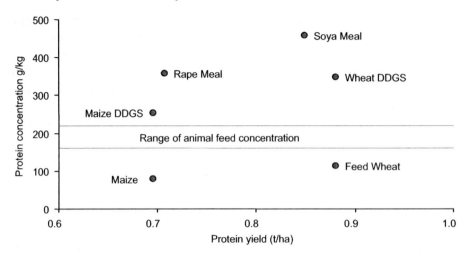

Figure 11. Protein content of animal feed

However, as can be seen in Figure 11, high concentration protein animal feed components can be obtained also by growing lower protein concentration crops, such as wheat and maize, and concentrating the protein. Low protein concentrations in cereal crops are concentrated by removing the starch to make bioethanol. Additionally, significant quantities of protein are produced during fermentation from non-protein nitrogen and starch to grow the yeast. This not only increases the protein concentration, but also the protein yield. The fermentation process therefore produces a protein concentration in DDGS that is high enough to replace soya meal for blending in animal feed.

Effective yield of biofuel crops

The effective yield of biofuels, such as cereals and rape, includes credit from the land area saved by using high protein co-product DDGS or seedcake to replace crops, such as feed cereals and soya, as animal feed. This credit has either been ignored completely in previous work on the evaluation of grain crops for biofuel production, e.g. Pimentel (9), or credit is taken only for the displacement of cereals, e.g. Searchinger (10).

EFFECTIVE BIOETHANOL YIELD OF WHEAT

Credit for the DDGS from wheat and maize, can be determined in various ways, depending on assumptions around which animal feed components are replaced by

DDGS, to which species the DDGS are fed, and where the replaced animal feeds are grown. DDGS protein may have a lower value than soya meal protein, due to degradation in the bioethanol process, and has a lower essential amino acid (EEA) content than some current animal feeds, such as soya. This makes little difference when DDGS are fed to ruminants, but limits the extent of DDGS use in feeds for monogastric animals, such as pigs and poultry. Analysis of data on feed trials for poultry using maize DDGS (27) shows slightly lower protein effectiveness. In order to take account of this, a DDGS protein effectiveness of 80% compared to soya meal protein has been assumed.

In the EU, feed wheat in excess of demand is exported and as shown in Appendix 2, soya meal imports are adjusted to meet the substantial EU demand for animal feed protein that is excess to internal EU supply. Feed wheat can therefore be regarded as the marginal animal energy feed and imported soya meal as the marginal high protein feed. It is assumed that DDGS will replace a mixture of feed wheat and soya meal imported from South America, to give the same metabolisable energy and effective amount of protein.

The simplest way of assessing the effective yield of bioethanol from wheat, is to compare two agricultural options, one which uses wheat for biofuel and the other which uses feed wheat and soya meal to match the animal feed value of DDGS. The comparison is summarised in Figure 12 and shown in detail in Appendix 4.

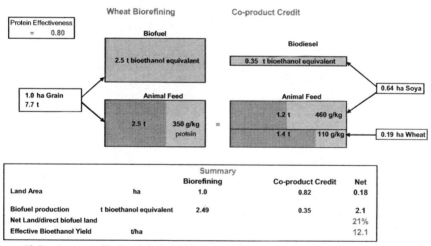

Figure 12. Land use and effective biofuel yield from scenarios using wheat for biofuel or using wheat and soya to match the animal feed value of DDGS

Scenario 1 – Using wheat for biofuel (Figure 12, left hand side)

- 1 ha of wheat is grown to produce bioethanol and DDGS for animal feed. This produces 2.5 t of bioethanol plus 2.5 t DDGS, with a protein content of 350 g/kg. The DDGS can replace a mixture of soya meal and feed wheat to give the same amounts of protein and metabolisable energy (ME) as the DDGS.

Scenario 2 – Use wheat and soya to achieve the same animal feed requirements (Figure 12, right hand side)

• To achieve the same energy and effective protein requirements, wheat needs to be mixed with soya meal in a ratio of 1.4 t wheat to 1.2 t soya. This requires 1.4 t of wheat using 0.19 ha of land and 1.2 t of soya meal using 0.64 hectares of land.

• The co-product soya oil is assumed to be made into biodiesel and, after correcting for the higher energy of biodiesel compared to bioethanol, it is credited as equivalent bioethanol.

In both cases, the animal feed product will be blended with more feed wheat to give the desired animal feed composition.

Comparing the two cases, the effective bioethanol yield is determined by dividing the net extra bioethanol by the net extra land area. The effective bioethanol yield from wheat in this case is 12.1 t/ha, compared to the direct biofuel yield of 2.5 t/ha. The reason for this result is explained further in Figure 13.

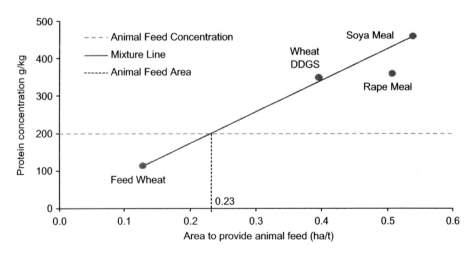

Figure 13. Area needed to provide animal feed

The mixture line between soya meal and feed wheat gives the land area needed to provide an animal feed at any concentration by blending these components. For example to supply animal feed with a protein content of 200 g/kg, the area is 0.23 ha/t feed. Using these data, the point for DDGS lies close to this mixture line. Therefore, the area needed to supply animal feed with a protein content of 200 g/kg from DDGS and feed wheat is the same as that of the blend of soya meal and feed wheat. Because the yield of biofuel from wheat is substantially higher than for soya bean, this extra fuel comes with no increase in land area.

It is claimed that some S American soya is grown on deforested land; therefore, the reduced EU soya requirement may lead to reduced deforestation.

EFFECTIVE YIELD OF OTHER BIOFUEL CROPS

A similar analysis has been done for other biofuel crops. The data are given in Appendix 4 and summarised in Figure 14.

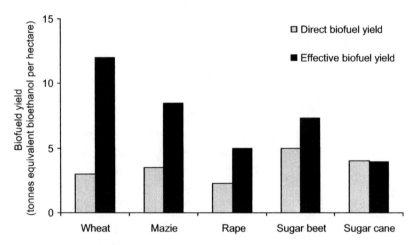

Figure 14. Effective biofuel yield of alternative crops

This shows that it is vital to take into account the credit for the biofuel co-products when comparing yields of biofuel crops. Although sugar beet has a high direct biofuel yield, there is little protein co-product, so the relative co-product credit is small.

Most plants producing bioethanol from sugar cane burn the bagasse to provide power, so there is no co-product credit (23). Although co-product molasses from the production of refined sugar is used as animal feed, the bioethanol yield assumes maximum sugar conversion. Although other co-products can be produced from sugar cane, or bagasse, these do not provide a land use credit.

Bioethanol production in EU

There are several ways in which the production of cereals can be increased within EU in order to provide feed for bioethanol production. These are:

- Increasing cereal crop yields - As shown in Figure 3, cereal yields in EU have been increasing steadily for many years. A more detailed analysis of these data is shown in Appendix 5.1. From these data it is reasonable to assume that yield increases in the original EU 15 countries will continue at the same rate of 1.5%/yr. The increased output in 2020, compared to current levels, will give approximately a further 48 Mt/yr

- Increasing Eastern EU productivity - In the period 1975-1982 cereal yields in Eastern EU countries were about 83% of the EU 15 countries, whereas current yields of cereals in Eastern EU countries are only 60% of the levels in EU15 countries. Yields in Eastern EU countries, therefore, have the potential to increase as more modern farming methods and science are applied. The nitrogen fertiliser usage per ha of arable crops in E Europe is less than half that in NW Europe (37). It is assumed that yields in the new EU 12 countries can be increased at a rate of 3%/yr to 2020. This is lower than the rate that both EU 15 and EU12 countries averaged between 1965 and 1985 and will give a further 38 Mt/yr of cereals

- Increased cereal land - The requirement for set aside land has been dropped in EU. It is assumed that cereal crops will be grown on half of this land. Together with a small amount of land being transferred from sugar beet, under the sugar reforms, this will provide 4 million ha of extra cereal land. Another 31 Mt/yr of cereals can be expected from this source.

The results of these increases in EU cereal production are shown in Appendix 5.2 and are summarised in Table 3 and Figure 15.

Table 3. Additional ethanol from cereals in EU

		Wheat	Maize	Barley	Total
Increase in EU 15 production by 2020	Mt/yr	26.4	9.5	11.8	48
Increase in EU 12 production by 2020	Mt/yr	17.6	14.2	6.2	38
Additional crop from extra land	Mt/yr	13.3	17.3	0.0	31
Impact of non biofuel consumption	Mt/yr	-16.2	3.3	3.3	-10
Additional cereals crop available	Mt/yr	41.0	44.3	21.3	107
Cereal displaced by DDGS co-product	Mt/yr	9.3	13.5	7.5	30
Additional cereals bioethanol crop	Mt/yr	50.4	57.8	28.8	137
Bioethanol production in EU	Mt/yr	16.2	19.4	8.2	44
Reduction in soya meal import	Mt/yr	7.7	5.7	4.4	18

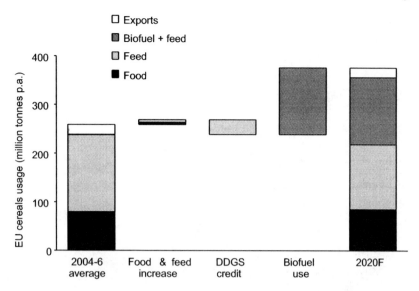

Figure 15. EU cereals balance for biofuels

Increase in demand for food and animal feed up to 2020 will give a small increase in cereal demand. However, this increase will be more than offset by the cereals that will be freed up by the DDGS co-product from cereal refining.

This analysis shows that there is considerable potential for extra cereal to be grown in the EU, which after accounting for increased cereal demand for food and animal feed, will give the potential for about 137 million tonnes of cereals for biofuel by 2020. This will allow a total production of 44 Mt/yr of bioethanol, within the EU, which will be equivalent to more than 8% of the energy demand for all EU transport fuels in 2020.

Assuming that increased EU rape and sunflower for biodiesel production can meet the remaining 2% EU energy target, the total target can be met by EU grown crops. The current trade position for cereals will not be changed, so the EU could neither be accused of causing higher food prices in the rest of the world by importing biofuels, nor of stifling food production in developing countries by increasing food exports. For a biofuels target above 10% in 2020, it is likely that the EU would need to import biofuels or include biofuels from waste materials.

The high protein co-product from the production of ethanol from cereals within the EU will reduce the increase in imports of soya meal (mainly from S America) by 18 Mt/yr by 2020. This will give a substantial improvement in the security of supply of non-GM animal feed in the EU.

The reduced EU demand for soya meal will avoid the use of about 6 million ha of new land in S America, which would come from destruction of forest or from cerrado grassland. Avoiding the destruction of these habitats should more than offset the environmental concerns of the re-use of 3.5 milllion ha of rotational set-aside land in the EU.

Technology developments

Technology development is required in several areas:

- Higher yielding strains of cereal
- Bioethanol plant technology
- Quality of DDGS
- Profile of essential amino acids

HIGHER YIELDING STRAINS OF CEREAL

New cereal strains continue to be developed to give higher yields and increased disease resistance. Further work needs to be done to find strains that are better suited to more marginal land and to give high yields in Eastern Europe. Although it is an advantage for wheat used for bioethanol to have higher starch content, this is not an overriding incentive as long as proper credit is given for the protein content in the DDGS

BIOETHANOL PLANT TECHNOLOGY

Starch utilisation from cereals in modern bioethanol plants is very good, but work needs to be done to develop yeasts, or staged fermentation, to operate at high ethanol concentrations and hence reduce energy consumption.

QUALITY OF DDGS

The effective yield of bioethanol depends on the quality of the protein in the DDGS, compared to that in soya meal and hence the ratio of feed wheat and soya meal replaced by the DDGS. In some bioethanol plants, protein can be degraded during the distillation and drying stages, such that some protein becomes degraded and is less effective. The relationship between the effective bioethanol yield from wheat in NW Europe and protein effectiveness is shown below.

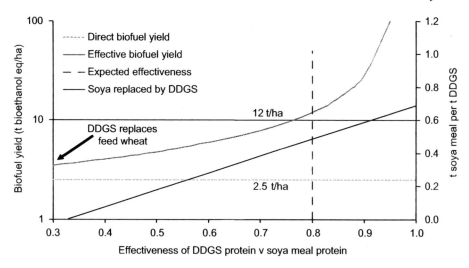

Figure 16. Effective biofuel yield from wheat

The direct bioethanol yield is 2.5 t/ha. If DDGS co-product simply replaces feed wheat as animal feed, to give the same metabolisable energy, the net land usage for biofuel is lower and the effective yield is 50% higher at 3.7 t/ha. Taking into account the higher protein value in DDGS, compared to wheat, DDGS actually replaces a mixture of wheat and soya meal as animal feed. Since soya has a much lower yield than wheat, the net land usage for biofuel reduces and effective yield increases. If the effective protein yield per hectare of DDGS is high enough that it can provide the same amount of animal feed per ha as soya meal, then the effective yield of bioethanol becomes infinite.

Further developments will be needed to avoid degradation of protein in the fermentation and DDGS drying process and to ensure consistency of the DDGS product.

PROFILE OF ESSENTIAL AMINO ACIDS

Animal feed must meet the required level of each essential amino acid (EAA) as well as the overall protein level. The EAA levels in various crops compared to the requirements for cattle are shown in Figure 17.

The first two bars in each section represent the EAA profile in beef and milk (22) and therefore give a good indication of the EAA demands for beef and dairy cattle. The other bars show the EAA content in alternative animal feed crops (22) and show how effectively the protein in different crops can be utilised by the animals. Where there is shortfall of EAA, it must be made up either by blending or addition of synthetic EAA. If there is a surplus, the EAA is broken down and used to build other proteins. It can be seen that the EAA levels in protein from cereals and oil seed meals match fairly closely the requirements for beef and dairy cattle. The exceptions are low levels of lysine and threonine in wheat and maize, tryptophan in maize, and methionine in soya meal. There is some degradation of lysine and other EAAs during DDGS drying. Synthetic lysine and threonine are readily available and are widely used as additives to compound feeds.

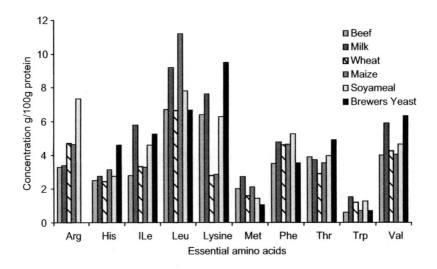

Figure 17. Essential amino acid profile of various crops compared to requirements for beef and dairy cattle

About 10% of the protein in DDGS is from the yeast and DDGS will contain the EAAs from the yeast that is grown during fermentation as well as the EAAs from the wheat. Brewers' yeast (24) has significantly higher levels of lysine, and yeast can be modified to produce higher amounts of EAAs, such as lysine, where there is a shortage in the cereal.

Ligno-cellulosic energy crops

There has been widespread promotion of the benefits of producing bioethanol from ligno-cellulosic energy crops, such as miscanthus and SRC willow (where the crop is used only to make biofuel), compared to cereals using arguments such as:

•   bioethanol from cereal crops competes with food; bioethanol from energy crops does not

- cereal crops require high nitrogen inputs which lead to high GHG emissions for biofuel production
- yields of biofuels from ligno-cellulosic feedstocks are significantly higher than from food crops, so energy crops should be used for biofuel
- savings in GHG emissions are higher for biofuels from energy crops than for biofuels from grain crops

These proposed benefits fail to give any credit to the high protein co-product animal feeds from grain crops, despite the amount of co-product being similar to the amount of biofuel production. These issues are discussed below.

COMPETITION BETWEEN FOOD AND FUEL

Current biofuel crops grown in the EU, such as cereals for bioethanol and rapeseed and sunflower for biodiesel, can be used for either food or biofuel production or a mixture of the two. Because energy crops produce cellulose that cannot be digested by humans, it has been argued that they do not compete with food. However, this argument misses the point. The important issue is whether or not energy crops are grown on land that can be used for food crops. If energy crops, such as miscanthus or SRC willow, are grown on land that could grow food crops, the biofuel product is competing with food just as much as biofuel from wheat or rape.

While some energy crops **can** be grown on marginal land that is not currently being used to grow food crops, they only relieve pressure on land if they actually **are** grown on marginal land. Certainly energy crops are currently being grown in the UK on land that was previously used for growing food crops.

Although some marginal land may currently not be needed for growing food, it does not mean that it is best to use that land for energy crops. It may be better to grow crops to provide food and fuel, even though the yields on this land are lower than on prime agricultural land. In order to justify using energy crops rather than cereals to produce bioethanol, it needs to be shown that energy crops will give higher effective yields of biofuel, or greater carbon savings per unit land area, than producing biofuels from cereal crops.

NITROGEN INPUTS

Substantial GHG emissions are associated with nitrogen fertiliser for growing cereals, both in the CO_2 and N_2O emissions from N fertiliser manufacture and also in the N_2O emissions from land.

In crops such as wheat, maize and rape, nitrogen from fertiliser is converted to nitrogen in the grain in the form of protein. All this protein goes into the DDGS or meal co-product. The nitrogen mass balance and conversions for the different crops, using the RTFO default figures (2), are shown in Table 4.

Table 4. Applied nitrogen utilisation in different crops

		UK wheat	*French maize*	*UK rape*
Raw grain yield	t/ha/yr	7.76	8.52	3.03
N fertiliser use	kgN/ha/yr	183	170	185
N fertiliser use	kgN/t grain	23.6	20.0	61.1
DDGS/meal yield	kg/kg grain	0.33	0.31	0.57
DDGS or meal protein content	g/kg	380	290	360
Nitrogen in DDGS/meal	kgN/t grain	20.4	14.5	32.7
N in grain/N in applied fertiliser	kg/kg	0.87	0.73	0.54

In Table 4, the applied nitrogen inputs are compared to the nitrogen output in protein per tonne of grain. Table 4 shows that cereal crops, such as wheat and maize are very efficient in converting applied nitrogen into protein and that the amount of nitrogen in protein in wheat DDGS is equal to 0.87 of the nitrogen that is applied to these crops in fertiliser.

The high nitrogen inputs to cereal crops are therefore being used to produce protein in co-product animal feed, not to produce bioethanol. Since DDGS and meal are used as animal feed, these nitrogen inputs still go into the food chain.

COMPARISON OF PRODUCT YIELDS

The overall efficiency of conversion of plant primary energy to biofuel has been determined, using data in Tables 1 and 2, and data from Refs 14-17, for the conversion of plant components to biofuels. The data are set out in Appendix 6 and are summarised in Figure 18.

Cellulose and hemicellulose will be converted to bioethanol using so called "Second Generation" technology. The white bars show the likely current state of technology (16); the grey bars are for technology targets (15); the black bars represent the Biomass to Liquids (BTL) route, which is the production of diesel and naphtha via pyrolysis, gasification, Fischer Tropsch synthesis and hydrocracking. Development work on second generation technology is progressing slowly because there are lots of problems and the technology is expensive. It is difficult to obtain a true picture of current progress.

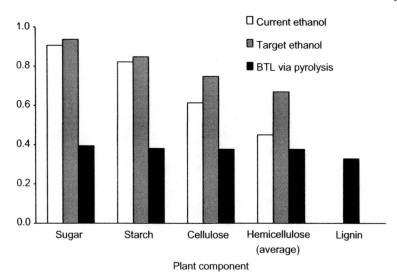

Figure 18. Biofuel energy efficiencies

Figure 18 shows that the energy conversion of sugar and starch, using first generation technology is good. Conversion of cellulose and hemi-cellulose, using currently available second generation technology is poor. The target energy conversion efficiency of cellulose and hemi-cellulose is lower than can currently be achieved by cattle. Also, the timescale for achieving the targets that have been set for second generation technology are unclear, but these could easily be 10 or 15 years away. This is discussed further in Appendix 6. It is not envisaged that it will become possible to convert plant lignin to ethanol.

Cereal crops such as wheat and maize have straw or stover that can be recovered to produce bioethanol. It is assumed that if technology becomes economic for making bioethanol from ligno-cellulosic crops such as SRC willow and miscanthus, it will also be economic to produce bioethanol from wheat straw and maize stover. Using typical crop yield and composition data, the total primary energy utilisation of some crops is shown in Appendix 6 and summarised in Figure 19.

The primary energy utilisation for SRC willow and miscanthus grown in the UK is similar to sugar beet and wheat. This indicates that these crops all utilise similar amounts of sunlight. The energy utilisation for maize is higher because it is grown in countries with a sunnier climate than UK. The split of crop components is different between food crops and energy crops, with food crops having a much higher level of sugar or starch, which give higher conversion to bioethanol. The effect of this is shown in Appendix 6 and Figure 20.

No account has been taken in Figure 20 of the displacement of soya by wheat and maize.

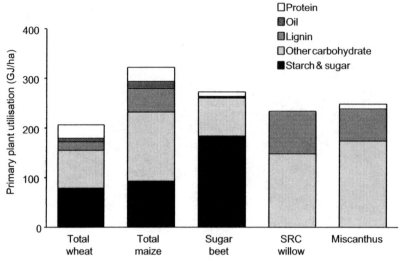

Figure 19. Utilisation of primary plant energy

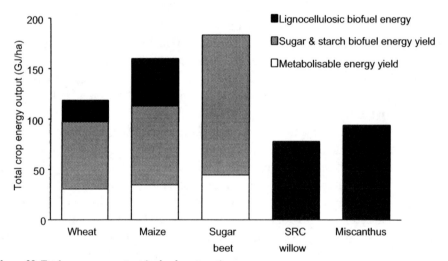

Figure 20. Total crop energy output (technology target)

Figure 20 shows that even using target technology performance for second generation technology, the energy output yield of energy crops, such as SRC willow and miscanthus, will be significantly lower than for current crops such as sugar beet, wheat and maize. This is because the efficiency of converting lignin, cellulose and hemicellulose to useful energy is significantly lower than for sugar and starch.

With improved crops, the yield from energy crops, such as SRC willow, poplar and miscanthus in the UK may rise significantly from the current 10-12 t/ha. However, yields of cereals are also increasing steadily and this is likely to continue.

Farmers are reluctant to tie up land to grow perennial energy crops, such as miscanthus and SRC willow rather than annual crops, because they may miss out on highly profitable years for annual crops. There are also problems that these perennial crops need investment and time to become established and it can be difficult to remove roots and return land to annual crops at the end of the energy crop life.

There is, therefore, no case for growing energy crops on arable land in order to obtain higher bioethanol yields.

Comparison of GHG emission savings

Due to the concern that the drive for biofuels will lead to a shortage of land, it is important to ensure that the GHG savings from biofuels are achieved as efficiently as possible from the land area available. The metric that needs to be compared is therefore the GHG saving per unit land area.

This has been calculated for some biofuel crops. The data used are given in Appendix 7.2 and the results are shown in Figure 21.

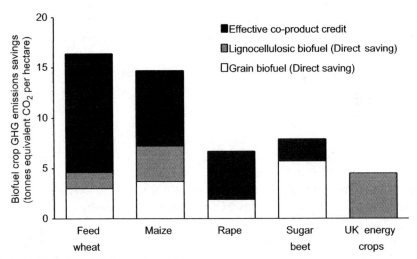

Figure 21. Biofuel crop GHG emissions savings

Estimates of GHG savings for biofuels include credit for co-product DDGS and seed cake, which are used as animal feed. DDGS replaces a mixture of feed wheat and soya meal, so that more arable land is released to grow food or more biofuel crops. The calculation of direct GHG savings (in the UK RTFO and JEC methodologies;

Refs 2 and 10), uses a substitution approach for the co-product. This gives a credit for the GHG emissions used to grow the soya bean and feed wheat replaced by the co-product. However, in a land limiting environment, the GHG credit for co-products should be calculated as the GHG savings from growing further biofuel crops, such as maize, on the displaced land. When this is taken into account, the effective GHG emission savings from making biofuels from grain crops are much higher than the direct GHG savings. Although sugar beet and sugar cane have higher direct GHG savings per ha than grain crops, they have little or no animal feed co-product to offset their land use. As a result, the effective biofuel yields from sugar cane and sugar beet are lower than for cereal crops.

It is important when, as proposed in UK and Germany, biofuel incentives are related to GHG savings, that the GHG credit for co-products gives proper credit for the protein. This will encourage the most efficient use of land for growing high yield energy plus protein crops, such cereals and rapeseed.

With improved technology for making bioethanol from ligno-cellulosic feeds, the GHG savings from using energy crops to make bioethanol will probably be increased to 100%, so the GHG savings per ha will increase. However, the effective GHG savings of bioethanol from wheat (taking into account the DDGS co-product), will still be substantially higher than those of bioethanol from energy crops. There is therefore no case for growing energy crops on arable land in the UK in order to produce bioethanol.

This analysis has been based on mixed farming in a temperate climate and there may be a case for using energy crops to produce biofuels, in other situations:

- countries with warmer climates, giving higher energy crop yields
- areas where there is no market for co-product animal feed from cereal crops.

A similar analysis should be done also for grassland, comparing alternative grass crops and their use for forage, or bioethanol plus fodder, or bioethanol only.

Plants can convert sunlight more efficiently to form sugar, starch and oil than to form lignin, so higher biomass yields are not obtained by growing ligno-cellulosic crops rather than food crops. Also, because both first and second generation biofuel processes will convert sugar, starch and oil to biofuels more efficiently than cellulose and lignin, there is no point in growing ligno-cellulosic crops for biofuel production.

References

1) Developments of biofuels - Study by the Royal Society - Evidence provided by Ensus Limited, Aug 2007, peer reviewed by Jeremy Woods, Imperial College, January 2008

2) Renewable Fuels Agency (2008) Carbon and sustainability reporting within the Renewable Transport Fuel Obligation, Technical guidance, Part 2. [Online] Jan 2008. http://www.dft.gov.uk/rfa/_db/_documents/ RFA_Technical_Guidance_Part_2_v1.2.pdf.

3) CONCAWE, EUCAR and JRC (2007) Well-To-Wheels Analysis of Future Automotive Fuels and Powertrains in the European Context. Well-to-Tank Report Version 2c. European Commission Joint Research Centre.

4) EEA (2008) Annual European Community GHG Inventory 1990-2006 and inventory report 2008, Technical Report No 6. European Environment Agency.

5) HGCA (2006) Research review 61 - Wheat as a feedstock for alcohol production. [Online]. http://www-dev.hgca.com/document. aspx?fn=load&media_id=3194&publicationId=3588.

6) Lee, D., Owens, V.N., Boe, A. and Jeranyama, P. (2007) Composition of Herbaceous Biomass Feedstocks. Report SGINC1-07, South Dakota State University.

7) Waliszewska, B. (2002) Chemical Composition of 2 and 4 yr old samples of willow varieties. In *Wood Structure and Properties '02.* (Eds. J. Kúdela and S. Kurjatko) pp21-23. Arbora Publishers, Zvolen, Slovakia.

8) A Whole Systems Approach to Bioenergy demand and Supply, TSEC-Biosys, TSEC website

9) Pimentel, D. and Patzek, T.W. (2005) Ethanol Production Using Corn, Switchgrass, and Wood; Biodiesel Production Using Soybean and Sunflower. Natural Resources Research 14, 65-76.

10) Searchinger, T., Heimlich, R., Houghton, R., Dong, F., Elobeid, A., Fabiosa, J., Tokgoz, S., Hayes, D., Yu, T. (2008) Use of U.S. croplands for biofuels increases greenhouse gases through emissions from land-use change. Science, 319, 1238-1240.

11) EC (2007) Economic Impact of Unapproved GMOs on EU Feed imports and Livestock Production. DG Agri, European Commission, Brussels.

12) Penning de Vries, F. W. T., Brunsting, A. H. M. and Van Laar, H. H. (1974). Products, requirements and efficiency of biosynthesis: a quantitative approach. Journal of Theoretical Biology, 45, 339–377.

13) Phillips, D.A. (1980) Efficiency of Symbiotic Nitrogen Fixation in Legumes, Ann Rev. Plant Physiol. 31, 29-49.

14) Wooley, R., Ruth, M., Sheehan, J., Ibsen, K., Majdeski, H. and Galvez, A. (1999) Lignocellulosic biomass to ethanol process design and economics utilizing co-current dilute acid prehydrolysis and enzymatic hydrolysis: Current and futuristic scenarios. NREL/TP-580-26157. Natl. Renewable Energy Lab., Golden, CO.

15) Aden, A., Ruth, M., Ibsen, K., Jechura, J., Neeves, K., Sheehan, J., Wallace, B., Montague, L., Slayton, A. and Lukas, J. (2002) Lignocellulosic ethanol process design and economics utilizing co-current dilute acid prehydrolysis and enzymatic hydrolysis. NREL TP-510-32438. Natl. Renewable Energy Lab., Golden, CO.

16) Private communication Imperial College. December 2007

17) Nexant (2007) The Feasibility of Second Generation Biodiesel Production in the UK prepared for National Non-Food Crops Centre.

18) Defra (2006) British Survey of Fertiliser Practice 2004 – 2006.

19) Strategie Grains, 12 April 2007

20) FEFAC (2005) Feed & Fuel Statistical Yearbook.

21) Nix, J. (2008) Farm Management Pocketbook, 38th edition, The Pocketbook, Melton Mowbray.

22) National Research Council (2001) Nutrient Requirements of Dairy Cattle. 7th rev. ed. Natl. Acad. Sci., Washington D.C.

23) Seebaluck, V., Mohee, R., Sobhanbabu, P.R.K., Rosillo-Calle, F., Leal, M.R.L.V. and Johnson, F.X. (2008) Bioenergy for sustainable development and global competitiveness: The case of cane sugar in S Africa. CARENSA/SEI 2008-2, Stockholm Environment Institute, Stockholm.

24) Pozo-Dengra et al, Screening of autolytic yeast strains for production of L-amino acids, Enzyme and Microbial Technology, 40 (2006) 46-50.

25) Jenssen & Kongshaug, Energy Consumption and GHG emissions in Fertiliser Production, IFS proceedings No 509

26) S J Del Grosso, AR Mosier, W J Parton, D S Ojima, Daycent Model Analysis of past and contemporary soil N2O and net GHG flux for major crops in the USA, 11 Jan 2005

27) Mahmoud K Masadeh et al, Dried Distillers Grains with Solubles in Laying Hens Ration, Feedinfo News Service, 14 Feb 2008

28) NNFCC. An assessment of the opportunities for sugarbeet production and processing in the UK. [Online] 2007. http://www.nnfcc.co.uk/metadot/index.pl?id=5309&isa=DBRow&field_name=file&op=download_file

29) EU Renewable Energy Directive, version 15.4, 23/1/2008

30) Annex to the (RED) Impact Assessment, SEC (2008) 85, 27 Feb 2008

31) DG Agri. Prospects for Agricultural Markets and Income in the European Union 2007-14. Brussels : European Commission, March 2008. http://ec.europa.eu/agriculture/publi/caprep/prospects2007b/fullrep.pdf

32)   FAO. FAOSTAT Production database. [Online] http://faostat.fao.org/default.
      aspx.
33)   Premier Nutrition Products Ltd. Premier Atlas 2008. [Online]
34)   Fediol, Our Industry, http://www.fediol.org/2/index.php
35)   CQS wheat analysis. HGCA. 2007.
36)   Yeasts for the Production of Fuel Alcohol. W. M. Ingledew, The Yeasts
      2nd Edition Vol 5 Yeast Technology pp 245-291 edited by AH Rose and JS
      Harrison Academic Press London 1993.
37)   FAO. FAOSTAT Resources database. [Online] http://faostat.fao.org/default.
      aspx.
38)   FAO. FAOSTAT Trade database. [Online] http://faostat.fao.org/site/342/
      default.aspx

Appendix 1 - Crop Yield Data

Plant energy conversion

Component	Wt product/ wt glucose	Combustion energy (LHV)	Primary energy for conversion	Plant energy conversion efficiency
	kg/kg	MJ/kg product		MJ product/MJ substrate
Soluble C6 sugar	1.0	13.8	13.8	1.00
Sucrose	0.826	14.9	16.7	1.00
Starch	0.826	16.1	16.7	0.97
Oil	0.33	37.2	41.7	0.89
Cellulose	0.826	16.0	16.7	0.96
Lignin	0.465	24.7	29.6	0.83
Proteins (available N)	0.51	22.1	27.0	0.82

Energy needed to produce protein

		Fixed N	Synthetic N
Plant energy (available)	MJ/MJ protein	1.22	1.22
Primary plant energy to	MJ/MJ protein	1.70	
Mineral energy	MJ/MJ protein		0.34
Total energy	**MJ/MJ energy**	**2.92**	**1.56**
Energy efficiency		0.34	0.64

Notes

- Data for primary plant energy requirements are taken from Refs. 12 and 13.

- Data for biofuel conversion efficiencies are taken from Ref. 2

- Crop yields for N W Europe are from Ref 32 and are the weighted average yields for UK, Germany, France, Ireland, Belgium, Denmark and Netherlands from 2004 -6.

Average NW Europe crop yields 2004-6

		Maize	Barley	Rye	Oats	Rape	Soya bean	Sunflower	Sugar beet	Broad beans	Feed wheat	Milling wheat
Yield NW Europe	t/ha	8.7	6.12	5.3	5.0	3.5	2.5	2.3	66.9	3.9	7.75	7.1
Composition (g/kg moist)												
Reference		(33)	(33)	(33)	(33)	(33)	(33/34)	(33/34)	(28)	(33)	(5/35)	(5/35)
Water		130	130	130	130	90	130	90	760	140	146	146
Protein		80	110	100	91	200	360	180	50	240	114	124
Lipid (B)		40	30	23	68	430	195	450	10	22	23	23
Carbohydrate		739	711	729	687	244	265	251	210	568	701	691
Ash		12	22	18	24	36	50	34	3	30	17	17
Starch + sugar		650	550	600	383			393	162	393	618	
Total check		1000	1000	1000	1000	1000	1000	1000	1000	1000	1000	1000
Protein content use	g/kg DM	92	126	115	105	220	414	192	20	279	133	145
Protein yield	t/ha	0.70	0.67	0.53	0.46	0.71	0.91	0.40	0.32	0.94	0.88	0.88
Primary energy usage	MJ/kg	16.1	15.9	15.8	16.7	27.4	22.3	27.7	3.7	16.9	15.7	15.8
Primary energy usage	GJ/ha/yr	140	98	84	84	97	57	64	244	66	122	112

Wheat

- The yield of feed wheat is 8.5% higher than that of milling wheat (9) and wheat grown in the EU is about 50:50 feed wheat : milling wheat (30), so the yield of feed wheat is taken as 4.25% higher and the yield of milling wheat 4.25% lower than average NW Europe wheat yields.

- Protein content for wheat is normally reported and quoted for the milling industry as N x 5.7. This has been converted to N x 6.25, which is the standard used for other crops and for the animal feed industry

- Feed wheat protein is average 2005 – 7 for Nabim groups 3 & 4 in the UK (13)

UK wheat protein - average 2005-7

	Avg moisture content 146 g/kg			
	Protein = N x 5.7		*Protein = N x 6.25*	
	DM (g/kg)	*Moist (g/kg)*	*DM (g/kg)*	*Moist (g/kg)*
All wheat	125	109	138	
Milling wheat	129	113		124
Feed wheat	119	104		114

Useful primary energy utilisation

		GJ/ha/yr				
		Sugar beet	*Wheat*	*Maize*	*Rape*	*Soya bean*
Protein	27.0	36.2	25.3	22.3	18.7	27.4
Oil	41.7	1.6	6.6	12.0	64.8	21.1
Carbohydrate	16.7	234	87.2	104.4	12.8	12.8
Total		272	119	139	96	61

Appendix 2 - Animal Feed Data

EU animal feed supply

Animal feed component	Volume used 2006/7	Protein concentration (g/kg)	Self sufficiency (%)	Total protein (Mt/yr)
	Ref 19	*Ref FAOStat*	*Ref 20*	
Wheat	52.5	98	100	5.1
Maize	39.1	77	90	3.0
Barley	38.9	110	100	4.3
Other cereals	17.3	110	100	1.9
Total cereals	148			
Maize gluten feed	3.5	230	48	0.8
Distillery by-products	0.5	320	50	0.2
Rape and sun seeds	1.4	220	50	0.3
Rapeseed meal	8.3	340	72	2.8
Soya cake and meal	32.7	480	2	15.7
Sunflower cake and meal	4.2	375	31	1.6
Other oilseed cake and meal	4.6	250	57	1.2
Pulses	2.4	270	93	0.6
Fish meal	0.9	650	57	0.6
Tapioca	0.9	100	0	0.1
Other materials (6)	0.9	250	23	0.2
Total	**208**		**50**	**38**

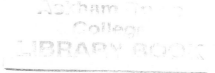

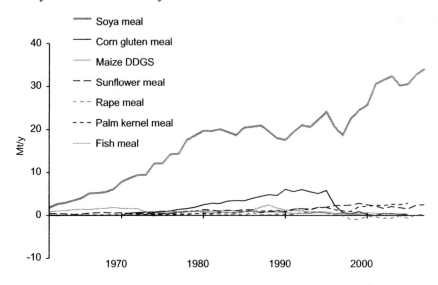

EU 27 Net imports of high protein animal feed (Source FAOSTAT (Ref 38))

Appendix 3 – Biofuel Processing Data

3.1 BIOFUEL CONVERSION AND ENERGY YIELDS

Bioethanol stoichiometry

					Efficiency
	Glucose		Ethanol		
	$C_6H_{12}O_6$	=	$2 \times C_2H_6O$	$+ 2*CO_2$	
Mass	180		92	88	0.511
Energy MJ/kg	13.8		26.8		
Energy MJ	2478		2466		0.99
	Sucrose				
	$C_{12}H_{22}O_{11}$ $+H_2O$	=	$4 \times C_2H_6O$	$+ 4*CO_2$	
Mass	342		184	176	0.538
Energy MJ/kg	14.9		16.8		
Energy MJ	5102		4931		0.97
	Starch		Ethanol		
	$C_6H_{10}O_5$ $+H_2O$	=	$2 \times C_2H_6O$	$+ 2*CO_2$	
Mass	162	18	92	88	0.568
Energy MJ/kg	16.1	0.0	26.8		
Energy MJ	2615		2466		0.94

Plant primary energy and biofuel conversion

	Within plant		*Biofuel processes*			
Component	*Plant energy conversion efficiency MJ/MJ*	*Extract efficiency*	*Process conversion efficiency mol/mol*	*Stoichiometric conversion efficiency MJ/ MJ*	*Biofuel energy conversion efficiency MJ/MJ*	*Overall energy efficiency MJ/MJ*
C6 sugar	1.0	1.0	0.92	0.99	0.92	0.92
Sucrose e.g. beet	1.0	0.97	0.92	0.97	0.86	0.86
Starch - cereals	0.97	0.985	0.92	0.94	0.85	0.83
Oil - oilseeds	0.89	0.80-0.96	0.95	1.00	0.90	0.80

Notes

- Plant energy conversion is from Appendix 1.

- Extraction efficiency is the amount of biofuel raw material that can be extracted from the crop. Data for starch from cereals are from Refs 5 and 36.

- Data for sugar beet are from Ref 28.

- The oil extraction efficiency from oil seeds varies from 0.80 for expelling to 0.96 using solvent extraction. Data are from Refs 33 and 34.

- Process conversion inefficiencies are due to by-product formation: some sugar is converted to yeast and non bioethanol products and there are oil refining losses for vegetable oils. Data references are:

Vegetable oil:	Ref. 2.
Bioethanol from cereals:	Refs 5 and 36
Bioethanol from cane sugar:	Ref 23

- The stoichiometric process energy inefficiencies are due to exotherms in the ethanol and trans-esterification reactions and are shown in the previous table.

3.2 BIOFUEL PRODUCT AND CO-PRODUCT YIELDS

Notes

- Input data has a shaded background

- Bioethanol yields from cereals are typically 0.90 to 0.93 of theoretical (15). An average of 0.915 is used

- Soya bean yield for Latin America is a weighted average for Brazil and Argentina

Biofuel process yield data

						value			Source
Theoretical bioethanol yield from starch					kg/kg	0.568			5
Typical bioethanol yield/theoretical yield						0.915			36
Biodiesel yield from vegetable oil					kg/kg	0.95			2

	Crop region	Feed wheat NW Eur	Maize NW Eur	Barley NW Eur	Rape seed NW Eur	Soya bean Lat Am	Sugar beet NW Eur	Sugar cane Brazil	Source
Crop yields									
Crop yield avg 2004-6	t/ha	7.75	8.7	6.1	3.5	2.36	66.9	74.0	32
Moisture content	g/kg grain	146	130	130	90	130			33
Protein content (Nx6.25)	g/kg grain	114	80	110					33/35
Sugar + starch	g/kg grain	618	646	551					33
Metabolisable energy	GJ/t DM	13.6	13.8	13.2					21
Metabolisable energy yield	GJ/ha	90	104	70					calc
Biofuel output									
Oil from grain	t/t grain				0.41	0.175			34
Biofuel from crop	t/t grain	0.321	0.336	0.286	0.69	0.166			calc
Biofuel from crop	t/t crop						0.078	0.064	2/17
Biofuel from crop	t/ha	2.49	2.92	1.75	1.37	0.39	5.20	4.70	calc
Biofuel heat value	GJ/t bf	26.8	26.8	26.8	37.2	37.2	26.8	26.8	2
Biofuel energy yield	GJ/ha	66.7	78.3	47.0	51.1	14.6	139	126	calc
Biofuel yield	t eq be/ha	2.49	2.92	1.75	1.91	0.54	5.20	4.70	calc
Animal feed output									
Animal feed moisture	g/kg	100	100	100	100	115	90	N/A	33
Animal feed yield	t/t crop	0.326	0.316	0.412	0.557	0.786	0.058	0	calc, 17
Protein	g/kg	350	250	270	360	460	75		calc, 33
Animal feed yield	t/ha	2.53	2.75	2.52	1.97	1.85	3.90		calc
Metabolisable energy	GJ/t DM	13.5	14.0	12.2	12.0	13.4	12.5		21
Metabolisable energy	GJ/ha	30.7	34.6	27.7	21.3	22.0	44.4		calc
Protein content	g/kg crop				200	360	4.4		calc
Protein yield	t/ha	0.88	0.70	0.67	0.71	0.85	0.26		calc

Appendix 4 – Effective Biofuel Yields from Food/Fuel Crops

Calculation of effective yields uses average NW Europe crop yields and a conservative estimate that DDGS protein is 0.80 as effective as soya protein.

All the data below are derived from the biofuel process yield data in Appendix 3.

The balances were obtained by solving simultaneous equations for energy and protein balances.

Effective yield of wheat bioethanol

Protein effectiveness of DDGS		*0.80*					
			Co-product replacement				
Crop use		*Wheat refining EU*	*Wheat feed EU*	*Soya refining Lat Am*	*Total*	*Net biofuel*	*Net area*
Land area	ha	1.0	0.19	0.64	0.82		0.18
Outputs							
Grain biofuel	t eq be	2.49		0.35		2.1	
Animal feed	t	2.53	1.44	1.18			
Metabolisable energy	GJ	30.7	17	14.0	30.7		
Effective protein	t	0.70	0.16	0.54	0.70		
Effective biofuel yield	t eq be/ha						12.1

Using similar balances for other crops:

Effective yield for biofuels

		Feed wheat	*Maize*	*Rape seed*	*Sugar beet*	*Sugar cane*
Protein effectiveness		0.80	0.80	0.80	0.80	
Direct biofuel yield	t eq be	2.49	2.92	1.91	5.20	4.55
Area of soya displaced	ha soya/ ha bf	0.64	0.464	0.56	-0.32	0
Metabolisable energy from soya	GJ/ha bf	14.0	10.2	12.4	-6.9	
Area of cereal feed displaced	ha feed/ ha bf	0.19	0.234	0.10	0.57	0
Biofuel from soya	te eq be/ ha bf	0.35	0.25	0.31	-0.17	
Effective biofuel yield		12.1	8.8	4.8	7.2	4.5

Appendix 5 – EU cereal balance for biofuels

5.1 CEREAL YIELD INCREASES

Yields and historic rates of cereals yield increases in the EU are shown below, using data from FAOSTAT (32).

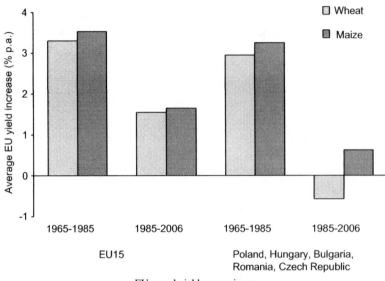

EU cereal yield comparisons

Yield increases of wheat and maize in Eastern European countries: Poland Hungary, Bulgaria, Romania and Czechoslovakia from 1965 to 1985 were similar to those of the EU 15 countries at levels higher than 3%/yr. This was a period of high real prices of cereals. However, in the period from 1985 to 2006, when real prices were substantially lower, yield increases were lower at approximately 1.5%/yr in EU 15 and lower in E European countries, with a yield decrease for wheat.

EU crop yields

Avg grain yield 2004-6		*Wheat*	*Maize*
NW Eur	t/ha	7.44	8.75
EU15	t/ha	6.00	8.98
EU27	t/ha	5.28	6.89
EU12	t/ha	3.78	5.15
Pol, Hun, Bul, Rom, Cz	t/ha	3.83	5.09
Ratio EU5/EU15		0.64	0.57

Avg grain yield 1975-82			Wheat	Maize
EU15	t/ha		3.58	5.23
Pol, Hun, Bul, Rom, Cz	t/ha		3.31	3.88
Ratio EU5/EU15			0.92	0.74

The average yields in E European countries in the period from 1975 to 1982 were similar to those in EU 15 countries – 92% in the case of wheat. However, due to the low rates of yield increase since this period, relative yields have fallen to levels that are substantially lower than EU15 countries – 64% for wheat.

This illustrates that E European yield potentials are substantially higher than yields achieved at present, given the necessary development and investment.

On the basis of this historic information, it is assumed that with higher cereal prices giving a positive return to farmers, yield increases in EU 15 countries will continue at 1.5%/yr and the new EU 12 countries can attain yield increases of 3%/yr that were being attained in the period 1965 -85.

5.2 ADDITIONAL BIOETHANOL FROM CEREALS IN THE EU

The base data and derivation of the data for Table 3 and Figure 15 are:

Additional bioethanol from cereals in EU

							Source
EU transport fuel demand 2020	Mt/yr	330					Ref 30
EU set-aside land avg 2005-7	Mha	7.0					Ref 31
Re-use of set-aside land	Mha	3.5					
Land from reduced sugar beet targets	Mha	0.5					Ref 31
Extra land available for cereals	Mha	4.0					

		Wheat	Maize	Barley	Total	
Avg EU 27 cereals production 2004-6	Mt/yr	137	64	58.4	256	FAOStat
Avg EU 27 crop yield 2004-6	t/ha	5.3	6.9	4.2		FAOStat
EU crop area	Mha	25.8	9.2	13.9	49	

Additional bioethanol from cereals in EU (contd)

		Wheat	*Maize*	*Barley*	*Total*	*Source*
W Europe (E15) increase in yield	per yr	1.5%	1.5%	1.5%		
New EU (E12) increase in yield	per yr	3%	3%	3%		
Average output E15/ EU27 2004-6		77%	60%	81%		FAOStat
Increase in EU 15 production by 2020	Mt/yr	26.4	9.5	11.8	48	
Increase in new EU 12 production by 2020	Mt/yr	17.6	14.2	6.2	38	
Extra land available	Mha	2.0	2.0	0	4.0	
Additional crop from extra land	Mt/yr	13.3	17.3	0.0	30.5	
Increase in non-biofuel consumption	% yr	0.9%	-0.4%	-0.5%		Ref 31
Impact of non-biofuel consumption	Mt/yr	-16.2	3.3	3.3	-10	Ref 31
Additional cereals crop available	Mt/yr	41.0	44.3	21.3	107	
Cereal displaced by DDGS co-product	Mt/yr	6.4	6.9	3.3	17	App 4
Additional cereals bioethanol crop	**Mt/yr**	**47.4**	**51.1**	**24.6**	123	
Bioethanol yield 2020	t/t	**0.33**	**0.34**	**0.30**	0.33	
Bioethanol production in EU	Mt/yr	**15.8**	**17.5**	**7.4**	**41**	
Potential bioethanol production in EU	Mt/yr				26	
Potential bioethanol/ total transport fuel					7.9%	
Reduction in soya meal import	Mt/yr	8.4	5.8	4.4	19	
Reduced land use from lower soya imports	Mha				10.0	

Additional bioethanol from cereals in EU in 2020

						Source
EU transport fuel demand 2020	Mt/yr	330				Ref 30
EU set-aside land avg 2005-7	Mha	7.0				Ref 31
Re-use of set-aside land for bioethanol	Mha	3.5				see text
Land from reduced sugar beet targets	Mha	0.5				Ref 31
Extra land available for cereals	Mha	4.0				

		Wheat	*Maize*	*Barley*	*Total*	
Avg EU 27 cereals production 2004-6	Mt/yr	137	64	58.4	259	Ref 32
Avg EU 27 crop yield 2004-6	t/ha	5.3	6.9	4.2		Ref 32
EU crop area	Mha	25.8	9.2	13.9	49	
W Europe (E15) increase in yield	per yr	1.5%	1.5%	1.5%		see text
New EU (E12) increase in yield	per yr	3%	3%	3%		see text
Average output E15/ EU27 2004-6		77%	60%	81%		Ref 32
Increase in EU 15 production by 2020	Mt/yr	26.4	9.5	11.8	48	
Increase in EU 12 production by 2020	Mt/yr	17.6	14.2	6.2	38	
Extra land available	Mha	2.0	2.0	0	4.0	
Additional crop from extra land	Mt/yr	13.3	17.3	0.0	30.5	
Increase in non-biofuel consumption	% yr	0.9%	-0.4%	-0.5%		Ref 31
Impact of non-biofuel consumption	Mt/yr	-16.2	3.3	3.3	-10	Ref 31
Additional cereals crop available	Mt/yr	41.0	44.3	21.3	107	

Additional bioethanol from cereals in EU in 2020 (contd)

		Wheat	Maize	Barley	Total	
Cereal displaced by DDGS co-product	Mt/yr	9.3	13.5	7.5	30	App 4
Additional cereals bioethanol crop	**Mt/yr**	**50.4**	**57.8**	**28.8**	137	
Bioethanol yield 2020	t/t	**0.32**	**0.34**	**0.29**	0.32	App 4
Bioethanol production in EU	Mt/yr	**16.2**	**19.4**	**8.2**	**44**	
Bioethanol production in EU	Mt/yr				**28**	
Boethanol/total transport fuel					8.5%	
Land area saving					**Land area**	
Re-use of set aside land	Mha				3.5	
Reduction in soya meal import	Mt/yr	7.7	5.7	4.4		18
Latin America soya yield growth	%/yr					3.6%
Reduced land use from lower soya imports	Mha				5.6	
Latin America soya oil yield	t/ha					0.39
Mal/ind palm oil yield	t/ha					3.3
Palm oil area to replace lost soya oil	Mha				0.7	
Net decrease in land use	Mha				**1.5**	

Notes

- The area split between wheat, maize and barley is assumed to stay the same, but in fact the move from barley to higher yielding wheat and maize is likely to continue.

- The bioethanol yield per unit of grain is expected to increase by about 5% from current best practice, due to the use of crop varieties with higher starch content and starch conversion to sugar, and the use of improved enzymes and yeasts to give higher sugar conversion to alcohol.

Appendix 6 - Biofuels from Energy Crops and Lignocellulosic Biomass

Bioethanol yield from biomass

Conversion status	Current	Intermediate conversion			Target conversion		
Reference	16	14	14	14	15	15	15
Component	Net molar conversion to EtOH	Molar conversion to sugarg	Molar sugar to EtOH yield	Net molar conversion to EtOH	Molar conversion to sugar	Molar sugar to EtOH yield	Net molar conversion to EtOH
C6 sugar	0.92	1.00	0.92	0.92	1.00	0.95	0.95
Sucrose	0.89	0.97	0.92	0.894	0.97	0.95	0.95
Starch	0.91	0.988	0.92	0.909	0.99	0.95	0.939
Cellulose	0.70	0.80	0.92	0.736	0.90	0.95	0.855
Hemicellulose							
Xylan	0.50	0.75	0.85	0.638	0.90	0.85	0.765
Arabinan	0.50	0.75	0.00	0.00	0.90	0.85	0.765
Mannan, Galac	0.70	0.75	0.00	0.00	0.90	0.85	0.765
Lignin	0.00	0.00	0.00	0.00	0.00	0.00	0.00

Conversions for ligno-cellulosic feedstocks to bioethanol are from Refs. 14 – 16.

Other data are from Appendices 1 and 3.

BTL energy efficiency

Pyrolysis	0.77
Gasification	0.89
FT synthesis	0.72
Hydrocracking	0.80
Overall	0.395

Conversions for ligno-cellulosic feedstocks to FT biodiesel from Ref. 17

No enzyme is available commercially for the fermentation of C5 sugars, so current conversions are uncertain. Current second generation technology for cellulose and hemicellulose must be run at low ethanol concentrations of 2-5% ethanol compared to 15-20% for conversion of starch. This results in a much higher cost and energy usage to evaporate excess water.

Bioethanol yield from plant primary energy

Component	Plant energy conversion MJ/MJ	Process molar conversion efficiency mole/mole		Process energy efficiency MJ/MJ	Contamination loss Ref 15	Overall bioethanol energy efficiency MJ/MJ		BTL via pyrolysis MJ/MJ
		Current	Target			Current	Target	
C6 sugar	1.00	0.92	0.95	0.99	0.01	0.906	0.936	0.395
Sucrose	1.00	0.89	0.95	0.97	0.01	0.855	0.909	0.395
Starch	0.97	0.91	0.94	0.94	0.01	0.822	0.848	0.382
Cellulose	0.96	0.70	0.86	0.94	0.03	0.613	0.749	0.378
Hemicellulose avg	0.96	0.51	0.765	0.94	0.03	0.451	0.670	0.378
Lignin	0.83	0.00	0.00	0.00	0.00	0.00	0.00	0.329
Hemicellulose C5	0.96	0.50	0.765	0.94	0.03	0.452	0.691	
Hemicellulose C6	0.96	0.70	0.765	0.94	0.03	0.632	0.691	

Utilisation of primary plant energy

Plant component	Primary energy for conversion	Overall biofuel energy efficiency Current	Overall biofuel energy efficiency Target	Wheat grain	Wheat straw	Maize	Maize stover	Sugar beet	Total wheat	Total maize	SRC willow	Miscanthus
	MJ/kg	MJ/MJ	MJ/MJ	Plant composition (g/kg DM)								
C6 sugar	13.8	0.91	0.94	30		20			20	10		
Sucrose	16.7	0.85	0.91					689	0	0		
Starch	16.7	0.82	0.85	690		720			450	350		
Cellulose	16.7	0.61	0.75	40	380	30	380	60	160	210	410	430
Hemicellulose	16.7	0.45	0.69	80	290	60	260	80	150	160	240	240
Xylan (C5)	16.7	0.45	0.69	50	230	40	220		110	130	200	200
Arabinan (C5)	16.7	0.45	0.69		30		27	80	10	10	27	27
C6	16.7	0.63	0.69	20	20	20	22		20	20	16	16
Pectin	16.7	0.00?	0.00?					60	0	0		
Lignin	29.6	0.00	0.00	10	145	10	189	4	60	100	290	190
Oil	41.7			260		50		2	20	20		
Protein	27.0			133	38	92	47	20	100	70		30
Recoverable yield t DM/ha				**66.1**	**35**	**75.7**	**80**	**161**	**101**	**156**	**100**	**115**
Primary energy utilisation GJ/ha												
Starch & sugar				79	0	93	0	184	79	93	0	0
Other CHO				21	56	19	120	76	76	139	148	174
Lignin				2.0	15.0	2.2	44.8	1.9	17.0	47.0	85.9	64.7
Oil				7.3	0.0	14.5	0.0	1.7	7.3	14.5	0.0	0.0
Protein				23.8	3.6	18.8	10.2	8.9	27.4	28.9	0.0	9.3
Total primary energy utilisation GJ/ha				**133**	**74**	**148**	**175**	**273**	**207**	**323**	**233**	**248**
Conversion to ethanol - current GJ/ha				**72**	**21**	**83**	**47**	**177**	**93**	**130**	**60**	**72**
Conversion to ethanol - target GJ/ha				**76**	**28**	**87**	**62**	**195**	**104**	**149**	**78**	**94**

Notes

- Wheat composition data are for low protein, high starch wheat for animal feed from Ref 5.

- Composition for ligno-cellulosic feed composition is from Refs. 6 and 7.

- Yield data for NE Europe grain crops are from Ref 32

- Yield data for UK energy crops are from Ref. 8.

- Higher yields can be achieved for all crops during controlled testing or trials. For example: wheat yields of 10 t/ha are widely achieved in UK and yields up to 15 t/ha are possible; yields of 17 t/ha have been achieved for miscanthus. Higher yields of energy crops can be achieved in the US due to a warmer climate. The yields used are average UK yields for crops grown in the UK, or average NW Europe and US yields for crops grown elsewhere.

- Rape straw and soya straw are friable and difficult to collect, so they have not been included in the data for these crops.

Appendix 7 - GHG Savings Data

7.1 COMPARISON OF SYNTHETIC NITROGEN WITH NITROGEN FIXATION

The nitrogen needed to provide protein in high yielding crops, can either be supplied via synthetic nitrogen or fixed nitrogen by the plant. When land is unlimited, the use of nitrogen fixation reduces N_2O emissions.

However, in a land-limited scenario, which is envisaged with the increase in biofuel production, the low efficiency of using primary plant energy for nitrogen fixation reduces total yield from the land. The calculation below compares GHG emissions for obtaining nitrogen within the plant by using synthetic nitrogen and by nitrogen fixation.

Benefit from using synthetic nigrogen

		Synthetic N	*Fixed N*	*Refs*
GHG emissions from synthetic N e.g. wheat				
CO_2 emissions from manufacture	kg CO_2/kg N	1.90		25
N_2O emission (no abatement)	Kg CO_2 eq/kg N	4.90		25
N_2O emission (80% abatement)	kg CO_2 eq/kg N	0.98		
Total GHG emissions from manufacture	**kg CO_2 eq/kg N**	2.88		
		Wheat	**Soyabean**	
Applied nitrogen - UK wheat	kg/ha/yr	197		18
Diesel for fertiliser spreading	kg CO_2 eq/ha	17		2, 21
N_2O emissions from land	kg CO_2 eq/ha	660	500	10, 26
Total N related GHG emissions	**kg CO_2 eq/kg ha**	**1246**	**500**	
Avg protein yeild NW Europe	t/ha	0.80	0.88	FAOStat
Nitrogen yield	kg/ha	128	141	
GHG emissions to obtain plant N	**kg CO_2 eq/kg N**	**9.7**	**3.5**	
GHG cost from lower biofuel yield				
Primary plant energy to fix N	MJ/kg N		234	13
Primary plant energy to make CHO	MJ/MJ CHO		1.21	Table 3.2
Increase in biofuel production	MJ bf/kg N		194	
Mineral fuel GHG emissions	kg CO_2 eq/GJ		85	2

Benefit from using synthetic nigrogen (contd)

		Synthetic N	Fixed N	Refs
Increase in mineral fuel emission	kg CO$_2$ eq/kg N		16	
Losses in biofuel processing			20%	
GHG cost from lower biofuel yield	**kg CO$_2$ eq/kg N**		**13.2**	
Total GHG emissions	**kg CO$_2$ eq/kg N**	**9.7**	**16.7**	
Benefit factor from synthetic nitrogen	**kg CO$_2$ eq/kg N**	**1.7**		

The quoted figures for GHG emissions for synthetic nitrogen in ammonium nitrate production are high, due to N$_2$O emissions from associated nitric acid plants. However, the returns of N$_2$O abatement on nitric acid plants are high compared to other means of reducing GHG emissions, and it has been assumed that N$_2$O abatement will continue to progress rapidly in the EU.

The GHG emissions needed to obtain plant nitrogen are determined by comparing the nitrogen related GHG inputs for wheat and soya. Total GHG emissions from producing N in wheat are 9.7 kg CO$_2$ eq/kg compared to 3.6 for soya. It is assumed that the primary plant energy that is used to fix nitrogen could otherwise be used to produce plant products such as starch or fat, which could be used to produce biofuels. The biofuels would be burnt instead of mineral fuels to reduce GHG emissions. The biofuel yield lost due to fixing N is 13.2 kg CO$_2$ eq/ kg of fixed N. Thus, in a land-limited scenario, the total GHG emissions associated with fixing N are 1.7 times higher than those associated with the use of synthetic N.

7.2 COMPARISON OF BIOFUEL FROM GRAIN CROPS AND ENERGY CROPS

GHG emission savings of biofuels

GHG emissions of mineral fuels							Ref
Petrol	kg CO_2eq/MJ	0.085					2
Diesel	kg CO_2eq/MJ	0.086					2
Coal	kg CO_2eq/MJ	0.112					2

Biofuel GHG emissions savings		*Feed wheat*	*Maize*	*Rape*	*Sugar beet*	*UK energy crops*	
Biofuel heat value (LHV)	GJ/t	26.8	26.8	37.20	26.8		
Grain biofuel saving c.f. mineral fuel		54%	56%	44%	48%		29
Direct grain biofuel yield	t/ha	2.49	2.92	1.37	5.20		
Direct grain GHG saving	**t CO_2eq/ha**	**3.1**	**3.7**	**1.9**	**5.7**		
Effective biofuel yield	t/ha	12.1	8.8	4.8	7.2		App 3
Effective graine GHG saving	t CO_2eq/ha	14.8	11.2	6.7	7.9		
Effective co-product credit	t CO_2eq/ha	11.7	7.5	4.8	2.2		
Lignocellulosic biofuel saving c.f. mineral fuel		87%	87%			80%	29
Lignocellulosic biofuel yield	GJ/ha	21.3	47.2			66	App 6
Lignocellulosic biofuel	**t CO_2eq/ha**	**1.6**	**3.5**			**4.5**	
Direct GHG saving	**t CO_2eq/ha**	**4.6**	**7.2**	**1.9**	**5.7**	**4.5**	
Effective GHG saving	**t CO_2eq/ha**	**16.4**	**14.7**	**6.7**	**7.9**	**4.5**	

Biofuel GHG savings compared to mineral fuels are typical values from the RED (Ref 29)

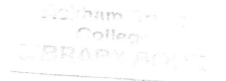

14

NUTRITIONAL AND ECONOMIC VALUE OF CO-PRODUCTS FROM BIOFUEL PRODUCTION

M. HAZZLEDINE

Premier Nutrition Products Limited, The Nutrition Centre, The Levels, Rugeley, Staffs, WS15 1R

Introduction

The biofuel industry produces a number of raw materials that can be used in livestock feeding. The production of ethanol from cereals results in distiller's grains and in distiller's solubles. These are normally combined, dried and sold as distillers dried grains and solubles (DDGS). Wet co-products are also available. Biodiesel production results in expeller rapeseed and in glycerol.

At the time of writing (September 2008) the supply of these materials into the UK at economic prices is limited. However early in 2009 Ensus will open a new bioethanol plant on Teeside. This will be the largest in the world, utilising some 1Mt of wheat and producing some 0.30-0.35 Mt/annum of dried wheat DDGS.

There are considerable published data on the nutritional value of maize DDGS and the performance of pigs fed on maize DDGS. However, there is little information on wheat DDGS, particularly that from modern biofuel plants. This chapter examines the analysis and the feeding value of DDGS from ethanol plants, with particular emphasis on wheat DDGS. It concludes with a commercial evaluation of wheat DDGS in a pig grower/finisher feed.

Ethanol production from cereals

Distillers dried grains with solubles (DDGS) is a co-product from the ethanol industry. It may be derived from any cereal grain (maize, wheat, barley, rye and sorghum have all been used). Maize predominates in the U.S. and the majority of published research is on maize DDGS. In the UK, wheat is likely to be the cereal of choice.

In the U.S., DDGS is defined as the product obtained after removal of ethyl alcohol by distillation from the yeast fermentation of a grain or a grain mixture by condensing and drying at least 75% of the resultant whole stillage by methods employed in the grain distilling industry (AAFCO, 2002).

The basic process for production of ethanol from cereals is relatively simple. The cereal is ground, cooked, liquefied and cooled. Yeast, nutrients and enzymes are added, and the mash is fermented and then distilled. A useful diagram of the process is given in Shurson, Spiehs and Whitney (2004).

It should be noted that exogenous enzymes and chemicals are prohibited from use in Scotch Whisky, and in grain whisky the enzymes are supplied from a small amount of germinated barley. In consequence residual starch levels in DDGS from whisky production are higher than those from bioethanol production.

Distillation produces ethanol and whole stillage. The stillage is centrifuged to yield wet distillers grains (spent grains) and thin stillage (draff). The thin stillage is then condensed into a syrup, or solubles. The condensed distiller's solubles and the distiller's grains may be sold wet, but in most cases are combined and dried resulting in DDGS. Some distillers solubles may be dried (distillers dried solubles, DDS) and sold separately as a feed ingredient.

There are a number of variations to this basic process. For example, the cereal may be milled to remove the germ and bran before fermentation in order to increase ethanol yield. The bran then may be added back to the DDGS to produce a higher starch material. Distiller's solubles can be burnt as a fuel source for the plant, so that dried distillers grains (DDG) alone are produced.

There is also considerable variation among bioethanol plants, in that older plants generally are less efficient in their fermentation technology. This results in more residual starch in the DDGS. Older plants may also have more aggressive dryers, potentially leading to a greater loss of nutritive value. Many papers point out that there are major differences in the nutritional quality of DDGS from "old" and "new" bioethanol plants. Generally ethanol producers are now more concerned about the quality of the DDGS they produce rather than simply getting rid of the material.

It is evident from the above that analysis of DDGS will depend upon the plant design and its operation, and that variation in DDGS analysis from plant to plant is likely to be high. Olentine (1986) suggested a total of 47 factors that influence the composition of distiller's co-products.

Analysis of DDGS

PROXIMATE ANALYSIS

Analysis of DDGS depends upon a large number of factors. It should be possible, however, to estimate the proximate analysis by considering that of the cereal used and the degree to which starch and sugars are removed during fermentation and distillation. In effect, the nutrients in the original cereal become more concentrated in the DDGS.

Stein (2007; Table 1) suggests an average of 73 g/kg starch (range of 38-114) in maize DDGS on a fresh weight basis.

Table 1. Concentration of carbohydrates in 46 samples of maize DDGS (g/kg; Unpublished data from the University of Illinois, cited by Stein, 2007)

	Mean	*Minimum*	*Maximum*	*S.D.*
Starch, total	73	38	114	14
Starch, soluble	26	5	50	12
Starch, insoluble	47	20	76	15
ADF	99	72	173	12
NDF	253	201	329	48

Sauvant, Perez, and Tran (2004; Table 2) categorised wheat DDGS as having less or more than 70g/kg starch, and found average levels of 42 and 138 g/kg DM in each category. It is likely that the higher starch material originated from bioethanol plants, where wheat is milled and the wheatfeed/bran added back after fermentation. Piron, Bruyer, Thewis, and Becker (2008) found a starch level of 44 g/kg DM in 11 samples of wheat DDGS from Western Europe.

Table 2. Composition of wheat DDGS

		Piron et al (2008)	*Sauvant et al (2004)*	
			<70 g/kg starch	*>70 g/kg starch*
n		11	64	25
Ether extract	g/kg DM		72	56
Crude protein (N*6.25)	g/kg DM	347	376	316
Crude Fibre	g/kg DM	69	102	61
NDF	g/kg DM	279	421	277
Starch	g/kg DM	44	42	138
Sugar	g/kg DM	11	9	38
Ash	g/kg DM	59	40	56
Gross energy	MJ/kg DM		21.4	20.4

Ethanol is not the only product of fermentation. Fermentation of sugar yields about 93% ethanol, 3% yeast, and 4% glycerol and other fermentation products (including acetaldehyde, ethyl acetate, methanol, C3-C5 alcohols and carboxylic acids). Most of these products remain in the DDGS, but the more volatile products escape into the ethanol. Thus, although the sum of oil (acid hydrolysis), protein, NDF, starch, sugar, ash and moisture approximates 1000 g/kg in grain, this is not the case in distillers products. The data from Sauvant *et al* (Table 2), based on ether extract oil, suggest a sum of 964 g/kg for low starch wheat DDGS and 887g/kg for high starch DDGS. The same authors reported an average sum of 909 g/kg, based on acid ether extract oil, for 1606 samples of maize distillers.

It should be noted that some published analyses show a total proximate of over 1000 g/kg. Although some excess values might be explained by analytical error, many analyses appear to have a disproportionately high NDF level. The original Van Soest method from 1991 can overestimate NDF in DDGS because some insoluble protein may be included. Using sodium sulphite within the analysis prevents this and yields lower NDF values (Shurson, 2008).

Taking residual carbohydrate and other fermentation products into account, the analysis of wheat DDGS can be estimated, assuming that the DDGS contains all of the solubles produced in the process, and that whole wheat is fermented. In an efficient plant, with a low level of residual starch and sugar in the DDGS, the nutrients in wheat DDGS would be expected to be approximately three fold higher than those in wheat (Table 3).

Table 3. Estimated analysis of low starch/sugar wheat DDGS assuming a threefold increase in analysis (dry matter basis)

		UK wheat	Estimated Wheat DDGS
Oil Ether extract	g/kg DM	17	51
Oil Acid ether extract	g/kg DM	26	78
Crude protein (N*6.25)	g/kg DM	126	378
Crude Fibre	g/kg DM	23	69
NDF	g/kg DM	98	294
Starch	g/kg DM	690	24
Sugar	g/kg DM	34	3
Ash	g/kg DM	20	60

The estimated analysis shows reasonable agreement with the analysis shown in Table 2. Some of the samples analysed will not contain all of the solubles, which might explain some of the discrepancies.

The mineral content of wheat DDGS has been estimated in a similar manner (Table 4). Analysed sodium levels appear higher than expected. In contrast, potassium levels are lower than expected.

In maize DDGS the most variable mineral has been suggested as sodium; Batal and Dale (2003) reported a range of 0.9-4.4 g/kg in 12 samples, with an average of 2.3 g/kg. Buffers may be used in yeast fermentation, which may account for some of this variation.

Table 4. Estimated and actual mineral levels in wheat DDGS (g/kg DM)

		Estimated*	Piron et al (2008)	Sauvant et al (2004)	
				<70 g/kg starch	>70 g/kg starch
n			11	64	25
Na	g/kg DM	0.1	4.1	0.6	0.5
K	g/kg DM	13.5	11.9	8.8	8.8
Ca	g/kg DM	1.5	1.1	3.7	2.1
Mg	g/kg DM	3.0	2.6	3.0	3.1
P	g/kg DM	9.5	9.0	7.4	8.9
S	g/kg DM	6	6.5		
Cl	g/kg DM	3.4	7.3	2.1	2.1
I2	mg/kg DM			0.2	0.2
Zn	mg/kg DM	80			
Cu	mg/kg DM	13			

* as a three-fold increase in wheat level

Digestibility of the phosphorus is higher in DDGS than in the originating cereal because some of the phytic acid is destroyed during fermentation. However, estimates vary widely, as do experimental protocols for determining phosphorus digestibility and availability. Stein (2006) suggested using an apparent total tract digestibility coefficient of 0.56 for maize DDGS.

Nyachoti *et al* (2005) determined apparent ileal digestibility coefficients of phosphorus in two samples of wheat DDGS to be 0.53 and 0.58, compared to wheat at 0.43. Values for calcium were 0.64 and 0.73 for the DDGS and 0.45 for the wheat. The faecal phosphorus digestibility coefficient in wheat DDGS was 0.50 and 0.55, suggesting that the large intestine does not play a significant role in phosphorus utilisation.

Energy

Sauvant *et al* (2004) suggested the following equation for determining the gross energy of wheat distillers:

$$GE = 17.3 + 0.0617 \, CP + 0.2193 \, EE + 0.0387 \, CF - 0.1867 \, Ash + 0.58$$

Where gross energy (GE) is expressed as MJ/kg DM; crude protein (CP), ether extract (EE), crude fibre (CF) and ash are expressed in % dry matter.

Nyachoti, House, Slominski and Seddon (2005) examined the digestibility of two samples of wheat DDGS in pigs of 30 kg initial body weight. Apparent ileal energy digestibility coefficients were 0.49 and 0.45; total tract energy digestibilities were 0.65 and 0.68. Ileal and faecal DE contents averaged 10.1 and 14.1 MJ/kg DM. Respective energy values for wheat were 14.4 and 15.8 MJ/kg DM.

Fastinger and Mahan (2006) determined the ileal energy digestibility coefficient, in pigs of 28 kg initial body weight, of 5 samples of maize DDGS as 0.68, 0.69, 0.67, 0.69 and 0.67.

Stein, Gibson, Pederson and Boersma (2006) examined ten samples of maize DDGS (Dakota Gold) in pigs of 30 kg initial body weight and found an average total tract energy digestibility coefficient of 0.66 (range 0.63-0.70), giving an average DE value of 14.9 MJ/kg DM (range 14.2-15.9 MJ/kg DM. Maize in the same trial had a DE value of 16.1MJ/kg DM.

Widyaratne and Zijlstra (2007), including 400 g/kg DDGS into a wheat control fed to 60kg pigs, determined that energy digestibility coefficients of wheat DDGS were 0.77 for total tract and 0.66 for ileal digestibility. Values for maize DDGS were similar, 0.79 for total tract and 0.67 for ileal, but wheat itself had a significantly higher total tract digestibility coefficient of 0.85. The wheat DDGS had an energy value of 16.8 MJ DE/kg DM, compared to wheat at 15.9 MJ/kg DM (maize DDGS 18.0 MJ DE/kg DM). The authors comment that the wheat DDGS "had a dark colour with slightly burnt odour, suggesting that it was overheated during the drying process". The sample also had a low lysine level and high NPN content which tends to confirm this observation.

Lan, Opapeju and Nyachoti (2008), using pigs of 82kg initial body weight, determined the apparent ileal energy digestibility coefficient at 0.73. The gross energy of the wheat DDGS was 19.9 MJ/kg DM, giving an apparent ileal DE of 14.5 MJ/kg DM.

The differences in faecal energy digestibility coefficients in the above trials are marked – as much as 0.12. Certainly the material itself will be a major contributor to this variation, but the age of pig and inclusion rate of DDGS into the feed might be areas for further investigation.

Amino acid concentration

Considering the process for production of DDGS, the amino acids in the protein might be expected to be similar to those of the cereal from which the DDGS is derived. However, the yeast will utilise some amino acids, presumably from the soluble protein fraction, and there will be some de novo synthesis of amino acids by yeast. There are possible losses due to thermal degradation. Finally, the amino acid profile of the DDGS will be influenced by the amount of solubles added back into the DDGS.

The amino acids in maize DDGS protein are indeed similar to those in maize itself (Degussa, 2006, 2007). Cystine, histidine, proline, arginine and lysine are found at lower concentrations in distillers protein compared to those of maize, although isoleucine, threonine, tryptophan and valine are at higher concentrations.

The amino acid profile of wheat DDGS is similar to that of wheat. However, there is notable reduction in lysine and tryptophan in the DDGS protein, and a smaller reduction in cysteine, arginine, and histidine.

Table 5. The amino acid profile (g/16gN) and coefficient of variation (%, in parenthesis) of maize and wheat and of DDGS (Degussa, 2006, 2007)

	Maize			*Wheat*		
	DDGS	*Grain*	*Ratio*	*DDGS*	*Grain*	*Ratio*
Number	409	765		49	165	
C.P. (g/kg as received)	263	84	3.13	320	103	3.11
Lysine	2.81 (13.0)	2.99 (10.2)	0.94	2.21 (16.5)	2.93 (6.5)	0.75
Methionine	1.93 (5.4)	2.01 (8.7)	0.96	1.49 (7.2)	1.57 (5.2)	0.95
Cystine	1.81 (6.0)	2.21 (6.9)	0.82	1.99 (5.1)	2.31 (5.2)	0.86
Met+cys	3.75 (4.9)	4.22 (6.7)	0.89	3.48 (5.6)	3.88 (4.5)	0.90
Threonine	3.75 (3.3)	3.55 (3.7)	1.06	3.07 (4.8)	2.92 (3.8)	1.05
Tryptophan	0.8 (13.3)	0.76 (7.9)	1.05	0.97 (1.7)*	1.29 (7.5)	0.75
Arginine	4.36 (7.1)	4.72 (7.7)	0.92	4.33 (9.2)	4.91 (4.6)	0.88
Isoleucine	3.67 (3.2)	3.29 (5.4)	1.11	3.49 (6.6)	3.31 (3.8)	1.05
Leucine	11.60 (3.8)	11.89 (6.4)	0.98	6.59 (5.2)	6.66 (2.4)	0.99
Valine	4.84 (3.1)	4.58 (4.8)	1.05	4.36 (6.9)	4.26 (4.3)	1.02
Histidine	2.61 (4.7)	2.9 (6.2)	0.90	2.11 (6.9)	2.35 (5.0)	0.90
Phenylalanine	4.92 (3.1)	4.83 (5.0)	1.02	4.52 (5.1)	4.54 (3.8)	1.00
Glycine	3.91 (3.1)	3.85 (7.3)	1.02	4.02 (3.0)	4.11 (4.2)	0.98
Serine	4.79 (3.3)	4.79 (4.1)	1.00	4.57 (4.8)	4.61 (3.2)	0.99
Proline	8.11 (9.1)	8.89 (10.0)	0.91	8.8 (11.9)	9.57 (7.0)	0.92
Alanine	7.25 (2.9)	7.33 (4.4)	0.99	3.78 (7.20)	3.65 (4.6)	1.04
Aspartic acid	6.59 (3.1)	6.56 (5.2)	1.00	5.11 (5.9)	5.18 (5.3)	0.99
Glutamic acid	17.27 (2.7)	17.97 (5.1)	0.96	26.52 (6.1)	27.52 (5.5)	0.96

* n=6

Piron *et al* (2008) reported lower values for lysine (1.75 g/16g N) and cysteine (1.72 g/16g N), although a higher value for tryptophan (1.07 g/16g N), in 11 samples of wheat DDGS of Western European origin. Sauvant *et al* (2004) reported an average lysine of 3.1g/16gN in low starch wheat DDGS and 2.0g/16gN in high starch. Furthermore, they reported a higher tryptophan concentration (1.5g/16gN, the same for both low and high starch materials) than the Degussa value of 0.97.

DDGS will contain some yeast protein and this can account for some of the discrepancies noted above. For example, yeast is relatively rich in threonine, and this amino acid is found at higher concentrations in DDGS than in the source material; yeast is low in cysteine, again as found in DDGS. However, yeast is particularly rich in lysine compared to cereals, and yet the concentration in DDGS is lower than in the originating cereal.

Table 6. The amino acid profile (g/16gN) of dried brewer's yeast (Degussa, 2006) and the ratio of amino acids in yeast to cereals

	Yeast (dried brewers)	Yeast: maize	Yeast: wheat
Lysine	6.57	2.2	2.2
Methionine	1.52	0.8	1.0
Cysteine	1.02	0.5	0.4
Met+cys	2.54	0.6	0.7
Threonine	4.61	1.3	1.6
Tryptophan	1.21	1.6	0.9
Arginine	4.67	1.0	1.0
Isoleucine	4.24	1.3	1.3
Leucine	6.68	0.6	1.0
Valine	5.18	1.1	1.2
Histidine	2.18	0.8	0.9
Phenylalanine	4.14	0.9	0.9
Glycine	4.34	1.1	1.1
Serine	4.92	1.0	1.1
Proline	4.47	0.5	0.5
Alanine	6.49	0.9	1.8
Aspartic acid	9.20	1.4	1.8
Glutamic acid	12.83	0.7	0.5

The low and variable levels of lysine, arginine and cysteine in DDGS are due to Maillard reactions. This is a chemical reaction between an amino acid and a reducing sugar. The reactive carbonyl group of the sugar reacts with the nucleophilic amino group of the amino acid, a process accelerated by heat and alkaline conditions. Fontaine, Zimmer, Moughan and Rutherford (2007) have looked at the effects of steamed autoclaving of extracted soya meal (468 g/kg crude protein) and maize DDGS (270 g/kg CP). In both cases lysine, cysteine and arginine are degraded appreciably by heat, but most of the other amino acids remain largely unchanged. The loss of lysine was considerably higher in DDGS than in maize and the authors suggested this is due to its higher sugar content.

Table 7. Effect of heat treatment of extracted soyabean meal and maize DDGS in a steamed autoclave at 135°C on lysine concentration

	Extracted soya meal		*Maize DDGS*	
Time (min)	*Lysine g/16g N*	*Lysine loss (%)*	*Lysine g/16g N*	*Lysine loss (%)*
0	6.18	0	2.99	0
15	5.62	9.0	2.40	19.7
30	4.87	21.1	1.97	34.2

Palm, Pederson, Simon and Stein (2007) suggested that the heat damage to lysine is mainly a result of the addition of solubles to distiller's grains. This may be because the solubles contain most of the sugar.

Maillard reactions produce compounds that are brown in colour; lysine results in the most colour due to its ϵ -amino group, whilst cysteine results in the least colour. Thus, colour may be an indicator of heat damage and poor nutritive value in DDGS.

As well as the mean amino acid levels in DDGS, their variability is also of interest to the commercial nutritionist (Table 5). In wheat the coefficient of variation (CV) of amino acid concentration in the protein is relatively low at 2.4-7.5% (although it should be noted that this is labelled "wheat 10.5% CP" in the Degussa tables and thus should be considered a subset). In maize the CV is similar to that in wheat, except for a higher variability in lysine (10.2%)

With the exception of lysine and tryptophan, the variation in the amino acid concentration in the protein of maize DDGS is generally lower than that of maize itself. This is in contrast to wheat DDGS, where amino acid concentration in the protein of DDGS is more variable than wheat for all amino acids. Lysine again shows the greatest variation, and is about 4-5 times higher than in extracted soya bean meal.

Both Adisseo and Evonik-Degussa apparently have NIR calibrations to measure total amino acids in maize DDGS, and Adisseo have one also for wheat DDGS. Evonik-Degussa is currently developing an NIR calibration for amino acids in wheat DDGS.

Amino acid digestibility

The standardised ileal digestibility coefficients of amino acids in 36 samples of maize DDGS, derived from various ethanol plants in the Midwest of the US, are shown in Table 8.

Table 8. Standardised ileal digestibility coefficient of maize and of 36 samples of US maize DDGS fed to growing pigs (DDGS data from Stein *et al.*, 2005, Palm *et al.*, 2006 a and b; Stein *et al.*, 2006; Urriola *et al.*, 2007; Maize data Degussa, 2006)

	Maize	Maize DDGS		
		Mean	Low	High
Protein		0.73	0.63	0.84
Lysine	0.76	0.62	0.44	0.78
Methionine	0.87	0.82	0.74	0.89
Cysteine	0.81	0.74	0.66	0.81
Threonine	0.80	0.71	0.62	0.83
Tryptophan	0.76	0.70	0.54	0.80
Arginine	0.88	0.81	0.74	0.92
Isoleucine	0.86	0.75	0.67	0.83
Leucine	0.89	0.83	0.75	0.91
Valine	0.86	0.74	0.66	0.82
Histidine	0.86	0.77	0.70	0.85
Phenylalanine	0.88	0.81	0.74	0.87

The digestibility coefficient of lysine in these samples averaged 0.62, with a range from 0.44 to 0.73. This is about 0.14 lower than that encountered in maize. Of the essential amino acids, lysine digestibility showed the greatest variability. The digestibility coefficients of all other amino acids were also lower in maize DDGS than in maize itself, with the average reduction being approximately 0.08.

Fastinger *et al* (2006) found the standardised ileal digestibility coefficient of lysine in 5 samples of maize DDGS to average 0.51 (0.38-0.61), cysteine 0.67 (0.57-0.72), threonine 0.67 (0.56-0.72), valine 0.74 (0.66-0.75), methionine 0.81 (0.73-0.83) and arginine 0.80 (0.75-0.82).

Widyaratne *et al* (2007) found the standardised ileal digestibility coefficient of amino acids in wheat and in maize DDGS to be similar (Table 9), but again lysine digestibility was much lower in the DDGS than in the originating grain. In this case the lysine digestibility coefficient in wheat DDGS was 0.14 lower than in wheat, with other amino acids 0.03-0.09 lower.

Pahm, Pederson, Hoechler and Stein (2008) reported standardised pig ileal digestibility coefficients for lysine in five samples of maize DDGS to be 0.73, 0.67, 0.67, 0.66 and 0.70. The digestibility of the other amino acids was similar for the 5 sources, except for leucine and glutamic acid. Additionally, they found that the lysine digestibility coefficient was significantly higher when the DDGS was from a beverage plant compared to an ethanol plant (0.69 vs. 0.65). The digestibility of amino acids in DDG were greater (P<0.05) than in DDGS, suggesting that amino acids in solubles may be less digestible.

Table 9. Standardised ileal amino acid digestibility coefficients of wheat and of wheat and maize DDGS in pigs of 30kg body weight. (Widyaratne *et al*, 2007)

	Wheat	*Wheat DDGS*	*Maize DDGS*	*Reduction in digestibility coefficient in wheat DDGS cf. wheat*
Lysine	0.783	0.641	0.666	0.142
Threonine	0.850	0.775	0.750	0.075
Methionine	0.884	0.842	0.860	0.042
Cysteine	0.884	0.792	0.804	0.092
Tryptophan	0.912	0.857	0.878	0.055
Arginine	0.922	0.880	0.886	0.042
Histidine	0.917	0.828	0.838	0.089
Isoleucine	0.891	0.814	0.813	0.077
Leucine	0.889	0.845	0.858	0.044
Valine	0.924	0.874	0.865	0.050
Phenylalanine	0.914	0.880	0.862	0.034

Shurson (2008) reported an average standardised ileal lysine digestibility coefficient for maize DDGS in pigs of 0.64 (14 samples, 0.56-0.78).

Lan *et al* (2008) determined the standardised ileal lysine digestibility coefficient in wheat DDGS to be 0.49, with methionine at 0.78, cysteine at 0.71 and threonine at 0.72.

Stein (2007) indicated that the maize DDGS samples that have the lowest concentration of lysine usually have the lowest digestibility, and that 60% of the variability in lysine digestibility can be explained by lysine concentration. He recommended that only samples with a lysine: CP ratio greater than 2.8 g/kg be used in pig feeds. However, such a relationship is not evident in 14 samples of maize DDGS reported by the University of Minnesota (Shurson, 2008).

It is evident that the digestibility of amino acids in DDGS is less than that in the originating cereal. This is particularly the case with lysine, probably due to heat damage (Cromwell, Herkelman and Stahly, 1993). The degree of heat damage in DDGS can be determined by measuring reactive lysine with either homoarginine or furosine (Fontaine *et al*, 2007). Both of these procedures have been shown to estimate lysine digestibility with an accuracy of around 70% (Stein, 2007). The furosine method is more suited to routine analysis.

Ergul (2003) demonstrated that Hunter L* and b* scores of maize DDGS were highly correlated with lysine and cysteine digestibility. Cromwell, Herkelman and Stahly (1993) found that the colour of maize DDGS was highly correlated with growth rate and feed conversion rate of chicks. Wheat DDGS is considerably darker than DDGS from maize and colour is likely to be less useful as a guide to nutritive value.

Evonik-Degussa have an NIR calibration for standardised ileal amino acid digestibility in maize DDGS.

Pig performance

As with laboratory analysis, much of the research into effects of DDGS on performance of pigs has been conducted in the U.S. using maize DDGS. Many of these trials involved graded levels of DDGS in maize/soya based diets. The formulations of many of these trial feeds do not take account of amino acid digestibility, the energy value of the DDGS is predicted from equations, and diets are formulated to metabolisable energy rather net energy. Furthermore, the majority of results are reported on a live-weight basis; DDGS is a high fibre raw material and with increasing dietary levels we would expect a lower killing-out percentage.

Whitney, Shurson, Johnston, Wulf and Shanks (2006) fed 0, 100, 200, or 300 g/kg maize DDGS to pigs of 29 kg initial body weight. Diets were maize and soya based, and formulated to total lysine. Although the pigs performed well with 100 g/kg DDGS, at higher levels performance deteriorated.

Table 10. Effect of maize DDGS on growth performance of finishing pigs (Whitney *et al.*, 2006)

	Maize DDGS inclusion (g/kg)			
	0	100	200	300
Intake (kg/day)	2.38	2.37	2.31	2.35
Live-weight gain (kg/day)	0.86[a]	0.86[a]	0.83[bc]	0.81[bd]
Feed Conversion Ratio	2.76[a]	2.76[a]	2.80[a]	2.92[b]
Final live weight (kg)	117[a]	118[a]	114[b]	112[b]

[a, b] Means within row with unlike superscripts are different (P<0.05)
[c, d] Means within row with unlike superscripts are different (P<0.05)

The authors concluded that poorer performance was probably due to formulating diets to total rather than digestible lysine. Killing- out percentage was 73.4, 72.8,

72.1 and 71.9 at the four levels of DDGS (P<0.1) and loin fat-depth was reduced significantly with higher levels of DDGS. However, there was no effect on backfat or carcass lean and DDGS level had no meaningful effect on pork muscle quality. Iodine number in belly fat increased linearly (66.8, 68.6, 70.6, and 72.0) with increasing inclusion of DDGS.

Fu, Johnston, Fent, Kendell, Usry, Boyd and Allee (2004) fed diets containing 0, 100, 200, and 300 g/kg maize DDGS to finishing pigs over a 92 day period. Diets were formulated to be isoenergetic and to contain equivalent amounts of ileal digestible lysine. Despite this, there was a reduction in feed intake and growth rate with increasing DDGS (Table 11).

Table 11. Effect of maize DDGS on growth performance of finishing pigs (Fu *et al.* 2004)

	Maize DDGS inclusion (g/kg)			
	0	*100*	*200*	*300*
Intake (kg/day)	2.56	2.53	2.44	2.41
Live-weight gain (kg/day)	1.03	1.01	0.99	0.98
Feed Conversion Ratio	2.47	2.50	2.46	2.47
Final live weight (kg)	124	122	121	119

Hastaad, Nelssen, Goodband, Tokach, Dritz, DeRouchey and Frantz (2005) conducted feed preference trials in growing pigs and showed a dramatic and linear reduction in intake of feed containing up to 300 g/kg maize DDGS.

Although the above trials suggest problems with feed intake at higher levels of maize DDGS, the majority do not. One of the most striking examples is that of Whitney and Shurson (2004) where feeding up to 250 g/kg of maize DDGS, for 35 days from weaning at 17 days of age, did not reduce feed intake over the entire trial period (Table 12).

Table 12. Effect of maize DDGS on growth performance of newly weaned pigs (Whitney *et al,* 2004)

Feed intake (kg/day)	*Maize DDGS inclusion (g/kg)*					
Days	0	50	100	150	200	250
0-14	0.40	0.39	0.39	0.39	0.39	0.38
14-35	0.99	0.99	1.0	0.97	1.06	1.04
0-35	0.76	0.75	0.76	0.74	0.79	0.78

Spiehs, Shurson, Johnston, and Seifert (2005) fed 500 g/kg DDGS to finishing pigs over a 16-week period and in only two, two-week periods, was feed intake lower than the control diet. DeDecker, Ellis, Wolter, Spencer, Webel, Bertelsen and

Peteron (2005), and Hansen, Libal, Pters, and Hamilton (1997) reported satisfactory results using up to 300 g/kg maize DDGS in finishing pigs.

More recently Guillou and Landeau (2008) examined eating behaviour of grower pigs of 10 weeks of age fed 100 g/kg wheat DDGS (replacing soya, sunflower, and rape) and 200 g/kg in finisher pigs (replacing wheat bran and peas). Pigs fed DDGS had a significantly higher feed intake (+2.2%, P<0.05). DDGS altered feeding behaviour; less visits to the feeder without eating (2.2 vs. 1.2 visits/day, P<0.05), longer time spent at the feeder during the finishing phase (55.2 vs. 63.2 min, P<0.05) and lower eating rate (41.8 vs. 38.0 g/min, P<0.05). Overall growth rate, feed conversion rate and carcass characteristics were not significantly affected, and the authors concluded that wheat DDGS is well accepted by pigs.

Maize DDGS has been fed successfully to lactating sows at inclusion rates of up to 300 g/kg (Shurson, 2006) without any reduction in appetite.

In summary, although overall feed intake normally does not decline with increasing inclusion rates of maize DDGS, it would appear that this can occur. Mycotoxins can be a problem in maize DDGS, and are concentrated up from the levels found in maize, and can of course reduce feed intake. This is unlikely to be such an issue in wheat DDGS, particularly in DDGS derived from UK wheat. Material that is over-dried is likely to be unpalatable. Diets containing higher levels of DDGS have higher crude protein contents, and increased heat increment may limit intake, particularly where pigs are kept in hot environments. DDGS is a high fibre raw material, so bulk may also limit intake, although only at higher levels of inclusion or if used with other fibrous feeds.

Pig meat quality

Soft carcass fat has been an issue in the U.S. when high levels of maize DDGS have been fed to finishing pigs. Sometimes these feeds additionally contained high levels of soya oil. In many European countries finishing pig feeds have a maximum linoleic acid constraint of 16 g/kg. This will prevent the problem of soft carcass fat (providing that other oils low in linoleic but high in other unsaturated fats, such as rapeseed and palm oil, are not also used). Wheat DDGS contains a lower level of linoleic acid and unsaturated fats than maize DDGS.

Pig health

It has been reported in young pigs that the inclusion of 100 g/kg of maize DDGS can positively affect gut health by reducing the prevalence and severity of lesions in the ileum and colon of pigs subjected to a moderate, but not a severe, Lawsonia intracellularlis challenge (Whitney, Shurson, Guedes, Gehart, Winkleman, 2003; Whitney, Shurston and Guedes, 2006).

Anti-nutritive factors

There are no reported anti-nutritive factors of significance in DDGS. However, Widyarante (2007) reported the soluble NSP level in wheat DDGS to be 77g/kg DM, and the insoluble 151 g/kg DM. This compares to wheat at 22 and 76 g/kg respectively. The soluble NSP reported in the same research for maize DDGS was only 14g/kg DM. Soluble NSP can have anti-nutritive properties in poultry and to a lesser extent in young pigs. The most common sugars in the soluble NSP of wheat DDGS are xylose (31g/kg DM), and arabinose (16g/kg DM). Enzymes are added to the mash pre-fermentation, but it is not known if these include xylanases. Should this be the case, and they would be useful potentially to reduce viscosity, then the choice of xylanase will be important because some can result in the production of free xylose. Free xylose is particularly reactive in Maillard reactions. Enzyme choice should be made in terms of not just ethanol yield, but also potential quality of DDGS.

Commercial pig feed formulations containing wheat DDGS

In order to highlight how wheat DDGS might feature in UK pig feeds, a formulation exercise was conducted using a typical pig growing/finishing feed (NE 9.8 MJ/kg, SID lysine 10g/kg) and costs for August 2008. The raw materials offered were those typically found in a compound feed mill; producers mixing their own feed frequently do not have available rape, biscuit and wheatfeed. The analysis of the wheat DDGS used in the evaluation is shown in Table 13, and the results of the evaluation are in Table 14.

It should be noted that for some time economics have dictated that amino acids have been used at maximum levels in UK pig finisher feeds. The maximum levels used are generally dictated by valine or tryptophan becoming limiting (sometimes isoleucine or histidine). Furthermore, in contrast to many other countries, the UK uses entire males pigs rather than castrates, has relatively low slaughter weights, and high penalties for fat pigs. Hence amino acid levels in feeds are high compared to most other countries.

Under the costs and constraints of this exercise, a wheat DDGS inclusion of 100 kg/t replaces largely wheatfeed and extracted soya meal. There is a significant increase in the use of lysine HCl, from 3.6 to 5.2 kg/t. Isoleucine in this formulation is limiting (as well as lysine, M+C, and threonine). Fat addition falls and there is a modest increase in the crude protein level of the feed.

Table 13. Composition of wheat DDGS used for formulation exercise (fresh weight basis)

				g/16 g N	*SID coeff.*
DM	g/kg	900	Lysine	2.20	0.64
Oil B	g/kg	67	Met	1.50	0.84
C.Protein	g/kg	333	Cys	2.00	0.79
Crude Fibre	g/kg	62	Thr	3.05	0.78
NDF	g/kg	260	Tryp	1.03	0.86
Ash	g/kg	54	Valine	4.30	0.87
GE	MJ/kg	18.8	Isoleuc	3.40	0.81
DE	MJ/kg	13.6	Hist	2.10	0.83
NE	MJ/kg	8.3			
Ca	g/kg	1.35			
P	g/kg	8.3			
DP	g/kg	5.0			

Table 14. Pig finishing feed formulations containing wheat DDGS (major ingredients, kg/t, costs August 2008)

Feedstuff	Control	Feeds with wheat DDGS		
DDGS	0	100	200	200
Wheat	441	460	438	500
Barley	150	150	150	85*
Wheatfeed	61	0	0	0
Biscuit	75	75	75	75
Extracted Rape meal	75	72	0	12
Extracted Soya meal	147	93	88	80
Fat	9	6	3	2
Lysine	3.7	5.2	6.1	6.2
Threonine	1.1	1.4	1.5	1.5
Methionine	0.3	0.3	0.4	0.4
Oil B g/kg	37.5	37.5	38.4	37.5
Crude protein g/kg	183	185	190	191
NDF g/kg	130	133	138	137

*Barley 150kg/t minimum removed

Increasing the inclusion rate to 200 kg/t, the additional 100g/kg of wheat DDGS largely replaces rape meal. Lysine inclusion has increased to 6.1kg/t and protein to 190 g/kg.

In the above formulations a minimum of 150kg/t of barley has been maintained, which is normal commercial practice in the UK in order to improve gut health. Because wheat DDGS may also have advantages in terms of gut health, the removal of this constraint may be justified and the effect of this is shown in the final formulation.

These formulations illustrate that to maximise the usage and value of wheat DDGS levels of lysine HCl will need to be higher than have been previously been encountered in commercial feed formulations. Yen, Kerr, Easter and Parkhurst (2004) reported that crystalline lysine and threonine were absorbed quicker than the amino acids when protein bound. This could result in a temporary imbalance or antagonism, reducing the efficiency of utilisation. It has been argued that this is an important consideration if pigs are fed once daily, but not if they are fed at least two meals a day, providing feeds are formulated using the ideal protein concept (Degussa, 2006b; Le Bellego *et al.*, 2001).

Increasing the use of wheat DDGS with higher levels of lysine HCL can lead to SID isoleucine and valine also becoming limiting (in addition to lysine, methionine + cystine, threonine, and often tryptophan).

A consequence of using DDGS is that as a result of the poor protein quality, the crude protein of the feed will increase. In this exercise the increase in crude protein is relatively modest. Under other scenarios increases of 10g/kg in crude protein per 100g/kg increase in DDGS inclusion have been evident. This may constrain DDGS in areas where nitrogen excretion is of concern.

Another consideration when using wheat DDGS is the maximum fibre constraint in finished feeds. Wheat DDGS has an NDF level similar to wheatfeed, approaching 300g/kg. Extracted rapeseed, which is normally attractively priced against extracted soya meal, is also quite high in NDF (approximately 220g/kg). Thus these three high fibre co-products will compete in pig feed formulations. Should they all remain relatively cheap in comparison to cereals and soya, then feeds of lower nutrient concentration are likely to be more cost-effective.

A particular consideration for the UK is that the majority of pigs are now housed in straw-based systems and eat considerable quantities of straw. Straw is known to reduce ileal amino acid digestibility. Thus U.S. trials incorporating maize DDGS into a low fibre maize and soya based diet, and fed to pigs on slats, may be of limited applicability to the UK.

Inclusion rates of wheat DDGS in pig feeds

There are few published recommendations on maximum inclusion rates of wheat DDGS in pig feeds, in contrast to maize DDGS. With maize DDGS, inclusion rates as high as 300 g/kg in finishing pigs and 500 g/kg for dry sows, have been suggested. In reality, the commercial nutritionist will be wary of using such high inclusion rates of wheat DDGS until variability is reduced and more pig performance data are available.

The financial value of a feed material declines with increasing inclusion rate and this is particularly the case with wheat DDGS. At low inclusion rates it tends to replace reasonable quantities of expensive extracted soya meal. However, as the above formulations illustrate, additional DDGS replaces less expensive rape meal and potentially raises other concerns. At low inclusion rates, wheat DDGS currently has a similar value in pig feeds and in cattle feeds. However, at higher inclusion rates the value is higher in cattle feeds. Because the availability of wheat DDGS is limited, this is a further factor that will influence inclusion rate of wheat DDGS in pig feeds.

DDGS and poultry feeds

The use of DDGS in poultry feeds was reviewed recently by Siatkiewicz and Koreleski (2008). They concluded that high quality DDGS may safely be fed at 50-80 g/kg in starter feeds for broilers and turkeys, 100-150 g/kg in grower/finisher feeds for broilers and turkeys, and 150 g/kg for layers. They point out that the major limitation for the use of DDGS in poultry feeds is its variability, particularly with regard to lysine, methionine, minerals, and energy level. They reported two trials where addition of NSP-hydrolysing enzymes reduced depressions in rate of lay and daily egg mass noted with higher levels of wheat and rye DDGS.

Conclusions and discussion

The composition of DDGS purchased on the open market is variable. This is inevitable considering differences in the design and operation of ethanol plants, and the relatively low priority of DDGS quality compared to ethanol yield. It is thus of paramount importance when purchasing DDGS that the source of the material is known, specifications supplied, and the product tested routinely. The higher the inclusion rate of DDGS being considered, the more thorough this process should be. Of course within-plant variation should be considerably less than between-plant variation. It may be that a very large modern operator can achieve a consistency of product approaching that of other processed feedstuffs, providing that DDGS quality is viewed as integral to the economics of the ethanol process.

Little research appears to have been conducted to examine the effects of variations in process conditions on the nutritive value of DDGS. For example, how does the strain of yeast influence amino acid yield? What enzymes are used and how do these influence residual NSP? How might we reduce Maillard reactions, thus preserving essential amino acids (e.g. residual sugar, pH)? To what extent does amino acid loss occur in DDGS drying compared to solubles evaporation? What buffers are used in the fermentation, and what influence do they have on DDGS quality?

It would appear that the loss of some essential amino acids is greater in wheat DDGS than in maize. The reasons for this are unclear. Tryptophan concentration in the protein of maize DDGS is similar to that of maize; in wheat it is lower, although marked variation in the tryptophan levels of wheat DDGS have been reported by several authors. The range in results suggests that this may be in part methodological. Tryptophan is limiting in many UK feeds for pigs up to 30 kg body weight and may become limiting in finishing feeds with increasing levels of DDGS.

Estimates of energy digestibility of DDGS vary markedly. Most published research concentrates on amino acids, but energy is a major determinant of the financial value of DDGS. For example, the difference in the financial value of wheat DDGS with a faecal energy digestibility coefficient of 0.65, compared to one of 0.80, is currently £15-45/t. Furthermore, DDGS with the higher energy coefficient will feature in young pig feeds, whereas inclusion of the poorer product will be limited. It may be that the age of pig and inclusion rate of DDGS in the test feed contribute more to the variation in energy digestibility than differences in the DDGS samples themselves.

The low lysine concentration in wheat DDGS protein necessitates higher inclusion rates of lysine HCL than are normal commercial practice. Providing that pigs are fed more than once a day, generally this should not result in a problem. This assumes that feeds are accurately formulated using SID amino acids (including valine, isoleucine, and histidine) and net energy. There has been some concern about the use of lysine HCL in wet feed systems, in that any fermentation may preferentially use the free lysine. The use of higher levels of lysine HCL leads also to a reduction in ionic balance (Na+K-Cl) and some nutritionists may wish to use sodium bicarbonate to restore this.

The use of wheat DDGS, particularly at higher inclusion rates, will increase both the protein and fibre levels in feeds. The influence of protein level on nitrogen excretion is well understood. Many of the effects of fibre are also well documented. However, there is little research comparing the nutrient requirements of pigs kept on straw (the majority in the UK) to those on slatted systems. Certainly pigs consume considerable quantities of fibre from straw and it is well documented that straw reduces amino acid digestibility. It may be, therefore, that when feeding pigs on straw-based systems we need either to more tightly constrain maximum fibre levels in the feed, or to increase amino acid concentration to take account of the reduction in digestibility as a result of straw consumption.

Finally, there are relatively high levels of NSPs in wheat DDGS, with the soluble NSP being at much higher levels than in maize DDGS. This may have some anti-nutritive properties, particularly in poultry. A number of enzyme manufacturers are investigating products for DDGS based feeds.

Acknowledgements

My thanks to:-

Dr Meike Rademacher – Evonik
Dr Simon Green – Adisseo
Dr Gary Partridge – Danisco
Dr John Sissins – AB Agri
Dr Huw Jones - Roquette

References

AAFCO (2002) Official publication of the Association of American Feed Control Officials, Inc.Oxford, IN.

Batal, A. and Dale, N.M. (2003) *Journal of Applied Poultry Research* **12**: 400-403.

Cromwell, G.L., Herkelman, K.L. and Stahly, T.S. (1993) *J. Anim Sci.* **71**:679-686.

DeDecker, J.M., M. Ellis, B.F. Wolter, J. Spencer, D.M. Webel, C.R. Bertelsen, and B.A. Peterson. (2005) *J. Anim. Sci.* **83** (Suppl. 2) p. 79. (2005 ASAS/ADSA Midwest Mtg. Abstract).

Degussa Feed Additives. (2006) AminoDat 3 Platinum vs. 1.0.0.34 Evonik Degussa GmbH, Feed Additives Division, Hanau, Germany.

Degussa (2007) Amino acid profiles of DDGS. Personal Communication

Degussa (2006b) *AminoNews*. **7**: 1-12.

Ergul, T., Martinez Amezcua, C., Parsons, C., Walters, B., Brannon, J and Noll, S.L. (2003) Poult. Sci. Assoc. meeting, Madison, WI.

Fastinger, N.D. and Mahan, D.C. (2006) *J. Anim. Sci.* **84**:1722-1728

Fontaine, J., Zimmer, U., Moughan, P.J and Rutherford, S.M. (2007) *J Agric Food Chem.* **55**: 10737-10743

Fu, S.X., Johnston, M. Fent, R.W., Kendall, D.C., Usry, J.L., Boyd, R.D and Allee, G.L. (2004) *J. Anim. Sci* **82** (suppl.2): 50

Guillou, D. and Landeau, E. (2008) 40eme Journees de la Recherche Porcine. Abstract. 5-6 Feb 2008

Hansen, E.L., Libal, G.W., Peters, D.N. and Hamilton, C.R. (1997) *J. Anim. Sci.* **75** (Suppl.1):194

Hastad, C.W., Nelssen, J.L., Goodband, R.D., Tokach, M.D, Dritz, S.S., DeRouchey, J.M. and Frantz (2005) *J. Anim. Sci.* **83** (Suppl. 2):73

Lan, Y., Opapeju, F.O., Nyachoti, C.M. (2008) *Animal Feed Science and Technology* **140:** 155-163

Le Bellego, L., Van Milgen, J., Dubois, S. and Noblet, J. (2001) *J. Anim. Sci.* **79**: 1259-1271.

Nyachoti, C.M., House, J.D., Slomainski, B.A. and Sheddon, I.R. (2005) *J. Sci. Food Agric* **85**:2581-2586

Olentine, C. (1986) Proceedings of the Distillers Feed Conference **41**:13-24

Pahm, A.A., Hoehler, D. and Stein, H. H. (2006a) *J. Anim. Sci.* **84** (Suppl. 1):285 (Abstr.)

Pahm, A.A., Pederson, C. and Stein, H.H. (2006b) *J. Anim. Sci.* **84** (Suppl. 2):121 (Abstr.)

Pahm, A.A., Pederson, C., Simon, d. and Stein, H.H. (2007) *J. Anim. Sci.* **85** (Suppl 1):513 (Abstr)

Pahm, A.A., Pederson, C. Hoechler, D. and Stein H.H. (2008) *J. Anim.S ci.* 86: 2180-2189.

Piron, F., Bruyer, D., Thewis, A. and Beckers, Y. (2008) Poster presented at the 42nd Nottingham Feed Conference, Nottingham University, Sutton Bonington. 3-4 Sept 2008.

Sauvant, D., Perez, J-M. and Tran, G (2004) "Tables de composition et de valeur nutritive des matieres premieres destiness aux animaux d'elevage" INRA, ISBN 2-7380-1158-6

Shurson, G., Spiehs, M and Whitney, M (2004) animalscience.com Reviews (2004) No 9 *Pig News and Information* **25** (2), 75N-83N.

Shurson, J. (2006). 67th Minnesota Nutrition Conf., St. Paul, MN. Sep 19-20, 2006.

Shurson, J (2008) Distillers grain by-products in livestock and poultry feeds. July 29 2008 www.ddgs.umn.edu/profiles.htm

Spiehs, M., Shurson, G., Johnston, L. and Seifert, K (2005) *J. Anim. Sci.* **83** (Suppl.2) p. 62.

Stein, H.H., Gibson, H.L., Pederson, C. and Boersma, M.G. (2006) *J. Anim. Sci.* **84**:853-860

Stein, H.H., Pederson, C. and Boersma, M.L. (2005) *J.Anim.Sci.* **83** (Suppl. 2):79 (Abstr.)

Stein, H.H. (2007) HHS-SwineFocus-001.2007 Department of Animal Sciences, College of ACES, University of Illinois.

Swiatkiewicz, J., Koreleski, J. (2008) *Worlds Poultry Science Journal,* **64**, 257-265

Urriola, P.E., Hoehler, D., Pederson, C., Stein, H.H., Johnston, L.J. and Shurson, G.C. (2007) *J. Anim. Sci.* **85** (Suppl. 2):XX (Abstr.) IN PRESS

Whitney, M.H., Shurson, G.C., Guedes, R.M., Gebhart, C.J. and Winkleman, N.L. (2003) *J. Anim. Sci.* **81** (supplement 2): 70.

Whitney, M.H. and Shurson, G.C (2004) *J.Anim.Sci.* **82**:122-128

Whitney, M.H., Shurson, G.C. and Guedes, R.C. (2006) *J. Anim. Sci.* **81**: 1870-1879

Whitney, M.H., Shurson, G.C., Johnston, L.J., Wulf, D. and Shanks, B (2006) *J. Anim. Sci.* 84: 3356-3363.

Widyarante, G.P. and Zijlstra, R.T. (2007) *Can. J. Anim. Sci.* **87**:103-114

Yen, J.T., Kerr, B.J., Easter, R.A. and Parkhurst, A.M. (2004) *J. Anim. Sci.* **82**:1079-1090

15

VARIABILITY OF QUALITY IN BIOFUEL CO-PRODUCTS

R.T. ZIJLSTRA[1] AND E. BELTRANENA[1,2]
[1]Department of Agricultural, Food and Nutritional Science, University of Alberta, Edmonton, Alberta, Canada T6G 2P5 and [2]Alberta Agriculture and Rural Development, Edmonton, Alberta, Canada T6H 5T6

Introduction

Fossil fuels are the main transportation energy source for human activity. However, the resulting release of 'greenhouse gases' has also been related to climate change (Grubb *et al.*, 1999). Considerable demand thus exists to replace fossil fuels with renewable fuel sources such as biodiesel and ethanol, even though the debate continues as to whether or not this is a worthwhile exercise (e.g., Farrell *et al.*, 2006). Biofuel production can be divided into two principal categories: (1) ethanol production and (2) biodiesel production.

Ethanol is currently produced at a commercial scale via the enzymatic breakdown of starch and yeast-driven fermentation of glucose into ethanol. Ethanol production based on cellulose is currently in the development phase. A number of grain starch sources can be used; however, maize is predominantly used globally with regional efforts in Canada and Europe geared towards using wheat or other small grains as a feedstock. Distillers' dried grain and solubles (DDGS) is the predominant co-product from ethanol production in North America, although wet feeding of the solubles or combined distiller's grain and solubles is also practiced.

Biodiesel is currently produced at a commercial scale via the conversion of oil extracted from oilseeds such as soyabean and canola or rapeseed or animal fat. In large-scale extraction plants, the oil from oilseeds is usually extracted using hexane and a protein meal is the resulting co-product. In medium- and small-scale plants, the oil can be extracted using an expeller or screw-press, respectively; expeller meal or press cake are then the resulting co-products, respectively. Subsequent transesterification of the extracted oil into biodiesel also produces crude glycerol as a co-product.

Co-products, by the fact that they have been processed, will be feedstuffs with more nutrient variability than the feedstock of origin. Apart from the inherent variability in feedstock composition, additional variability is introduced due to processing required to produce biofuels. A feedstock that has a limited compositional variability, such as hybrid maize, contrasts to massive variability in the DDGS co-product, due to processing, including milling, fermentation, drying, and removal or addition of specific fractions (Stein, 2007). Co-products should therefore be sourced from specific plants and not specific geographical regions to limit variability in feedstuff due to processing. Biofuels plants are not necessarily built to optimize co-product quality. Addressing co-product variability may therefore be an afterthought after commissioning and reaching top biofuel production.

Biofuel co-products

Production of biofuels and therefore co-products is quickly expanding. However, a few co-products such as DDGS, oilseed meal and cake, and glycerol are now common feedstuffs.

Distillers' Dried Grain and Solubles. DDGS is a co-product from the cereal grain-based ethanol and alcohol beverage industries (Newland and Mahan, 1990). With the rapid growth of the ethanol industry, increasing quantities of DDGS are available for livestock feeding. Maize DDGS is largely produced in the USA and eastern Canada, whereas wheat DDGS is produced in Europe and western Canada. In general, DDGS has higher concentrations of nutrients such as protein, fat, vitamins, minerals, and fibre than its parent grain stock. These nutrients are concentrated due to conversion of most of the cereal starch to ethanol and carbon dioxide during the fermentation process (Weigel *et al.*, 1997).

The process of production of ethanol and DDGS follows several typical steps (Patience *et al.*, 2007) in most ethanol plants: dry milling of grain, fermentation, distillation of ethanol, and drying of the distillers' grains. In the latter stage, the soluble components that have been separated before for distillation are blended back with the distillers' grains containing most of the solids during the final drying. Recently, additional steps have been added to remove grain fractions prior to fermentation. Germ, oil and hulls (fibre) are sometimes removed upfront firstly to, target specific markets, and secondly to enhance the efficiency of the fermentation process. Each single step or a combination of steps, however, introduces more variability in the nutritional quality (profile and availability) of DDGS in the global market place.

Oilseed meal and cake. For the purpose of this chapter, the focus of oilseed meal and cake will be on canola. Variability of soyabean meal quality has been described elsewhere (Van Kempen *et al.*, 2002) and canola is probably the most important source of biodiesel in Europe. Canola meal is produced using solvent-extraction with hexane (Thacker, 1990). Therefore, canola meal has a low content of residual oil. Canola expeller meal is generated following heat conditioning of the seed and crushing in the expeller press operated to optimise oil extraction that may generate temperatures up to 135°C for the brief period that seed is passing through the press. Some plants operate double- or triple-pass systems where seed cake is reprocessed to increase oil recovery. Oil may also be extracted using a cold, screw press, where seed is not pre-conditioned prior to oil extraction, and temperatures up to 65°C are generated by the screw pressing against the chamber merely by frictional force. Therefore, canola expeller meal will have a higher residual oil content than solvent-extracted canola meal, with even higher residual oil content for cold-pressed cake (Leming and Lember, 2005; Spragg and Mailer, 2007). Cold pressing of canola does not require as high a capital investment, and might be preferred for local extraction of oil for biodiesel production (Bender, 1999).

Crude glycerol. To produce biodiesel, the oil extracted from oilseeds undergoes transesterification using an alcohol and a catalyst, thereby producing methyl esters for biodiesel production and crude glycerol as a resulting co-product (Kerr *et al.*, 2007). The production of one litre of biodiesel may yield 79 g of crude glycerol (Thompson and He, 2006). Glycerol forms the backbone of triglycerides and is involved in phospholipid synthesis in hepatic and adipose tissues (Mourot *et al.*, 1994). In the small intestine of pigs, ingested fats are broken down into three compounds: two free fatty acids and a monoglyceride. Following absorption, these compounds are transported to the liver, and the monoglyceride is broken down into glycerol and a third free fatty acid. Dietary glycerol can then be converted to glucose via gluconeogenesis or oxidized as a source of energy via glycolysis and the citric acid cycle. Thus, dietary glycerol may provide energy (Mourot *et al.*, 1994; Lammers *et al.*, 2008), be stored as glycogen, or be used to form body fat (lypogenesis). Processing methods used for the production of biodiesel may result in varying levels of impurities. Alcohol, salts and heavy metals can be found in crude glycerol (Doppenberg and Van der Aar, 2007; Johnson and Taconi, 2007). Future use of crude glycerol in livestock feeds may be subject to feed regulations.

Variability of quality in DDGS

A major source of variation in the quality of DDGS is the botanical origin of the feedstock (Widyaratne and Zijlstra, 2007). Maize contains more starch and oil and less protein and fibre than wheat (CVB, 2006; Sauvant *et al*, 2004). Following starch conversion to ethanol and carbon dioxide during fermentation, the DDGS reflects the original feedstock in a concentrated form (approximately 3x). Co-fermentation, the combined fermentation of two or more feed stocks (e.g. maize and wheat), is currently common practice in western Canada (Table 1). Alterations in the ratio of co-fermented feedstocks will add to variability in the quality of DDGS.

Table 1. Chemical characteristics of wheat, and maize, wheat/maize, and wheat distiller's dried grains with solubles (g/kg DM)[1]

Variable	Wheat	Distiller's dried grains with solubles		
		Maize	Wheat/maize[2]	Wheat
Moisture	118	118	80	81
Crude protein	198	303	424	445
Non-protein nitrogen	46	54	124	102
Crude fat	18	128	47	29
Ash	21	48	50	53
Acid detergent fibre	27	146	195	211
Neutral detergent fibre	94	312	306	303
Crude fibre	24	70	78	76
Amino acid				
Cysteine	4.8	7.0	8.9	9.6
Lysine	5.2	8.3	7.2	7.2
Methionine	3.2	6.1	6.7	6.9
Threonine	5.4	10.9	12.2	12.8
Tryptophan	2.3	2.3	3.7	4.4
Total	194.8	283.2	372.5	402.1

[1]Source: Widyaratne and Zijlstra (2007).
[2]Derived from the combined fermentation of wheat and maize in a 4:1 ratio.

Similar to other chemical characteristics, phosphorus is concentred in maize and wheat DDGS (Table 2). Intact phytate, i.e., inositol hexaphosphate (IP6), undergoes transformations during the fermentation and drying process, and is partially converted into lower forms of phytate, ranging from IP2 to IP5. Arabinoxylans are found in higher quantities in wheat DDGS than in maize DDGS, making them a theoretical candidate for xylanase supplementation of pig feeds, although a beneficial effect has not been observed to date (Widyaratne *et al.*, 2008).

The energy and amino acid digestibilities of wheat and maize DDGS have rarely been compared directly (Widyaratne and Zijlstra, 2008). Even though wheat DDGS has a higher crude protein content than maize DDGS, lysine content and quality were higher in the maize DDGS (Table 3) because older fermentation and drying technologies prepared the batch of wheat DDGS. Maize DDGS has a higher digestible energy content, because it has a higher fat content. Without exception, phosphorus digestibility, and therefore digestible phosphorus content, is higher in DDGS than the parent grain.

Table 2. Content (g/kg DM) of inositol phosphates and non-starch polysaccharides (NSP) of wheat, and maize, wheat/maize, and wheat distiller's dried grains with solubles[1]

		Distiller's dried grains with solubles		
Variable	*Wheat*	*Maize*	*Wheat/maize[2]*	*Wheat*
Phosphorus	4.0	8.6	10.2	11.0
Inositol phosphates				
Inositol diphosphate (IP2)	0.0	0.0	0.0	0.8
Inositol triphosphate (IP3)	0.0	0.9	0.9	0.9
Inositol quadraphosphate (IP4)	0.0	1.9	1.8	2.8
Inositol pentaphosphate (IP5)	0.0	4.5	3.3	6.4
Phytate (IP6)	13.9	9.2	6.2	8.1
Total NSP	97	192	219	229
Xylose	34	62	81	81
Arabinose	23	43	47	49

[1]Source: Widyaratne and Zijlstra (2007)
[2]Derived from the combined fermentation of wheat and maize in a 4:1 ratio

Table 3. Standardized ileal digestible amino acid content (g/kg DM), ileal and total tract digestible energy (MJ/kg DM) and total tract digestible P (g/kg DM) contents in wheat, and maize, wheat/maize, and wheat distiller's dried grains with solubles measured in grower-finisher pigs[1]

		Distiller's dried grains with solubles		
Variable	*Wheat*	*Maize*	*Wheat/maize[2]*	*Wheat*
Amino acid				
Cysteine	4.1[d]	4.9[c]	6.6[b]	6.9[a]
Isoleucine	5.7[d]	8.4[c]	11.6[b]	12.2[a]
Lysine	3.7[bc]	4.5[a]	4.0[b]	3.4[c]
Methionine	2.7[c]	5.1[b]	5.6[a]	5.6[a]
Threonine	4.1[c]	7.3[b]	9.2[a]	9.3[a]
Tryptophan	2.0[c]	1.8[c]	2.9[b]	3.5[a]
Valine	7.3[d]	12.4[c]	15.5[b]	16.0[a]
Digestible energy				
Ileal	13.48[ab]	14.13[a]	13.18[ab]	12.59[b]
Total tract	15.91[a]	16.30[a]	14.74[b]	14.83[b]
Phosphorus	0.6[b]	5.8[a]	6.8[a]	6.8[a]

[1]Source: Widyaratne and Zijlstra (2008).
[2]Derived from the combined fermentation of wheat and maize in a 4:1 ratio.
[a-d]Within a row, means without a common letter differ ($P < 0.05$).

Overall, factors including the type of cereal grain used for fermentation, method of fermentation (batch or continuous), completeness or duration of the fermentation process, drying temperature and duration, and the amount of solubles blended with distiller's dried grains can affect the chemical, physical and nutritional characteristics of DDGS (Spiehs *et al.*, 2002). The nutrient composition of DDGS should still reflect the nutrient content of original cereal grain, with a higher concentration of remaining nutrients following starch conversion and removal as ethanol and carbon dioxide (Mustafa *et al.*, 1999).

Maize DDGS has been available in large quantities for a decade in North America. The existence of a large variability in quality of maize DDGS is well known in the industry. Gradually the ranges in quality are being described in the scientific literature, but reports remain mostly descriptive in nature, whereas the underlying causes for the variability remain largely unexplored. Ten ethanol plants in a narrow geographical location (Minnesota and South Dakota) each submitted 12 maize DDGS samples at 2-month intervals. Means (g/kg DM) and coefficients of variation among all plants were 302 and 6.4% for crude protein, 109 and 7.8% for crude fat, and 162 and 28.4% for acid-detergent fibre (Spiehs *et al.*, 2002). Among the amino acids analyzed, lysine was the most variable (CV = 17.3%), followed by methionine (CV = 13.6%). Ranges in quality were not reported. This research by the University of Minnesota clearly demonstrated that variability in DDGS quality exists within and among ethanol plants, even among plants using the same fermentation and processing technology.

Some maize DDGS is marketed in the USA under specific brand names, suggesting above average and a more consistent quality. Quality control generally occurs via monitoring of macronutrient profile, in particular crude protein content. In 10 such samples, crude protein content had a range from 246.0 to 290.7 g/kg on an as-is basis, and total lysine ranged from 4.4 to 5.9 g/kg (Stein *et al.*, 2006). The coefficient of standardized ileal digestibility of lysine ranged from 0.439 to 0.630. The coefficient of apparent total tract digestibility of gross energy ranged from 0.627 to 0.705 among the 10 samples of maize DDGS. The largest range was found for lysine, which may be a result of heat damage during drying in some samples of maize DDGS. The measured ranges in quality were not related to any physical or chemical characteristic; however, other research suggests that specific samples of maize DDGS that are much darker, have a reduced digestibility of amino acids (Fastinger and Mahan, 2006).

In addition, 10 samples of maize DDGS were collected from a narrow geographical range in South Dakota from 10 ethanol plants (Pedersen *et al.* 2007). On an as-fed basis, content of crude protein ranged from 259 to 324 g/kg and ether extract ranged from 86 to 124 g/kg. The coefficient of apparent total tract digestibility of gross energy ranged from 0.739 to 0.828 and, combined with the range in gross energy content, resulted in a range in DE content from 14.42 to 16.55 MJ/kg, as fed. The range in DE content could be predicted accurately from the concentrations of ash, ether extract,

ADF, and GE (Pedersen *et al.*, 2007) and was not related to changes in colour of the DDGS samples. The existence of a range in DDGS quality, in particular ileal amino acid digestibility, was confirmed recently (Pahm *et al.*, 2008).

For heat-treated protein feedstuffs, a critical quality characteristic is the amount of intact (bioavailable) lysine instead of total lysine. The amount of intact lysine can be measured using the reactive lysine analysis (Fontaine *et al.*, 2007). In 80 samples of maize DDGS, reactive (intact) lysine content of crude protein ranged from 10 to 27 g/kg. Interestingly, total lysine content of crude protein ranged from 20 to 35 g/kg, and followed a similar pattern (Fontaine *et al.*, 2007) when graphed against the loss of reactive lysine as a proportion of crude protein. These results indicate that total lysine per unit of crude protein might also be a good predictor of lysine quality among samples of maize DDGS.

Fractionation of maize prior to fermentation results in maize DDG of a different composition (Widmer *et al.*, 2007). The maize can be dehulled and degermed, and if the solubles are not added back to the DDG at drying, the resulting product has a higher crude protein content than regular maize DDGS. The high protein DDG contained 411 g/kg of crude protein and 37 g/kg of ether extract (Widmer *et al.*, 2007). The coefficient of apparent total tract digestibility of gross energy was 0.882 and, combined with the gross energy content, resulted in a DE content of 18.43 MJ/kg, as fed. The high protein DDG thus has a higher energy content than regular maize DDGS.

From experience in our laboratory, major contributors to DDGS variability are the amount of concentrated solubles added back and the drying process. Processing plants prefer to add back as much solubles (stillage) as possible during the drying process; otherwise they have to sell another liquid, less uniform co-product. Adding back the solubles, creates lumps when a viscous liquid comes in contact with the drying, mash distillers' grain. A way to dissolve the lumpiness of DDGS and prevent caking in storage bins thereafter is overdrying. However, the intensity of heat, the extent of, the speed of and the equipment used for drying can cause amino acid damage. Protein damage generally becomes evident as an increasingly darker product. However, improper fermentation and excess solubles can confer a dark colour to DDGS deepen by improper drying (Beltranena and Zijlstra, 2008). In contrast to protein damage, the ethanol and DDGS production processes increase mineral bio-availability, apparently by releasing phytate-bound ions (Pedersen *et al.*, 2007; Widyaratne and Zijlstra, 2007).

Variability in quality of canola meal

Obviously, large quality difference exists between rapeseed meal and canola meal due to the genetically reduced content of the anti-nutritional factors, mainly glucosinolates and erucic acid, in canola. These changes in quality will not be addressed, because mostly canola, not rapeseed, is used for oil production. Hexane extraction of canola oil from seed is efficient; therefore, residual oil is not expected to change much. In contrast, the protein content of canola meal ranged as much as 82 g/kg (Bell and Keith, 1991; Fan *et al.*, 1996). This value might be an underestimation for the entire range that exists in protein content for canola meal, based on reported ranges in protein and oil content among analyzed canola seed samples. However, greater uniformity was obtained among samples collected from a specific plant (Bell and Keith, 1991), indicating that specific sourcing of ingredients might reduce variation in nutritional quality of purchased canola meal. Gums removed early in the processing process are typically added back into the meal, causing further changes in fat content and thus quality (Spragg and Mailer, 2007). A direct comparison of digestible and available lysine has not been made among canola meal samples, but available lysine ranged from 19.8 to 23.7 g/kg among canola meal samples (Bell and Keith, 1991). Processing conditions have a major impact on lysine content and digestibility, as measured in poultry (Newkirk *et al*, 2003). Amino acid digestibility has been positively correlated to protein content and negatively to NSP (Fan *et al.*, 1996), suggesting that NSP in canola meal may interfere with protein digestion (Bell, 1993). Relationships of other anti-nutritional factors in canola meal, e.g., glucosinolates and tannins, with variation in amino acid digestibility have not been reported.

Variability in quality of expeller meal and press cake

Canola expeller meal and canola press cake differ in quality due to the process used to extract the oil. With the additional heat provided prior to expelling instead of merely cold–pressing, extra oil is removed; therefore, less residual oil remains in expeller meal; 116 versus 178 g/kg (Leming and Lember, 2005). Expeller extracted meals do vary in oil content; in 41 samples the oil content ranged from 85 to 170 g/kg (Spragg and Mailer, 2007). Not surprising, the difference in efficiency of oil extraction results in large difference in crude protein content among samples of expeller meal (316 to 417 g/kg), with obvious implications for amino acid content. In oil extraction via expelling, less heat is provided than with solvent extraction. Content of residual glucosinolates ranged from 24 to 89 g/kg, but were overall higher than for canola meal (53 vs. 17 g/kg; Spragg and Mailer, 2007). The implications of the residual glucosinolate content on animal performance are less clear.

Variability in quality of crude glycerol

Specific research describing the variation in dietary energy content among samples of crude glycerol appears not to have been published to date. Glycerol content was

869.5 g/kg in one sample of crude glycerol obtained from a biodiesel facility in the USA (Lammers *et al.*, 2008). This specific sample also contained 1.2 g crude fat/kg, 0.28 g methanol/kg, 31.9 g ash/kg, 12.6 g sodium/kg, and 18.6 g chloride/kg, indicating that some crude glycerol samples used in animal experiments contains low amounts of impurities (Lammers *et al.*, 2008). However, the realities of commercial production of crude glycerol might be starkly different. Indeed, seven samples of crude glycerol obtained from commercial production facilities in Europe ranged from 252 to 887 g glycerol/kg, 2 to 492 g crude fat/kg, and 48 to 187 g ash/kg (Kijora and Kupsch, 1996), indicating that crude glycerol might differ in quality among commercial production facilities and that quality should therefore be monitored. The crude fat content was 156 g/kg in a sample of crude glycerol obtained from Canada (Zijlstra *et al.*, 2009), providing further evidence that quality differences occur.

Feeding of crude glycerol may present practical problems beyond an error in estimated energy content. Methanol content should not exceed 150 ppm in glycerol used as a feedstuff. Higher levels may cause metabolic acidosis, vomiting, blindness, and gastrointestinal problems (Kerr *et al.*, 2007). An increased NaCl content may limit dietary inclusion of glycerol to avoid that dietary Na and Cl levels exceed recommendations. Finally, glycerol is a viscous gel, which may present problems for feed mixing and flow (Kerr *et al.*, 2007). Oxidation of residual oil in crude glycerol possesses concerns regarding the long-term stability unless antioxidants are added.

Managing ingredient variability

Precision diet formulation is becoming increasingly important to maintain competitive and sustainable of pork production systems. Animal models and proximate analyses have been used as evaluation methods for decades to describe the energy value of feedstuffs for pigs. Using these methods, average 'book' values for feedstuffs have been established (e.g., CVB, 2003; Sauvant *et al.*, 2004), and are commonly used for diet formulations. However, these book values and evaluation methods do not allow for immediate changes in diet formulation following changes in quality of batches of co-products arriving at feed processing plants. Furthermore, the physical and proximate analyses used to support trade of feedstuffs are not the best predictors for energy values, either due to lack of repeatability among laboratories or time required to complete the analyses.

Rapid methods for estimation of energy values of feeds are required to support quick and correct decisions. Near infra-red reflectance spectroscopy (NIRS) is one of such methods. Separately, in vitro digestibility methods have been progressively developed. These in vitro methods mimic the successive digestive processes, e.g., in the porcine gastro-intestinal tract. In vitro methods are considered rapid by some, but their main advantages are that the total extent of energy digestibility can probably be predicted more accurately than with proximate analyses and that only a few grams of feedstuff are required. Following proper validation, in vitro digestibility methods can then entirely replace in vivo determination of energy values (Regmi *et al.*, 2008). The in vitro analyses to measure total extent of digestibility subject feedstuffs samples sequentially to a mimicked gastric and small intestinal digestion, generally using purified digestive enzymes or enzyme cocktails. Variations in the methodology exist, including methods that include a partial mimic of degradation of the non-starch polysaccharide fraction in feedstuffs. With collected samples spanning the entire quality range within a feedstuff, in vitro digestibility analyses have been able to explain more than 95% of the measured variation in energy value. The relative error of the analyses is generally less than for in vivo digestibility measurements (Regmi *et al.*, 2008).

The advantage of the NIRS method is that it can be used as a non-invasive analysis. Samples are scanned across a wavelength spectrum (e.g., 400 to 2500 nm) by sending light into the sample. Reflected light is measured and, by difference, absorption can be determined across the entire spectrum. The changes in absorption spectra are caused by changes in chemical bonds, and these changes can be statistically related to changes in energy values or digestible nutrient content. As such, calibrations to predict the nutritional characteristics of importance for diet formulations can be developed (Van Barneveld *et al.*, 1999). Following the collection of a robust set of samples spanning the entire range of nutritional characteristics and with a sufficient variation in quality, calibrations with a standard error of prediction of 1% can be achieved (Zijlstra *et al.*, 2006). Following the effort of calibration development and validation, subsequent predictions of quality on new samples can be completed within one minute. Scans with differing profiles from maize DDGS samples seem promising for the development of calibration to predict their nutritional quality (Figure 1).

Recommendations

Biofuel co-products are feedstuffs that provide an opportunity to reduce feed cost. However, one risk of biofuel co-products is the large variation in quality introduced due to processing among co-product samples. As second risk is the use of feed quality evaluation methods that do not properly quantify the nutritional content and bio-availability of co-products high in fibre and protein. Specific procedures to manage both risks should be implemented to ensure that biofuel co-products can be used effectively to achieve predictable animal performance.

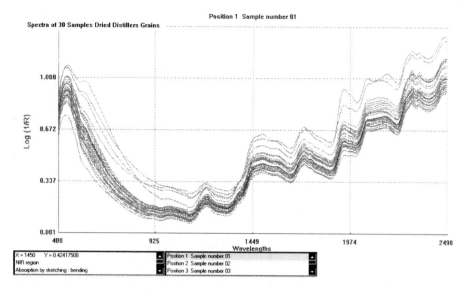

Figure 1. Near infra-red reflectance spectroscopy scans from 30 maize DDGS samples.

References

Bell, J.M. (1993) Factors affecting the nutritional value of canola meal. *Can. J. Anim. Sci.* **73**, 679-697.

Bell, J.M. and Keith, M.O. (1991) A survey of variation in the chemical composition of commercial canola meal produced in Western Canadian crushing plants. *Can. J. Anim. Sci.* **71**, 469-480.

Beltranena, E. and Zijlstra, R.T. (2008) Containing feed cost using biofuel coproducts. Advances in Pig Production. Proc. Banff Pork Seminar. pp. 263-273.

Bender, M. (1999) Economic feasibility review for community-scale farmer cooperatives for biodiesel. *Bioresource Technol.* **70**, 81-87.

CVB (Centraal Veevoeder Bureau). (2003) "Veevoedertabel" (Table of feeding value of animal feed ingredients). CVB, Lelystad, The Netherlands.

Doppenberg, J. and Van der Aar, P. (2007) The nutritional value of biodiesel by-products. Part 2: Glycerine. Feed Business Asia Mar/Apr: 42–43.

Fan, M.Z., Sauer, W.C. and Gabert, V.M. (1996) Variability of apparent ileal amino acid digestibility in canola meal for growing-finishing pigs. *Can. J. Anim. Sci.* **76**, 563-569.

Farrell, A.E., Plevin, R.J., Turner, B.T., Jones, A.D., O'Hare, M. and Kammen, D.M. (2006) Ethanol Can Contribute to Energy and Environmental Goals. *Science* **311**, 506-508.

Fastinger, N.D. and Mahan, D.C. (2006) Determination of the ileal amino acid and energy digestibilities of corn distillers dried grains with solubles using grower-finisher pigs. *J. Anim. Sci.* **84**, 1722-1728.

Fontaine, J., Zimmer, U., Moughan, P.J. and Rutherford, S.M. (2007) Effect of heat damage in an autoclave on the reactive lysine contents of soy products and corn distillers dried grains with solubles. Use of the results to check on lysine damage in common qualities of these ingredients. *J. Agric. Food Chem.* **55**, 10737-10743.

Grubb, M., Vrolijk, C. and Brack, D. (1999) The Kyoto protocol - A guide and assessment. Royal Institute of International Affairs, London, UK.

Johnson, D.T. and Taconib, K.A. (2007) The glycerin glut: options for the value-added conversion of crude glycerol resulting from biodiesel production. *Environ. Prog.* **26**, 338–348.

Kerr, B.J., Dozier, W.A., III and Bregendahl, K. (2007) Nutritional value of crude glycerine for nonruminants. In *Proc. 23rd Carolina Swine Nutrition Conference.* pp. 6–18. Carolina Feed Industry Assoc., Raleigh, NC, USA.

Kijora, C. and Kupsch, R.-D. (1996) Evaluation of technical glycerols from "Biodiesel" 213 production as a feed component in fattening of pigs. *Fett/Lipid* **98**, 240–245.

Lammers, P.J., Kerr, B.J., Weber, T.E., Dozier, W.A., III, Kidd, M.T., Bregendahl, K. and Honeyman, M.S. (2008) Digestible and metabolizable energy of crude glycerol for growing pigs. *J. Anim. Sci.* **86**, 602–608.

Leming, R. and Lember, A. (2005) Chemical composition of expeller-extracted and cold-pressed rapeseed cake. *Agraarteadus* **16**, 103-109.

Mourot, J., Aumatire, A., Mounier, A., Peinau, P. and Francois, A.C. (1994) Nutritional and physiological effects of dietary glycerol in the growing pig. Consequences on fatty tissue and post mortem muscular parameters. *Livest. Prod. Sci.* **38**, 237–244.

Mustafa, A.F., McKinnon, J.J. and Christensen, D.A. (1999) Chemical characterization and in vitro crude protein degradability of thin stillage derived from barley- and wheat-based ethanol production. *Anim. Feed Sci. Technol.* **80**, 247–256.

Newkirk, R.W., Classen, H.L., Edney, M.J. (2003) Effects of prepress-solvent extraction on the nutritional value of canola meal for broiler chickens. *Anim. Feed Sci. Technol.* **104**, 111-119

Newland, H.W. and Mahan, D.C. (1990) Distillers by-products. In *Nontraditional feed sources for use in swine production* (Eds. P.A. Thacker and R. N. Kirkwood). pp. 161–173. Butterworths, Stoneham, MA, USA.

Pahm, A.A., Pedersen, C., Hoehler, D. and Stein H.H. (2008) Factors affecting the variability in ileal amino acid digestibility in corn distillers dried grains with solubles fed to growing pigs. *J. Anim. Sci.* doi:10.2527/jas.2008-0868.

Patience, J.F., Leterme, P., Beaulieu, A.D. and Zijlstra, R.T. (2007) Utilization in swine diets of distillers dried grains with solubles derived from corn or wheat used in ethanol production. In *Biofuels: implications for the feed industry* (Eds. J. Doppenberg and P. van der Aar). pp 89–102 Wageningen Academic Press, Wageningen, The Netherlands.

Pedersen, C., Boersma, M.G. and Stein H.H. (2007) Digestibility of energy and phosphorus in ten samples of distillers dried grains with solubles fed to growing pigs. *J. Anim. Sci.* **85**, 1168-1176.

Regmi, P.R., Sauer, W.C. and Zijlstra, R.T. (2008) Prediction of in vivo apparent total tract energy digestibility of barley in grower pigs using an in vitro digestibility technique. *J. Anim. Sci.* **86**, 2619-2626.

Sauvant, D., Perez, J.M. and Tran, G. (2004) Tables of composition and nutritional value of feed materials: pigs, poultry, cattle, sheep, goats, rabbits, horses, fish. Wageningen Academic Publishers, Wageningen, The Netherlands and INRA Editions, Versailles, France.

Spiehs, M.J., Whitney, M.H. and Shurson, G.C. (2002) Nutrient database for distiller's dried grains with solubles produced from new ethanol plants in Minnesota and South Dakota. *J. Anim. Sci.* **80**, 2639–2645.

Spragg, J. and Mailer, R. (2007) Canola meal value chain quality improvement. Final Report for AOF and Pork CRC.

Stein, H.H. (2007) Distillers dried grains with solubles (DDGS) in diets fed to swine. Swine Focus #001. http://www.livestocktrail.uiuc.edu/uploads/porknet/papers/DDGS%20in%20Swine%20Diets-Stein.pdf [Accessed Aug 8, 2008]

Stein, H.H., Gibson, M.L., Pedersen, C. and Boersma, M.G. (2006) Amino acid and energy digestibility in ten samples of distillers dried grain with solubles fed to growing pigs. *J. Anim. Sci.* **84**, 853-860.

Thacker, P.A. (1990) Canola meal. In *Nontraditional feed sources for use in swine production* (Eds. P.A. Thacker and R. N. Kirkwood). pp. 69–78. Butterworths, Stoneham, MA, USA.

Thompson, J.C. and He, B.B. (2006) Characterization of crude glycerol from biodiesel production from multiple feedstocks. *Appl. Eng. Agr.* **22**, 261–265.

Van Barneveld, R.J., Nuttall, J.D., Flinn, P.C. and Osborne, B.G. (1999) Near infrared reflectance measurement of the digestible energy content of cereals for growing pigs. *J. Near Infrared Spectrosc.* **7**, 1-7.

Van Kempen, T.A., Kim, I.B., Jansman, A.J., Verstegen, M.W.A., Hancock, J.D., Lee, D.J., Gabert, V.M., Albin, D.M., Fahey, G. C., Jr, Grieshop, C.M. and Mahan, D. (2002) Regional and processor variation in the ileal digestible amino acid content of soybean meals measured in growing swine. *J. Anim. Sci.* **80**, 429-439.

Weigel, J.C., Loy, D. and Kilmer, L. (1997) Feed co-products of the dry corn milling process. pp. 2–4. Renewable Fuels Association and National Corn Growers Association. Washington, DC and St. Louis, MO, USA.

Widmer, M.R., McGinnis, L.M. and Stein, H.H. (2007) Energy, phosphorus, and amino acid digestibility of high-protein distillers dried grains and corn germ fed to growing pigs. *J. Anim. Sci.* **85**, 2994-3003.

Widyaratne, G.P., Patience, J.F., and Zijlstra, R.T. (2008) Effect of xylanase supplementation of wheat distiller's dried grains with solubles on energy, amino acid and phosphorus digestibility and growth performance of grower-finisher pigs. *Can. J. Anim. Sci.* (Submitted).

Widyaratne, G.P. and Zijlstra, R.T. (2007) Nutritional value of wheat and corn distiller's dried grain with solubles: digestibility and digestible contents of energy, amino acids and phosphorus, nutrient excretion and growth performance of grower-finisher pigs. *Can. J. Anim. Sci.* **87**, 103–114.

Widyaratne, G.P. and Zijlstra, R.T. (2008) Erratum. Nutritional value of wheat and corn distiller's dried grain with solubles: digestibility and digestible contents of energy, amino acids and phosphorus, nutrient excretion and growth performance of grower-finisher pigs. *Can. J. Anim. Sci.* **88**: 515-516.

Zijlstra, R. T. (2006) Rapid methods for estimation of energy values of feedstuffs for pigs. In *Proc. Net energy systems for growing and fattening pigs', Pre-Symp. 10th Int. Symp. Digestive Physiology in Pigs.* pp. 74–80. May 24, Vejle, Denmark.

Zijlstra, R.T., Menjivar, K., Lawrence, E., and Beltranena, E. (2009) The effect of crude glycerol on growth performance and nutrient digestibility in weaned pigs. *Can. J. Anim. Sci.* (In Press).

16

USE OF DRIED DISTILLERS GRAINS WITH SOLUBLES (DDGS) CO-PRODUCTS IN COMMERCIAL PIG FEEDING PROGRAMMES

JOSEPH LOUGHMILLER
SCA Nutrition, USA

Introduction

The recent growth of grain-based ethanol production has dramatically increased the availability of Dried Distillers Grains with Solubles (DDGS) products in pig feeding programmes. Rapid adoption of these ingredients as cost-effective alternatives has challenged the pig nutrition industry to provide accurate, cost-effective diet formulations. As with any new ingredient, there are significant unanswered questions about feeding quality and ingredient characteristics. Current market conditions dictate a higher risk tolerance and greater use of these relatively new products while questions regarding composition, variability, palatability, and relative nutritional merits are under debate. Furthermore, DDGS supply continues to change as ethanol manufacturing margins are reduced. The reduced margins stimulate development of higher value co-product uses via fractionation, extraction, or other technologies that separates the constituent components for refinement and higher-value use. Thus, the purpose of the current chapter will be to review current DDGS feeding strategies with pigs while recognizing that current recommendations are changing as the DDGS supply changes.

Feed compounding issues with increased DDGS use

Maize DDGS preferred for pig diets is from newer, dry-grind production systems (Whitney, Shurson, Johnston, Wulf, and Shanks, 2006). These ethanol production facilities grind the dry grain prior to liquefying, fermentation, ethanol distillation, followed by concentrating, blending and drying the final DDGS product. The resulting co-products are subjected to lower temperature drying, and less harsh manufacturing methods than previous wet-grind ethanol production methods (Urbanchuck, 2008). These newer products are higher in nutritional value than previous DDGS co-products (Stein, 2007; see Table 1). These newer, higher value DDGS products are lighter in colour and sweeter smelling than older, wet-milled products. The lighter, golden colour and fermented smell correlates well with a higher digestibility, primarily of amino acids and gross energy. This visual and olfactory inspection method is frequently used at feed manufacturing locations to check product acceptability. If the product is dark brown with burnt or charred particles, and smells burnt, it is typically rejected (Gaines, Kocher, and Wolter, 2007). This subjective quick check method is used in place of more objective, but slower, methods like proximate analysis and lysine/crude protein ratio (Stein, 2007). Objective tests are not rapid enough for real-time quality assurance sampling at commercial mills (Gaines *et al.*, 2007a). The subjective quick tests are often used in conjunction with other laboratory tests like Provimi's proprietary, in-house NIR determination of nutrient profiles to identify reliable DDGS suppliers. Because energy content is one of the primary drivers of DDGS use, these NIR tests help in providing a better estimate of the variability within and between DDGS suppliers (see Table 2). These laboratory tests are used to quantify the relative nutritional value of a specific DDGS source and help predict its relative merit. Following the initial assessment, clients are advised on proper colour and smell checks when they receive DDGS supplies. Continued, routine sampling and laboratory testing are imperative as it is commonly observed that DDGS samples vary greatly between plants, even those with identical construction and similar operating procedures (Dr. Neil Paton, Akey, personal communication).

Table 1. Recommended standards for dry-grind DDGS products.[1]

Nutrient	Minimum	Maximum
Crude Protein, g/kg	270	--
Fat (oil), g/kg	90	--
Phosphorus, g/kg	5.5	--
Lysine, g/kg of crude protein	28.0	--
Acid detergent fibre, g/kg	--	120
Neutral detergent fibre, g/kg	--	400

[1]Adapted from Stein (2007)

Mycotoxin contamination is a concern with DDGS supplies. Mycotoxins, like other remaining components after starch extraction, are concentrated three times higher in DDGS. Hofstetter and Pichler (2008) reported that, of 191 maize DDGS samples

Table 2. DDGS analyzed nutrient content summary.[1]

Component	Minimum	Maximum	SD
Moisture, g/kg	35	134	15
Crude Protein, g/kg	205	327	11
Fat (oil), g/kg	57	129	9
Ash, g/kg	9	78	6
Starch, g/kg	1	134	15
Acid detergent fibre, g/kg	51	250	21
Neutral detergent fibre, g/kg	204	406	24

[1]Summary of 1,381 samples from various North American ethanol production facilities from 2006 through 2008.

tested, 166 tested positive for zearalenone (mean 0.2 mg/kg); 134 tested positive for DON (mean 1.5 mg/kg); 168 tested positive for fumonisin (mean 0.8 mg/kg). Because of this risk, DDGS suppliers should have a verifiable mycotoxin control plan (Stein, 2007; Gaines *et al.*, 2007a). Many plants today supply mycotoxin testing results with their analytical laboratory results from internal product sampling (Gaines *et al.*, 2007a). United States pork producers vary in their use of mycotoxin control agents. Some prefer preventative control in breeding herd diets, while other similar accounts prefer to save diet cost and bear more risk.

Flowability concerns require special consideration when using DDGS in a commercial pig feeding programme. Bridging of DDGS in ingredient bins occurs primarily during warm, humid summer months. Flowability issues are primarily related to the moisture and oil content of the DDGS supply. Feed manufacturers and pork producers are occasionally required to reduce their DDGS use during summer months (Gaines *et al.*, 2007a). In addition, flowability agents like zeolite, limestone, and a commercial moisture migration control product all failed to significantly improve DDGS flowability and angle of repose with 90 and 116 g/kg moisture DDGS supplies (Johnston, Hillbrands, Shurson, and Goihl, 2008).

Pig feeding recommendations

Commercial pig feeding programmes in the United States are successfully utilizing higher levels of maize DDGS than recently thought practical. Much of this is driven by increased raw material costs and lower pork production returns. Nonetheless, most nutritionists and producers have reported very few problems associated with higher DDGS feeding levels. Most issues relate to DDGS product quality, ingredient variation, and the associated effects on nutrient content. The increased variability has increased customer reliance upon their nutrition suppliers to balance cost savings with increased risks like feed refusal, reduced growth performance, reduced carcass yield and fat quality. Additional issues relating to feed bulk density, and feed intake variation in gestating and lactating brood sows, and mature, working boars require attention. Current feeding recommendations by phase are listed in Table 3, and the recommendations are discussed below.

Table 3. Typical dietary maize or sorghum DDGS inclusion.

Production phase	Body weight range, kg	Typical Usage, g/kg	Usage Range, g/kg
Early Nursery	5 – 10	0	0 - 100
Late Nursery	10 – 20	50 -100	0 - 300
Grow-Finish	20 – 120	75 - 200	0 - 200
Developing Gilts	20 - 140	75 - 200	0 - 200
Breeding Herd	--	100 - 200	0 - 300

NURSERY PIGS (10 TO 20 kg BW)

Feeding maize DDGS to nursery pigs has increased within the last 24 months. Recently, several trials have demonstrated the nutritional merit of feeding DDGS to pigs from 7 to 20 kg (see Table 4). Commercial and university research results indicate that moderate levels of DDGS can be fed to nursery pigs from 10 kg BW and heavier with minimal growth performance effects. Commercial nursery pig nutrition programmes in the United States contain up to 300 g DDGS /kg, primarily after 10 kg BW, with some starting as early as 7 kg BW (Dr. Kevin Soltwedel, Professional Swine Management, personal communication). Those using higher DDGS levels are more focused on diet cost savings than improved growth performance. Nutrition programmes that have consistent, higher growth performance typically utilize dietary levels of 50 to 150 g DDGS/kg.

GROW-FINISH PIGS (20 TO 120 kg BW)

Maize or sorghum DDGS is becoming a staple ingredient of grow-finishing pig feeding programmes. Commercial and university research has consistently shown that feeding no more than 200 g DDGS /kg from 20 to 120 kg BW is a practical alternative to typical US maize-soyabean meal feeding programmes (see Table 5). Commercial feeding of dietary DDGS levels higher than 200 g/kg is not practical

Table 4. Effects of dry-grind corn DDGS on pig performance from 7 to 20 kg.

Reference	DDGS Treatments	Results
Whitney and Shurson (2004)	0, 50, 100, 150, 200, 250 g DDGS/kg	Decreased growth performance from day 4 to 18. No growth performance effect from day 18 to 40.
Spencer *et al.*, (2007)	0, 75, 150 g DDGS/kg; DDGS level varied by phase in 4 phase program	No effect on pig growth rate at all DDGS supplementation rates.
Barbosa *et al.*, (2008)	0, 75, 150, 225 g DDGS/kg	No effect on pig growth rate in all phases.
Burkey *et al.*, (2008)	0, 50 or 300 mg/kg dietary DDGS for 14 days followed by 0 or 300 mg/kg dietary DDGS for 20 days	300 g/kg in final 20 days had no effect on pig performance. Pigs fed DDGS during earlier phase had reduced growth performance.
Seabolt *et al.*, (2008)	Exp 1 – 0, 100, 200, 300 mg DDGS/kg preference test Exp 2 - 0, 300 g/kg good colour and smell DDGS, 300 mg/kg bad colour and smell DDGS dietary supplementation	Exp 1 – Linear decrease in diet preference as DDGS inclusion increased. Exp 2 - No effect on pig growth rate.

as reduced growth performance is often observed. In addition, pigs typically need a transition phase to diets that contain more than 100 g DDGS /kg. Experience shows that pigs provided 75 to 100 g DDGS /kg for 2 weeks can successfully be transferred to diets up to 200 g DDGS /kg with little or no growth performance loss. When feeding DDGS levels above 100 g DDGS /kg, it is imperative to have an accurate energy estimation of the DDGS source as significant variation exists between sources (see Table 2).

Carcass characteristics like backfat depth and *longissimus* muscle area are typically unaffected when DDGS are used in the feeding programme (Stein, 2007; Gaines *et al.*, 2007a). In contrast, carcass yield or dressing percent is typically at risk when feeding DDGS, especially at levels above 100 g DDGS /kg (see Table 6). Although a few recent trials did not observe yield loss when higher levels of DDGS were fed, a significant majority of recent research have measured yield loss. The yield loss in Table 6 is variable, averaging 0.3% per 100 g DDGS /kg. Practical experience shows risk of yield loss is very low with dietary DDGS levels at or below 100 g/kg. Feeding dietary DDGS levels above 100 g/kg typically results in economically significant yield loss. Yield loss has been successfully countered with strategies like feeding 5 mg ractopamine/kg and/or reducing or removing dietary DDGS during the last 3 to 4 weeks before slaughter, feeding natural ingredients that improve growth performance, or marginally extending days to market. Whatever the strategy used, carcass yield loss needs to be economically accounted for when valuing higher DDGS levels in feeding programmes.

Table 5. Effects of dry-grind corn or sorghum DDGS on pig growth performance from 20 to 120 kg.

Reference	Treatments	Results
Cook *et al.*, 2005	0, 100, 200, 300 g DDGS /kg	No differences in growth performance. Mortality decreased linearly as DDGS use increased.
Whitney *et al.*, 2006	0, 100, 200, 300 g DDGS /kg in 3 pig BW classifications.	No weight by dietary DDGS interactions. Pigs fed 200 and 300 g DDGS/kg had lower ADG than pigs fed 0 or 100 g DDGS/kg.
Feoli *et al.*, 2007	0, 400 g high energy maize DDGS /kg, 400 g moderate energy maize DDGS /kg and 400 g moderate energy sorghum DDGS /kg	Higher ADG for 0 versus all DDGS sources.
Gaines *et al.*, 2007b	0, 300 g DDGS /kg, enzyme + 300 g DDGS/kg	No differences in growth performance.
Gaines *et al.*, 2007c	0, 300 g DDGS/kg removed from diet 0, 3, and 6 weeks before slaughter.	No ADG performance differences. 300 g/kg and no withdrawal had lower G:F versus 0 g DDGS/kg or 300 g/kg with 6 week withdrawal.
Lineen *et al.*, 2007	Exp. 1 - 0 or 150 g DDGS/kg Exp. 2 - 0, 100, 200, 300 g DDGS/kg Exp. 3. - 0, 50, 100, 150, 200 g DDGS/kg	1. No growth performance differences. 2. Decreased ADG and ADFI above 100 g DDGS/kg. 3. Lowest ADG at 200 g/kg, decreased ADFI linearly with increasing DDGS.
Xu *et al.*, 2007	0, 100, 200, 300 g DDGS/kg	No effect on ADG. Reduced ADFI and F:G at 200 and 300 g/kg.
Augspurger *et al.*, 2008	DDGS substitution by phase, 0 or 300 gDDGS/kg.	Removal or addition of DDGS in any phase did not affect growth performance.
Dutlinger *et al.*, 2008	25 g glycerol/kg with or without 200 g DDGS/kg	No glycerol by DDGS interaction. No ADG effect of DDGS. Increased ADFI with DDGS.
Feoli *et al.*, 2008a	0, 400 g DDGS/kg with or without 50 g/kg tallow or 50 g palm oil/kg	400 g DDGSkg without added fat had reduced ADG and ADFI versus 0 g DDGS/kg

Table 5. Contd.

Reference	Treatments	Results
Feoli *et al.*, 2008b	0, 400 g DDGS/kg with or without 50 g stearate/kg or 50 g coconut oil/kg.	0 g/kg with fat DDGS had highest ADG.
Hill *et al.*, 2008	0, 100, 200, 300 g DDGS/kg. DDGS withdrawn from 200 and 300 g DDGS/kg at 30 days before slaughter.	No meaningful growth performance differences.
Jacela *et al.*, 2008	Solvent extracted, low-oil DDGS source at 0, 50, 100, 200, 300 g/kg. Diets balanced for ME and SID lysine from previous experiment.	Linearly decreased ADG & ADFI with increasing DDGS, worst at or above 200 g DDGS/kg.
Weimer *et al.*, 2008	0, 0 plus oil, 100, 200, 300 g DDGS/kg	Tended towards lower ADG and G:F at 200 and 300 g DDGS/kg.
Widmer *et al.*, 2008	0, 100, 200 g DDGS/kg; 0, 200, 400 g High protein, Low-fat DDGS /kg 50, 100 g dietary maize germ /kg.	No performance differences in any DDGS source or level. Higher final BW in corn germ fed pigs.
Williams *et al.*, 2008	Low protein control (0 g DDGS/kg), high protein control (0 g DDGS/kg, high protein with 300 g DDGS/kg	Excess crude protein in high protein with 300 g DDGS/kg had lower ADG and ADFI than low protein control. High protein control did not differ from low protein control.
Xu *et al.*, 2008	0, 150, 300 g DDGS/kg with 0, 3, 6, 9 week DDGS withdrawal before slaughter.	300 g DDGS/kg with no withdrawal had lower ADG versus 0 g/kg control.

BREEDING HERD

Recently, DDGS have provided significant ration cost savings in both gestation and lactation feeding programmes. Concerns about mycotoxins, ingredient variability and quality, and the associated risks to sow and boar productivity had made many producers reluctant to use higher dietary DDGS levels when other alternatives provided similar ration cost. Recent research and practical experience have shown that DDGS levels up to 300 g/kg can successfully be fed in commercial breeding herd rations (see Table 7). Most commercial producers are currently using 100 to 200 g DDGS /kg in breeding herd rations.

Table 6. Effects of dry-grind maize or sorghum DDGS on pig carcass yield at slaughter.[1,2]

Reference	Treatments	Results
Cook et al., 2005	0, 100, 200, 300 g DDGS/kg	DDGS reduced carcass yield 0.39% per 100 g/kg dietary DDGS on average.
Whitney et al., 2006	0, 100, 200, 300 g DDGS/kg in 3 pig BW classifications.	DDGS reduced carcass yield by 0.36% per 100 g DDGS/kg.
Feoli et al., 2007	0, 400 g high energy maize DDGS/kg, 400 g moderate energy DGS/kg and 400 g moderate energy sorghum/kg	DDGS reduced carcass yield 0.18% per 100 g DDGS/kg on average.
Gaines et al., 2007b	0, 300 g/kg, enzyme + 300 g DDGS/kg	DDGS reduced carcass yield 0.25% per 100 g DDGS/kg on average.
Gaines et al., 2007c	0, 300 g DDGS/kg removed from diet 0, 3, 6 weeks before slaughter.	No withdrawal DDGS reduced yield 0.4% per 100 g DDGS/ kg on average. 3 week DDGS withdrawal recovered half of yield loss. 6 week DDGS withdrawal recovered all of yield loss.
Dutlinger et al., 2008	25 g glycerol/kg with or without 200 g DDGS/kg	DDGS reduced carcass yield 0.3% per 100 g DDGS/kg in diets without glycerol.
Feoli et al., 2008a	0, 400 g DDGS/kg with or without 50 g tallow/kg or 50 g palm oil/kg	DDGS reduced carcass yield 0.5% per 100 g DDGS/kg.
Feoli et al., 2008b	0, 400 g DDSG/kg with or without 50 g stearate/kg or 50 g coconut oil/kg.	DDGS reduced carcass yield 0.5% per 100 g DDGS/kg.
Hill et al., 2008	0, 100, 200, 300 g DDGS/kg. DDGS withdrawn from 200 and 300 g DDGS/kg diets at 30 days before slaughter.	No carcass yield differences were observed.
Jacela et al., 2008	0, 50, 100, 200, 300 g Solvent extracted, low-oil DDGS /kg. Diets balanced for ME and SID lysine from previous experiment.	DDGS reduced carcass yield 0.25% per 100 g DDGS/kg on average.
Widmer et al., 2008	0, 100, 200 g DDGS/kg; 0, 200, 400 g High protein, Low-fat DDGS /kg; 50, 100 g maize germ/kg.	No carcass yield differences were observed.
Williams et al., 2008	Low protein control (0 g DDGS/ kg), high protein control (0 g DDGS/kg, high protein with 300 g DDGS/kg.	DDGS reduced carcass yield 0.23% per 100 g DDGS/kg on average.

[1] Carcass yield is calculated as hot carcass weight, kg/live weight, kg * 100.
[2] Carcass yield loss averages ~0.30% per 100 g DDGS/kg.

Table 7. Effects of dry-grind maize or sorghum DDGS on brood sow and litter performance.

Reference	Treatments	Results
Song *et al.*, 2007	0, 100, 200, 300 g DDGS/kg lactation diet. Evaluating effect on sow and litter performance during 1 lactation.	No differences in litter performance or sow subsequent wean to estrus interval. Sows fed 300 g DDGS/kg had the greatest body weight loss during lactation.
Greiner *et al.*, 2008	0, 100, 200, 300 g DDGS/kg lactation diet following 100 g DDGS/kg in gestation.	No differences in sow ADFI with increasing dietary DDGS. Increased sow weight gain, increased percent bred back in 7 days, and decreased wean to service interval with increasing dietary DDGS. Subsequent reproductive performance was best in sows fed 300 g DDGS/kg with no change in litter performance from DDGS feeding level.
Hill *et al.*, 2008	Two experiments testing 0 and 150 g DDGS/kg lactation diets on sow and litter performance.	No differences in sow or litter performance were associated with including DDGS in lactation diets.

Finally, when feeding any co-product to limit-fed pigs with a volumetric feed dispenser, changes in feed bulk density need to be addressed. Since maize DDGS is bulkier than maize and soyabean meal, each 100 g increase in DDGS/kg increases diet volume by 30 g/kg (Stein, 2007).

References

Augspurger, N.R., G.I. Petersen, J.D. Spencer, and E.N. Parr. (2008) Alternating dietary inclusion of corn distillers dried grains with solubles (DDGS) did not impact growth performance of finishing pigs. *Journal of Animal Science,* **86 (E-suppl. 2)**, 523.

Barbosa, F.F., S.S. Dritz, M.D. Tokach, J.M DeRouchey, R.D. Goodband, and J.L. Nelssen. (2008) Use of distillers dried grains with solubles and soybean hulls in nursery pig diets. *Journal of Animal Science*, **86 (E-suppl. 2)**, 446.

Burkey, T.E., P.S. Miller, R. Moreno, S.S. Shepherd, and E.E. Carney. (2008) Effects of increasing levels of distillers dried grains with solubles (DDGS) on growth performance of weanling pigs. *Journal of Animal Science*, **86 (E-suppl. 3)**, 50.

Cook, D., N. Paton, M. Gibson. (2005) Effect of dietary level of distillers dried grains with solubles (DDGS) on growth performance, mortality, and carcass characteristics of grow-finish barrows and gilts. *Journal of Animal Science*, **83 (suppl. 1)**, 335.

Duttlinger, A.W., M.D. Tokach, S.S. Dritz, J.M. DeRouchey, J.L. Nelssen, R.D. Goodband, and K.J. Prusa. (2008) Effects of increasing dietary glycerol and dried distillers grains with solubles on growth performance of finishing pigs. *Journal of Animal Science*, **86 (E-suppl. 2)**, 607.

Feoli, C., J.D. Hancock, C. Monge, T.L. Gugle, S.D. Carter, and N.A. Cole. (2007) Effects of corn and sorghum based distillers dried grains with solubles on growth performance and carcass characteristics in finishing pigs. *Journal of Animal Science*, **85 (suppl. 2)**, 95.

Feoli, C., J.D. Hancock, S. Issa, T.L. Gugle, and S.D. Carter. (2008a) Effects of adding beef tallow and palm oil to diets with sorghum based distillers dried grains with solubles on growth performance and carcass characteristics in finishing pigs. *Journal of Animal Science*, **86 (E-suppl. 3)**, 52.

Feoli, C., J.D. Hancock, D.H. Kropf, S. Issa, T.L. Gugle, and S.D. Carter. (2008b) Effects of adding stearic acid and coconut oil to diets with sorghum based distillers dried grains with solubles on growth performance and carcass characteristics in finishing pigs. *Journal of Animal Science*, **86 (E-suppl. 3)**, 53.

Gaines, A.M., M. Kocher, and B. Wolter. (2007a) Practical aspects of feeding distillers dried grains with solubles (DDGS) to swine. In *Proceedings of the 2007 Carolina Nutrition Conference*, 1-5.

Gaines, A.M., G.I. Petersen, J.D. Spencer, and N.R. Augspurger (2007b) Use of corn distillers dried grains with solubles (DDGS) in finishing pigs. *Journal of Animal Science*, **85 (suppl. 2)**, 96.

Gaines, A.M., J.D. Spencer, G.I. Petersen, N.R. Augspurger, and S.J. Kitt. (2007c) Effect of corn distillers dried grains with solubles (DDGS) withdrawal program on growth performance and carcass yield in grow-finish pigs. *Journal of Animal Science*, **85 (suppl. 1)**, 438.

Greiner, L.L., X. Wang, G. Allee, and J. Connor. (2008) The feeding of dry distillers grain with solubles to lactating sows. *Journal of Animal Science*, **86 (E-suppl. 3)**, 63.

Hill, G.M., J.E. Link, D.O. Liptrap, M.A. Giesemann, M.J. Dawes, J.A. Snedegar, N.M. Bello, and R.J. Tempelman. (2008) Withdrawal of distillers dried grains with solubles (DDGS) prior to slaughter in finishing pigs. *Journal of Animal Science*, **86 (E-suppl. 3)**, 52.

Hill, G.M., J.E. Link, M.J. Rincker, D.L. Kirkpatrick, M.L. Gibson, and K. Karges. (2008). Utilization of distillers dried grains with solubles and phytase in sow lactation diets to meet the phosphorus requirement of the sow and reduce fecal phosphorus concentration. *Journal of Animal Science*, **86**, 112-118.

Hofstetter, U. and E. Pichler. (2008) An international survey on the occurrence of mycotoxins in dried distillers grains with solubles (DDGS). *Journal of Animal Science,* **86 (E-suppl. 2)**, 194.

Jacela, J.Y., J.M. DeRouchey, S.S. Dritz, M.D. Tokach, R.D. Goodband, J.L. Nelssen, J.M. Benz, K. Prusa, R.C. Thaler, and D. E. Little. (2008) Effect of deoiled corn dried distillers grains with solubles (solvent extracted) on growth performance and carcass characteristics of growing and finishing pigs. *Journal of Animal Science,* **86 (E-suppl. 2)**, 522.

Johnston, L.J., A.M. Hildebrands, G.C. Shurson, and J. Goihl. (2008) Selected additives do not improve flowability of dried distiller's grains with solubles (DDGS) in a commercial system. *Journal of Animal Science,* **86 (E-suppl. 3)**, 54.

Linneen, S.K., M.D. Tokach, J.M. DeRouchey, S.S. Dritz, R.D. Goodband, J.L. Nelssen, R.O. Gottlob, and R.G. Main. (2007) Effects of dried distillers grain with solubles on grow-finish pig performance. *Journal of Animal Science,* **85 (suppl. 2)**, 96.

Seabolt, B.S., E. van Heugten, K.D. Ange-van Heugten, and E. Roura. (2008) Feed preferences in nursery pigs fed diets containing varying fractions and qualities of dried distillers grains with solubles (DDGS). *Journal of Animal Science,* **86 (E-suppl. 2)**, 447.

Song, M., S.K. Baidoo, G.C. Shurson, and L.J. Johnston. (2007) Use of dried distillers grains with solubles in diets for lactating sows. *Journal of Animal Science,* **85 (suppl. 2)**, 97.

Spencer, J.D., G.I. Peterson, A.M. Gaines, and N.R. Augspurger. (2007) Evaluation of different strategies for supplementing distillers dried grains with solubles (DDGS) to nursery pig diets. *Journal of Animal Science,* **85 (suppl. 2)**, 96.

Stein, H.H. (2007) Distillers dried grains with solubles (DDGS) in diets fed to swine. Swine Focus #001, University of Illinois at Urbana-Champaign, Dept. of Animal Sciences, http://www.livestocktrail.uiuc.edu/uploads/porknet/papers/DDGS%20in%20Swine%20Diets-Stein.pdf

Urbanchuk, J.M. (2008) Feed ingredient availability and price expectations. In *2008 Proceedings of the American Association of Swine Veterinarians, San Diego CA,* 425-429.

Weimer, D., J. Stevens, A. Schinckel, M. Latour, and B. Richert. (2008) Effects of feeding increasing levels of distillers dried grains with solubles to grow-finish pigs on growth performance and carcass quality. *Journal of Animal Science,* **86 (E-suppl. 3)**, 51.

Whitney, M.H. and G.C. Shurson. (2004) Growth performance of nursery pigs fed diets containing increasing levels of corn distillers dried grains with solubles originating from a modern Midwestern plant. *Journal of Animal Science,* **82**, 122-128.

Whitney, M.H., G.C. Shurson, L.J. Johnston, D.M. Wulf, and B.C. Shanks. (2006) Growth performance and carcass characteristics of grower-finisher pigs fed high-quality distillers dried grain with solubles originating from a modern Midwestern plant. *Journal of Animal Science*, **84**, 3356-3363.

Widmer, M.R., L.M. McGinnis, D.M. Wulf, and H.H. Stein. (2008) Effects of feeding distillers dried grains with solubles, high-protein distillers dried grains, and corn germ to growing-finishing pigs on pig performance, carcass quality, and the palatability of pork. *Journal of Animal Science*, **86**, 1819-1831.

Williams, S.C., J.D. Hancock, C. Feoli, S. Issa, and T.L. Gugle. (2008) Effects of excess dietary crude protein from soybean meal and distillers dried grains with solubles in diets for finishing pigs. *Journal of Animal Science*, **86 (E-suppl. 2)**, 523.

Xu, G., S.K. Baidoo, L.J. Johnston, J.E. Cannon, and G.C. Shurson. (2007) Effects of adding increasing levels of corn dried distillers grains with solubles (DDGS) to corn-soybean meal diets on growth performance and pork quality of growing-finishing pigs. *Journal of Animal Science*, **85 (suppl. 2)**, 76.

Xu, G., S.K. Baidoo, L.J. Johnston, J.E. Cannon, D. Bibus, and G.C. Shurson. (2008) Effects of dietary corn dried distiller's grains with solubles (DDGS), and DDGS withdrawal intervals, on pig growth performance, carcass traits, and fat quality. *Journal of Animal Science*, **86 (E-suppl. 3)**, 52.

17

THE USE OF ENZYMES TO IMPROVE THE NUTRITIVE VALUE OF CO-PRODUCTS

MICHAEL BEDFORD

AB-Vista Feed Ingredients Ltd, Marlborough, Wilts. SN8 4AN

Introduction

The majority of feed enzymes used commercially have been specifically targeted at phytate, the major cereals and to a lesser extent soyabean meal, with few if any being designed specifically for other co-products used routinely in the animal feed industry. Perhaps the main reason for this is that only the target substrates mentioned above are used in volumes large enough to justify the cost for the toxicological and efficacy data requested and required for registration. Nevertheless enzymes have been routinely used in diets which may contain wheat and maize milling by-products, and oilseed meals other than soyabean meal. In many cases they have possibly increased the nutritive value of these products and hence the diets overall, but it is an inescapable fact that the reason for using such enzymes commercially is generally driven by the choice of the main cereal and/or soyabean meal component of the diet. This is beginning to change, however, with the advent of the ethanol industry which may in the future limit supply of some of the major cereals whilst simultaneously producing large quantities of co-products, principally maize and wheat dried distillers grains with solubles. There is increasing interest in determining how best to use these new co-products as the quantities available increase, with the use of enzymes being seen as one avenue to explore. This chapter will review the use of enzymes on co-products, starting with the wheat milling and oilseed industries, and then focussing on the more recent work on co-products from the ethanol industry.

Wheat milling products

In the early 1990s the nascent enzyme industry focussed a considerable amount of attention on the use of xylanases in wheat (and rye as a model for wheat) -based diets as a result of the considerable success of B-glucanases in barley-based diets (Bedford *et al.*, 1991; Choct and Annison, 1992; Barrier-Guillot *et al.*, 1995). It was clear at this time that wheat quality varied and the success of the use of such enzymes was inversely related to initial quality. The efficacy of such enzymes was related to their ability to reduce viscosity, partially degrade endosperm cell wall structures and produce fermentable xylo-oligosaccharides that encouraged more favourable intestinal microfloral populations (Campbell and Bedford, 1992; Annison, 1993; Simon, 1998). Wheat co-products from the milling industry are the result of removal of the starchy endosperm (ie flour) for human consumption. The remainder consists of the aleurone and bran layers with some minor quantities of starchy endosperm which escaped separation. From a simplistic viewpoint it may seem that the opportunities for responses on use of a xylanase on wheat milling co-products would be considerable; they contain significantly more insoluble arabinoxylans than whole wheat and the cell wall structure of the aleurone layer is significantly more robust than that of the endosperm and, as a result, is more resistant to digestion (Parkkonen *et al.*, 1997; Glitso *et al.*, 1998). Consequently some data suggest that there is potential for the use of xylanases in diets rich in wheat milling co-products although the variation in responses noted are large (Jaroni *et al.*, 1999; van der Meulen *et al.*, 2001; Yin *et al.*, 2004; Nortey *et al*, 2007).

In vitro and in vivo microscopy does show, however, that the destructive effect of xylanases on cell wall integrity is greater on the endosperm than the aleurone layer (Tervila-Wilo *et al.*, 1996; Bedford and Autio, 1996; Parkkonen *et al.*, 1997), probably as a result of the fact that the aleurone cell walls are so much thicker and hence resistant to digestion. The digesta transit time in non-ruminants is limited, particularly in the younger animal, and there may not be sufficient time for exogenous enzymes to significantly degrade cell walls of the aleurone layer. This suggests that there is more to be gained through enzymatic digestion of complete wheat diets compared with its co-products which have reduced endosperm content (See fig 1).

Despite the 2-3 fold greater content of cell wall material in wheat bran and middlings compared with whole wheat, the water soluble, viscous arabinoxylan contents are not markedly different. This is because most of the additional NSP content in wheat co-products is insoluble cell wall material. As a result the viscosity of wheat co-products may not be any greater than that of wheat itself (Mathlouthi *et al.*, 2002). Research with intact wheat shows considerable variation in viscous polymer content. As a result it would be expected that similar variation in wheat milling co-product variation also exists, and thus response to xylanase use would also vary markedly as is evident in the literature

In summary, the use of xylanases on wheat co-products seems to result in responses of the same order of magnitude as that observed when used on wheat diets. This is not surprising given that viscosity may not be of any greater importance in co-products compared with whole wheat, and that the relative intransigence of the aleurone cell wall to degradation compared with the endosperm means that a long incubation time is required for them to be "punctured". In this regard wheat milling co-products may respond to xylanase treatment, more so in older compared with younger animals. As stated earlier, exact quantification of the effects of any enzyme on any wheat co-products is frustrated by the fact that in most studies the majority of the remainder of the diet consists of ingredients which may be equally responsive to the enzyme applied.

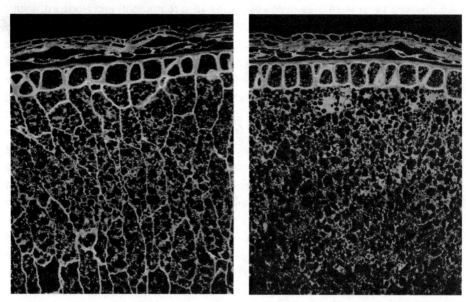

Figure 1. Wheat aleurone and endosperm cell wall structure before (left panel) and after (right panel) incubation with a Trichoderma xylanase

The aleurone layer is where the bulk of the phytic acid in wheat is found. Wheat co-products, by virtue of the fact that they concentrate the aleurone layer, concentrate the phytic acid and hence there has been interest in the use of phytases in conjunction with cell well degrading enzymes to accelerate phytic acid degradation and hence nutrient release. Work with diets containing wheat and/or wheat bran has demonstrated a potential synergy between these enzymes (Zyla *et al.*, 1999; Ravindran *et al.*, 1999; Selle *et al.*, 2001; Pourreza and Classen, 2001). Some authors have even suggested that the phytate may be structural and its hydrolysis therefore facilitates the breakdown of the aleurone cell walls.

Rapeseed meal

Rapeseed meal (or canola) is the product that remains following extraction of the oil for further purposes. Modern breeding has all but eliminated concerns regarding erucic acid or glucosinolate contents but there are still constraints with regard to the use of such meals which relate to fibre and phytic acid content. Furthermore, the process most often involves a final hexane extraction process to remove as much oil as possible. Considerable heat then needs to be applied to drive the contaminating hexane off, and often temperatures are reached which can result in denatured and damaged residual protein which is resistant to digestion.

Rapeseed meal is rich in fibre consisting of pectins, arabinoxylans, glucans, some mannans and cellulose (Slominski and Campbell, 1990). In vitro studies have shown that several NSP targeting enzymes are able to significantly degrade the cell wall material of rapeseed meal (Malathi and Devegowda, 2001; Meng *et al.*, 2006). However experience has shown that there is little value to be gained in attempting to extract energy from fibre through hydrolysis of the arabinoxylans to their constituent sugars and this is also likely true of the mannans and pectins. Not only is complete hydrolysis of the fibre fraction unlikely given the time constraints of feed residence within the tract of poultry and swine, but also release of some of the constituent sugars in significant quantities would likely prove to be detrimental (Schutte, 1990; Schutte *et al.*, 1991). Progress is most likely through selection of enzymes which facilitate cell wall fragmentation such that digestive enzyme are able to access the contents of those cells which have remained intact following the oil extraction process. Some data suggest that pectinase, cellulase and xylanases are able to break open rapeseed cell walls, and in the case of full fat rape, increase digestibility of the contents (Meng *et al.*, 2005; Meng *et al.*, 2006). However, the responses in complete diets often lead to results which are less pronounced and even non-existent (Kocher *et al.*, 2001; Kocher *et al.*, 2000; Meng and Slominski, 2005; Meng *et al.*, 2005; Meng *et al.*, 2006;Hoare *et al.*, 2003).

Some work has investigated the use of proteases in conjunction with fibre degrading enzymes in pre-incubation studies and, again, these data have shown that the feeding value of rapeseed meal could be improved (Bedford and Morgan, 1995; Guenter *et al.*,1995). However, the treatments were relatively harsh and when the same enzymes were used in vivo, the results were small and not significantly different from the control.

The lack of response when these enzymes or their combinations are used in more complete diets is likely due in large part due to the relatively low levels of rapeseed meal that can be gainfully employed. Even if rapeseed meal were to comprise as much as 200-250g/kg diet, the response of the meal to the enzyme would have to be very large if any benefit were to be seen as being significant. Moreover, there is great difficulty in ascribing the value of an enzyme towards rapeseed meal when the enzyme is often employed in a diet which contains large quantities of other ingredients which may be equally if not more so responsive to the enzyme.

Rapeseed meal is also rich in phytic acid compared with soyabean meal and this may be a significant antinutrient as has been discussed previously (Cowieson *et al.*, 2004, 2006). Although there have been numerous reports of the beneficial use of phytase in rapeseed meal containing diets (Leske and Coon, 1999; Newkirk and Classen, 2001; Ravindran *et al.*, 1999; Selle *et al.*, 2006; Zyla and Korelski, 1993) it has been noted that the phytic acid in rapeseed may not be as susceptible to hydrolysis as that from soyabean meal in vivo (Leske and Coon, 1999; Ravindran *et al.*, 1999) This may be due to inaccessibility of some of the phytate to hydrolysis (Newkirk and Classen, 1998). As such the opportunity to upgrade this ingredient may well be less than initially envisaged.

Nevertheless, it is clear that far greater advances can be made if the hexane extraction process is avoided in the first place. It is remarkable just how much damage is done to the value of the residual meal by the toasting process. As a result of the biodiesel drive it is clear that avenues for use of increasing amounts of rapeseed meal must be found. It is possible that there is not the capacity or desire to radically increase the use of the current product that is produced today. However there may well be considerable interest in the higher value products produced via methods which avoid hexane evaporation and hence result in highly digestible proteins. In process treatment of such meals with enzymes may prove far more effective than in vivo for increasing the nutritive value.

DDGS

Dried Distillers grains with solubles without doubt represents the co-product from the biofuel industry which has generated most interest in recent years. It is not clear whether producing ethanol from edible starch sources is sustainable and this has undoubtedly tempered enthusiasm for investigating "new" enzyme classes for use on such materials. Nevertheless, in the short to medium term the animal feed markets are going to be presented with ever increasing quantities of materials which it will find difficult to use unless solutions to its variability in digestibility are found.

Many of the comments raised with respect to use of enzymes on wheat milling co-products and rapeseed meal apply to that of DDGS. Since DDGS is a relatively new entrant into the non-ruminant nutrition market, the research is several years behind that of wheat or even rapeseed meal targeting products. One major problem is the variability of the product which creates great difficulties in designing a focused enzyme product. Table 1 below shows the results of some work by Ward *et al.* (2008), where 30 samples of DDGS were investigated. It is quite clear that the fibre contents and their constituent sugars vary much more markedly than would be expected for maize, suggesting that there are large differences in process of manufacture between ethanol plants. Until this variation is significantly reduced it will be difficult for the feed enzyme industry to offer a product which gives consistent results.

Nevertheless there are a number of feeding trials which suggest some measure or success in "improving the value" of DDGS containing diets. In truth the majority of such work leaves the reader unclear of whether the effect is due to activity of the enzyme towards the DDGS or, as is more likely, towards the other components in the ration. For example in 2 recently reported poultry trials, addition of cell wall degrading enzymes simply recovered the performance lost when DDGS was introduced (Pierce *et al.*, 2008; Jackson *et al.*, 2008).

Table 1. Nutritional and total fibre components from 30 samples of maize DDGS. Ward *et al.*, 2008

Component	Average (g/kg)	Std	CV%	Min	Max
Dry Matter	902.5	14.5	2	877.3	942.5
ADF	136.5	19.8	15	90.9	173.3
EE	111.7	20.9	19	31.8	135
CP	325.6	33.4	10	278	467.6
Rhamnose	0.8	0.1	13	0.5	0.0.9
Ribose	1.1	0.4	36	0.6	2
Fucose	0.6	0.4	67	0.1	1.8
Arabinose	49.8	4.9	10	40.9	60.8
Xylose	64.2	7.2	11	48.1	77.8
Mannose	16.2	4.3	27	11.6	24.4
Glucose	78.6	8.6	11	67.2	96.8
Galactose	16.1	1.9	12	11.9	20.8

More definitive work has shown that an enzyme which was capable of increasing the AME of a maize-soya diet for broilers by approximately 0.28 MJ/kg was equally effective in maintaining this benefit in a diet containing 150g high protein maize DDGS/kg (Gady *et al.*, 2008a). This suggests that the DDGS are at least as responsive as the maize. In layers, a similar trial showed that the same enzyme was increasingly effective in elevating the AME of a maize/wheat soya diet with incremental addition of maize DDGS. This suggests, in this case, that the enzyme was more effective on the DDGS than it was on the basal maize/wheat diet (Gady *et al,*, 2008b). There may be an effect of age within these results as the broilers were 22 d of age and the layers 38 weeks. Older animals have a more developed large intestine and as such may derive greater benefit from production of fermentable oligosaccharides which arise as a result of NSP enzyme activity.

In northern Europe it is most likely that wheat derived DDGS will be the co-product available for use. It differs substantially from maize DDGS as is clear from the data in table 2. The principal points of interest relate to the higher protein in wheat (principally from the aleurone layer), the lower fat and higher non phytate P content, all of which contribute to the value of the product.

Table 2. Comparison of composition of wheat (n=2) with maize (n=4) DDGS. Slominski *et al.*, 2008

	g/kg DM	
	Wheat	*Maize*
Protein	407	305
Total amino acids	370	304
Simple sugars	9	21
Starch	18	71
Fibre	332	355
NDF	273	326
Fat	45	107
NPP	8.5	6.2

Phytases have also been used in maize-soya diets containing DDGS. One problem with DDGS is that much of the phosphorus is non-phytate P, and as a result the diet will often contain more digestible phosphorus than expected. Recent data suggest that even for young broilers, the coefficient of bioavailability of phosphorus in DDGS was 0.67 (Martinez-Amezcua *et al.*, 2006). Addition of as much as 10,000 U/kg phytase to P deficient diets resulted in a small response in gain and a larger but still limited response in tibia ash suggesting limited phytate hydrolysis. Phytase alone did not influence AME.

In poultry, when phytases are used in combination with an NSP targeting enzyme, the effects on DDGS seem to be at least as great as they are on the maize (Moran and Lehman, 2008). The use of DDGS and phytase in sow diets showed that the combination resulted in no reduction in performance with significant reductions in phosphorus pollution compared with the maize-soya diet. In this regard DDGS can be an attractive ingredient when combined with phytase where phosphorus pollution is an issue. This may be particularly relevant in older animals that can utilise fibre more effectively.

Conclusions

Co-products offer a significant savings in non-ruminant diet formulations. If the nutrients they contain can be consistently retrieved then their use will likely increase as the costs of the major cereals increase. Development of effective enzymes is likely to play a significant role in this process, but more focussed research is necessary to accurately quantify the effects of such products on the co-product when they are routinely used in the background of other, more responsive ingredients.

References

Bedford, M.R. and Autio, K. (1996) Microscopic Examination of feed and digesta from wheat-fed broiler chickens and its relation to bird performance. *Poultry Science* **75** :14

Bedford, M. R. and Morgan, A. J. (1995) The use of enzymes in canola-based diets. European symposium on Feed Enzymes, II, 125-31.

Cowieson, A. J., Acamovic, T. and Bedford, M. R. (2004) The effects of phytase and phytic acid on the loss of endogenous amino acids and minerals from broiler chickens. *British Poultry Science* **45**, 101-08.

Cowieson, A. J., Acamovic, T. and Bedford, M. R. (2006) Phytic acid and Phytase: Implications for Protein Utilization by Poultry. *Poultry Science* **85**, 878-85.

Gady, C, P. Dalibard, and P. A Geraert (2008a) Nutritional evaluation of a high-protein corn distillers dried grains with solubles (HP corn DDGS) in broilers and evaluation of NSP-enzyme effect on energy digestibility. *Poultry Science* **87**, Supp 1, 112.

Gady, C, P. Dalibard, and P. A Geraert (2008b) Nutritional evaluation of corn distillers dried grains with solubles (DDGS) in layers and potential benefit of NSP-enzyme supplementation on energy digestibility. *Poultry Science* **87**, Supp 1, 112.

Guenter, W., *et al.* (1995) Potential for improved utilisation of canola meal using exogenous enzymes. Proc. 9th International Rapeseed Congress, Cambridge, 164-66.

Hoare, B., *et al.* (2003) The effect of non-starch polysaccharide enzymes on the nutritive value of rapeseed meal for growing and finishing pigs. *Irish Journal of Agricultural and Food Research* **42**, 255-63.

Jackson, M. E., Stephens, K.R. and Mathis, G. (2008) The effect of B-Mannanase (Hemicell Feed Enzyme) and high levels of distillers dried grains on turkey hen performance. *Poultry Science* **87**, Supp 1, 65-66.

Jaroni, D, Scheideler, S.E., Beck, M.M. and Wyatt, C. (1999) The effect of dietary wheat middlings and enzyme supplementation - II: Apparent nutrient digestibility, digestive tract size, gut viscosity, and gut morphology in two strains of leghorn hens. *Poultry Science* **78**, 1664-1674.

Kocher, A., *et al.* (2001) Effects of enzyme supplementation on the replacement value of canola meal for soybean meal in broiler diets. *Australian Journal of Agricultural Research* **52**, 447-52.

Kocher, A., *et al.* (2000) The effects of enzyme addition to broiler diets containing high concentrations of canola or sunflower meal. *British Poultry Science* **79**, 1767-74.

Leske, K. L. and Coon C.N. (1999) A bioassay to determine the effect of phytase on phytate phosphorus hydrolysis and total phosphorus retention of feed ingredients as determined with broilers and laying hens. *Poultry Science* **78**, 1151-57.

Malathi, V. and Devegowda, G. (2001) In vitro evaluation of nonstarch polysaccharide digestibility of feed ingredients by enzymes. *Poultry Science* **80**, 302-05.

Martinez-Amezcua, C., Parsons, C. M. and Baker, D. H. (2006) Effect of microbial phytase and citric acid on phosphorus bioavailability, apparent metabolizable energy, and amino acid digestibility in distillers dried grains with solubles in chicks. *Poultry Science* **85**, 470-75.

Meng, X, *et al.* (2006) The Use of Enzyme Technology for Improved Energy Utilisation from full fat oilseeds. Part 1: Canola seed. *Poultry Science* **85**, 1025-30.

Meng, X and B. A. Slominski. (2005) Nutritive values of Corn, Soybean meal, Canola meal and peas for broiler chickens as affected by a multicarbohydrase preparation of cell wall degrading enzymes. *Poultry Science* **84**, 1242-51.

Meng, X., *et al.* (2005) Degradation of cell wall polysaccharides by combinations of carbohydrase enzymes and their effect on nutrient utilization and broiler chicken performance. *Poultry Science* **84**, 37-47.

Moran, E. T. and Lehman, R. (2008) Response to combined amylase-phytase-protease-xylanase supplementation when 8 week broiler males had received corn-soybean meal feeds devoid of antimicrobials with/without alfalfa meal and/or DDGS. *Poultry Science* **87**, Supp 1, 158.

Newkirk, R.W. and Classen, H.L. (1998) In vitro hydrolysis of phytate in canola meal with purified and crude sources of phytase. Animal Feed Science and Technology 72, 315-27.

Newkirk, R.W. and Classen, H.L. (2001) The non-mineral nutritional impact of phytate in canola meal fed to broiler chicks. *Animal Feed Science and Technology* **91**, 115-28.

Nortey, T.N., Patience, J.F., Sands, J.S. and Zijlstra, R.T. (2007) Xylanase supplementation improves energy digestibility of wheat by-products in grower pigs. *Livestock Science* **109**, 96-99.

Parkkonen, T., Tervila-Wilo, A., Hopeakoski-Nurminen, M., Morgan, A.J., Poutanen, K. and Autio, K. (1997) Changes in wheat microstructure following in vitro digestion. *Acta Agric.Scand.* **47**, 43-47.

Pierce, J. L., *et al.* (2008) Effect of Allzyme® SSF on growth performance of broilers receiving diets containing high amounts of distillers dried grains with solubles. *Poultry Science* **87**, Suppl, 770.

Ravindran, V., *et al.* (1999) Influence of microbial phytase on apparent ileal amino acid digestibility of feedstuffs for broilers. *Poultry Science* **78**, 699-706.

Schutte, J.B. (1990) Nutritional implications and metabolizable energy value of D- Xylose and L-Arabinose in chicks. *Poultry Science* **69**, 1724-30.

Schutte, J.B., *et al.* (1991) Nutritional implications of D-xylose in pigs. *British Journal of Nutrition* **66**, 83-93.

Selle, P.H., *et al.* (2006) Influence of dietary phytate and exogenous phytase on amino acid digestibility poultry: A review. *Journal of Poultry Science* **43**, 89-103.

Slominski, B.A. and Campbell, L.D. (1990) Non-starch polysaccharides of canola meal: Quantification, digestibility in poultry and potential benefit of dietary enzyme supplementation. *Journal of the Science of Food and Agriculture* **53**, 175-84.

Tervila-Wilo, A., Parkkonen, T., Morgan, A.J., Hopeakoski-Nurminen, M., Poutanen, K., Heikkinen, P. and Autio, K. (1996) In vitro digestion of wheat microstructure with xylanase and cellulase from Trichoderma reesei. *J.Cereal Sci.* **24**, 215-225.

van der Meulen, J., Inborr, J. and Bakker, J.G.M. (2001) Effects of cell wall degrading enzymes on carbohydrate fractions and metabolites in stomach and ileum of pigs fed wheat bran based diets. *Archives of Animal Nutrition [Archiv fur Tierernahrung]* **54**, 101-115.

Yin, Y.L., Deng, Z.Y., Huang, H.L., Li, T.J. and Zhong, H.Y. (2004) The effect of arabinoxylanase and protease supplementation on nutritional value of diets containing wheat bran or rice bran in growing pig. *Journal of Animal and Feed Sciences* **13**, 445-461.

Zyla, K. and Korelski, J. (1993) In-vitro and in-vivo dephosphorylation of rapeseed meal by means of phytate-degrading enzymes derived from Aspergillus niger. *Journal of the Science of Food and Agriculture* **61**, 1-6.

18

IMPACT OF BIOFUEL CO-PRODUCTS ON CARCASS QUALITY

R.C. JOHNSON

Director of Pork Quality. Farmland Foods, Inc. Denison, IA.

Introduction

The cost associated with feeding pigs to reach a suitable market weight has increased as a result of competition for maize by the ethanol industry. Therefore, it has become necessary for pig producers to investigate and utilize alternatives to high-priced maize. Much of the maize replacement has focused on utilization of co-products of the ethanol industry; most specifically, feeding dried distillers grains with solubles (DDGS). Changes in the fatty acid profile of pork originating from pigs fed greater than 200g DDGS /kg diet can occur due to the relatively high concentration of unsaturated fat present in DDGS (Whitney *et al.*, 2006).

Fat present within and around muscle tissue plays a vital role in the ultimate assessment of meat quality as it influences product appearance, oxidative stability, palatability, texture and healthfulness (Nishioka and Irie, 2006). The old meat science mantra that "Fat = Flavour" has been confirmed many times in research projects evaluating the level of marbling in high quality chops and steaks. Indeed, the quality and fatty acid profile of adipose tissue present in muscle foods contributes to the palatability and distinctiveness of meat; this is what makes pork taste like pork and beef taste like beef. Thus, as alterations in the fat profile are generated that differ from what has become gastronomically acceptable or characteristic to a given meat product, so the level of acceptance of that product to the consumer will probably be compromised. Those responsible for dietary formulation of livestock feeds must therefore consider the lipid source if they are truly concerned with the ultimate eating quality of the final meat product. This concern is of great importance with regard to non-ruminant species of livestock.

The flavour of a meat product is the most important criterion for the repeat purchase of that particular product; if it tastes good, consumers are more likely to buy it again. However, the most important criterion for the initial purchase decision (made at the retail outlet) is the visual appearance of that product (Brewer and McKeith, 1999); if it looks "off", it will not be purchased. The ultimate success of the pork industry therefore comes down to 1) consumers like the appearance of pork (they buy it) and 2) they like the taste of the pork (they buy it often).

Wood (1984; as cited by Hugo and Roodt, 2007) described high quality pork carcass fat as firm and white, and poor quality fat as soft, oily, wet, grey and floppy, and indicated that flavour was also important when describing good and poor quality fat.

Carcass traits

Carcass yield and composition are not influenced consistently by the inclusion of DDGS in diets fed to growing-finishing pigs (Stein, 2008). However, belly firmness is reduced and fat iodine values are increased by the inclusion of DDGS in these diets. It may therefore be necessary to reduce the inclusion of these products in diets fed during the final 3 to 4 weeks prior to slaughter.

The concept of formulating diets on iodine value product (IVP) basis in order to influence the iodine value of fat of pigs has been used by several production systems (Matthews, 2005). The IVP is derived from the following formula:

IVP = (IV of the feed source fat) × (g fat / kg feed source) × 0.01

Table 1 illustrates how IVP is different among some selected feed sources. This table demonstrates not only how the iodine value of a fat source affects IVP, but also how the content of fat in the feed source affects the IVP. For example, an ingredient source such as maize has a low IVP although the fat/oil in maize has a relatively high IV because the oil is a small component of corn. Conversely, beef tallow has a lower IV, but contains 990g fat/kg; thus, it has a higher IVP than maize.

Loin quality

The principal criterion for fresh pork loins to qualify for the high quality Japanese export market are 1) dark red lean colour, 2) firm muscle, and 3) sufficient marbling. Two of these criteria are influenced by soft fat. The level of unsaturation will be effective at the muscle cellular level and may influence the firmness of the boneless loin. With regard to marbling, the transparency of unsaturated fat may make visualization of marbling more difficult and may give the cut surface of the loin chops a more soft and oily appearance.

Table 1. Iodine value product of selected feed ingredients

Ingredient	Iodine value of the fat	g fat/kg raw material	Iodine value product
Feed ingredients			
Maize	125	39	49
Soyabean meal	130	30	39
Wheat	125	16	20
Peanut meal	92	65	60
Maize distillers grain	125	79	99
Bakery product	86	73	63
Common fat sources			
Beef tallow	44	990	436
Choice white grease	60	990	594
Lard	64	990	634
Poultry fat	78	990	772
Restaurant grease	75	990	743
Alternative fat sources			
Maize oil	125	995	1244
Soyabean oil	130	995	1294
Coconut oil	10	995	100
Palm oil	50	995	498

Pork bellies/bacon

According to the USDA National Nutrient Database for Standard Reference, the average total lipid (fat) content of edible portion for pork, fresh, belly, raw is 530 g/kg and, for pork, cured, bacon, raw is 450 g/kg (http://www.nal.usda.gov/fnic/foodcomp/search/). Alterations to carcass fat will be noted most in this fatty, high-value cut of pork. Soft fat associated with bacon processing has the potential for problems when the common industry practice of high-speed slicing of bacon slabs is considered. This is particularly important considering the average slicing yield for retail bacon is nine slices per inch (approximately 3.5/cm) and food service is 13 slices per inch (approximately 15.5/cm; Mandigo, 1998). Firmer fat is an insurance policy that facilitates more even slicing and improves definition of the slices in the vacuum package (NPB, 2000). Soft bellies have the potential to produce bacon slices that flatten together or fold, can appear wet or oily, are more prone to more rapid spoilage (rancidity through oxidation), and the soft fat may be more likely to separate from the lean in the bacon slice (NPB, 2000). All these defects create an undesirable presentation that may be rejected by consumers at the point of purchase. In addition, prior to slicing, slabs of bacon are "pressed" to a more uniform shape to facilitate more rapid and consistent movement through the slicer. Softer bacon slabs may be more prone to fold during pressing which produces irregular strips of bacon. There is a good reason why these statements on the soft fat of fresh bellies generating these quality defects are presented. It is because several industry contacts state that soft bellies are not a problem going through the slicer. This is because the majority of bacon processors place bacon slabs in a tempering cooler (-4 °C) to facilitate optimal pressing and slicing. The -4 °C chill placed on the bacon slab effectively alleviates the slicing problems associated with soft fat.

Thus if this soft fat is not an issue with regard to bacon processing, this raises the question as to why is there such a large focus placed on, for example, the use of DDGS in finishing pig diets relative to changing the fat profile of bellies/ bacon. Initially, the "defects" are passed on to the consumer when they open the package. Once removed from the confines of the vacuum pack, the slices appear wet and oily, the fat separates from the lean, and, now exposed to oxygen, is more prone to rancidity. Furthermore, alteration of the fatty acid profile may change the flavour profile of the bacon in those products that have a more mild cure. Fatty acid profile alterations may not be the only fat-related factors to influence flavour. Fat soluble flavenoids, ethanol processing byproducts, and other volatiles may be incorporated into the fat tissue along with the lipid from the dietary source.

References

Brewer, M.S. and McKeith, F.K. (1999) Consumer-related quality characteristics as related to purchase intent of fresh pork. *J. Food Sci.* **64**, 171-174.

Hugo, A. and Roodt, E. (2007) Significance of porcine fat quality in meat technology: A review. Food Reviews International 23, 175-198.

Mandigo, R.W. (1998) National Pork Producers Council Lean Growth Modeling Study – Belly quality study update. Pages 239-248. In Proc. Pork Quality & Safety Summit. National Pork Board, Des Moines, IA.

Matthews, J.N. (2005) Fat Quality Literature Review. PSF Technical Report, Milan, MO.

NPB (2000) Pork Composition and Quality Assessment Procedures. National Pork Board, Des Moines, IA.

Nishioka, T. and Irie, M. (2006) Fluctuation and criteria of porcine fat firmness. *Animal Sci.* **82**, 929-935.

Stein, H.H. (2008) Feeding Distillers Dried Grains with Solubles (DDGS) to Pigs. Midwest ASAS Meetings. Des Moines, IA.

Whitney, M.H., Shurson, G.C., Johnson, L.J., Wulf, D.M. and Shanks, B.C. (2006) Growth performance and carcass characteristics of grower-finisher pigs fed high-quality corn distillers dried grain with soluble originating from a modern Midwestern ethanol plant. *J. Anim. Sci.* **84**, 3356-3363.

Wood, J.D. (1984) Fat deposition and quality of fat tissue in meat animals. In Fats in Animal Nutrition. (Ed. J. Wiseman) Butterworths, London.

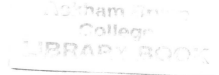

POSITIVE EFFECTS OF AN ENZYME COMBINATION ON THE PERFORMANCE AND BODY COMPOSITION OF BROILERS FED CORN-BASED DIETS CONTAINING DISTILLERS DRIED GRAINS WITH SOLUBLES

A. PÉRON[1], P. PLUMSTEAD[1] AND E.T. MORAN[2]

[1]Danisco Animal Nutrition, PO Box 777, Marlborough, SN8 1XN, UK
[2]Poultry Science Department, Auburn University, AL 36849, USA

The use of distillers dried grains with solubles (DDGS) in poultry feeds has increased with the growth of the bioethanol industry. However, because DDGS samples exhibit high variability in their nutritional quality, and they contain several anti-nutritional factors (e.g. fibre, Maillard reaction products), their utilisation remains a challenge for the feed formulator. Addition of appropriate feed enzymes offers an opportunity to improve nutritional value of diets containing DDGS. In the current study, 400 male Ross 708 broilers were placed at day-old in 16 floor pens with 25 birds / pen. Four dietary treatments were applied to 4 replicate pens from 0 to 56 days of age using a 3-phase feeding program of starter (0-21 days), grower (22-42 days) and finisher (43-56 days of age). All diets were based on maize / soyabean meal and contained 100g maize DDGS from a defined source/kg. The four treatments were 1. Positive Control (PC) that contained adequate levels of all nutrients and energy, or 2. Negative Control (NC) with Metabolisable Energy (ME) reduced by 0.33 MJ/kg, Calcium reduced by 1.2g/kg and Available Phosphorus reduced by 1.0g/kg versus PC. For treatments 3 and 4 both the PC and NC diets were supplemented with a combination of two commercial enzyme products containing xylanase, amylase and protease (300, 400 and 4000 U/kg feed respectively, Avizyme® 1502) and phytase (500 FTU/kg feed, Phyzyme® XP). All diets were pelleted (at 80°C) before feeding. Growth performance was determined between 0 and 56 days of age and, at the end of the trial, one half of the birds were taken at random for measurement of carcass parameters, including femur breaking strength. Results showed that the enzyme combination significantly (P<0.05) increased 0-56d body weight gain by 4.7 and 12.3% versus PC and NC, respectively. FCR body-weight-corrected value at 56d (FCR corrected to the same body weight gain as the Positive Control, using a factor of 3 points FCR per 100 g body weight gain) was improved by an average of 4.0% when the enzyme combination was added to the control treatments, however the result was not significant (P>0.05). Broilers fed the NC diet supplemented with enzymes showed significantly (P<0.05) higher carcass weight than the corresponding control and femur break strength value was significantly (P<0.05) increased by enzyme supplementation in both the PC and NC diets.

Corresponding author: Alexandre Péron. Email: alexandre.peron@danisco.com

COMBINATION OF PHYTASE AND XYLANASE ACTIVITIES IMPROVES ENERGY AND NUTRIENT DIGESTIBILITY IN PIGS FED CORN-BASED DIETS CONTAINING DISTILLERS DRIED GRAINS WITH SOLUBLES

A. PÉRON[1] AND P. PLUMSTEAD[1]
[1]*Danisco Animal Nutrition, PO Box 777, Marlborough, SN8 1XN, UK*

The use of distillers dried grains with solubles (DDGS) in pig feeds has increased with the growth of the bioethanol industry. However, because DDGS samples exhibit high variability in their nutritional quality, and they contain several anti-nutritional factors (e.g. fibre, Maillard reaction products), their utilisation remains a challenge for the feed formulator. The addition of appropriate feed enzymes offers an opportunity to improve the nutritional value of diets containing DDGS. For the current trial, the design was a repeated Latin square with four dietary treatments assigned to eight castrates (25-60 kg bodyweight, BW) each fitted with a T-shaped cannula at the terminal ileum. Pigs were housed individually in pens and fed each of four diets (mash) for a 7-day feeding period. The diets were based on maize / soyabean meal and contained 200g maize DDGS from a defined source. They were either unsupplemented (control) or supplemented with phytase (500 FTU/kg feed, Phyzyme® XP), xylanase (2000 U/kg feed, Porzyme® 9300) or both enzymes combined. Pigs were fed at 3 times their maintenance energy requirement (444 kJ Metabolisable Energy (ME) /kg $BW^{0.75}$, NRC, 1998). After a four-day acclimatisation to the diet, samples of faeces were collected on day 5 for determination of coefficient of total tract apparent digestibility (CTTAD) of gross energy, phosphorus and calcium. Ileal samples collected on days 6 and 7 were used for determination of coefficient of ileal apparent digestibility (CIAD) of protein and amino acids. The results showed that phytase and xylanase, when added individually, significantly ($P<0.05$) improved CTTAD for gross energy by up to 4.1% and CIAD for protein and amino acid by 3 to 7% versus the control treatment. In combination, phytase and xylanase activities significantly ($P<0.05$) improved CTTAD for gross energy by 5.6% and CIAD for protein and amino acid by 4 to 8%, versus the control treatment. The enzyme combination also had the greatest significant effects ($P<0.05$) on the CTTAD of calcium (+24%) and phosphorus (+135%).

Corresponding author: Alexandre Péron. Email: alexandre.peron@danisco.com

WHEAT-BASED DRIED DISTILLERS' GRAINS ARE VARIABLE IN CHEMICAL COMPOSITION

F. PIRON [1], D. BRUYER [2], A. THÉWIS [1] AND Y. BECKERS [1]

[1]*Gembloux Agricultural University, Gembloux, Belgium;* [2]*Beldem SA, Andenne, Belgium*

Introduction

There is worldwide increasing interest in producing ethanol from grains. Currently, maize is the main grain used in fuel ethanol production (particularly in the USA). However, in Western Europe and Canada, wheat is the main grain for ethanol plants. Barley, rye or combinations of grains are also used (Swiatkiewicz and Koreleski, 2008). The process of ethanol production from grains generates by-products (distillers' grains). Like maize distillers' grains, wheat distillers' grains have potential as an ingredient for livestock feed. Nevertheless, there is a lack of experience with distillers' grains and particularly with wheat-based by-products. Moreover, initial reports show that distillers' grains are highly variable (Patience *et al.*, 2007). In the near future (2010), about 2.4 million metric tons/ year of wheat distillers' grains will be produced in Benelux, France, Germany and United Kingdom (calculated from Ziggers, 2007). However uncertainties and expected variability in nutritional values are currently responsible for recommended inclusion rates that are relatively limited. Consequently, better knowledge of chemical composition of wheat distillers' grains is essential. The aim of the present study was to chemically characterise 11 batches of wheat-based dried distillers' grains purchased from some plants in Western Europe.

Material and methods

Samples of by-products were analysed for crude ash (550°C, 16h00), Na, K, Ca, Mg, P, S and Cl (microwaves mineralisation prior ICP-AES), nitrogen (Kjeltec 1035, Foss Tecator), amino acids (fluorimetric detection, AccQ-Tag, Waters, with performic oxidation for sulphur amino acids and alkaline hydrolysis for tryptophan), digestible and resistant starch (McCleary and Monaghan, 2002), sugars (mono-, di- and oligosaccharides of glucose and fructose measured with Megazyme kits K-MASUG and K-SUFRG), NDF (with amylase and without sulfite), ADF (separated analysis) crude fibre (FiberCaps, Foss Tecator).

email: piron.f@fsagx.ac.be

Results

Crude protein (6.25 N) varied among batches of wheat-based dried distillers' grains (Table 1). Starch was partly removed by ethanol production process. Consequently, crude protein and fibre were more concentrated in distillers' grains with regard to corresponded tabular value of wheat grain (Sauvant *et al.*, 2004). Ratios of distillers' grains to grain varied between 2.3 and 3.2 (protein), 1.6 and 2.7 (NDF) and 2.3 and 5.1 (ADF). Furthermore, heat treatment used during the production process of dried distillers' grains could cause destruction of significant amounts of some amino acids, especially lysine (Swiatkiewicz and Koreleski, 2008). Lysine varied among batches of wheat-based dried distillers' grains (Table 1). Moreover, ratios of lysine to crude protein also varied (between 0.011 and 0.029, mean = 0.018, CV = 27%). On the other hand, starch and sugars are incompletely eliminated and varied between batches of wheat-based dried distillers' grains (Table 1). For total starch (digestible + resistant), ratios of distillers' grains to tabular value of wheat grain (Sauvant *et al.*, 2004) varied between 0.02 and 0.23. Finally, production process (use of buffer) could cause differences in minerals contents (Table 1).

Table 1. Summary of chemical composition of wheat-based dried distillers' grains [1].

g / kg DM	Min.	Mean	Max.	CV (%)
6.25 N	274	347	389	11
Lys	3.7	6.1	8.0	20
Met	4.9	6.2	6.9	10
Met + Cys	8.1	12.2	14.7	19
Thr	8.3	10.4	11.5	10
Trp	2.7	3.7	4.4	13
Sugars [2]	3	11	29	65
Dig. starch	5	35	150	124
Res. starch	4	9	15	35
NDF	228	279	387	16
ADF	84	152	184	21
Crude fibre	53	69	129	30
Crude ash	47	59	83	19
Na	0.4	4.1	9.9	80
K	9.7	11.9	19.4	23
Ca	0.7	1.1	3.0	58
Mg	2.0	2.6	3.0	10
P	7.3	9.0	10.5	9
S	2.8	6.5	11.3	41
Cl	6.5	7.3	9.0	10

[1] : n = 11 ; [2] : mono-, di- and oligosaccharides of glucose and fructose.

Conclusions

Chemical composition of wheat-based dried distillers' grains is variable. More information is needed about digestibility and availability of these nutriments.

Acknowledgements

The research was funded by Beldem SA. Plants implicated in sample providing are kindly acknowledged. Technical contributions of B. Smets and S. Steels are greatly appreciated.

References

McCleary, B. V., Monaghan, D. A., 2002. *J AOAC Intern* **85**: 665-675.
Patience, J. F., Leterme, P., Beaulieu, A. D., Zijlstra, R. T., 2007. In Doppenberg, J., Van Der Aar, P. (*Ed.*). *Biofuels: implications for the feed industry.* Wageningen academic Publishers. pp 89-102.
Sauvant, D., Perez, J.-M., Tran, G., (*Ed.*), 2004. Tables de composition et de valeur nutritive des matières premières destinées aux animaux d'élevage. INRA Éditions. pp 80-81.
Swiatkiewicz, S., Koreleski, J., 2008. *World's Poultry Sci J* **64**: 257-265.
Ziggers, D., 2007. *Feed Tech* **11.8**: 14-16.

The forty-second University of Nottingham Feed Conference was organised by the following committee:

DR Z. DAVIES (*Defra*)
MR M. HAZZLEDINE (*Premier Nutrition*)
MR W. MORRIS (*BOCM PAULS Ltd*)
DR D. PARKER (*Novus International*)
MR M. ROGERS (*Volac International*)
DR M.A. VARLEY (*Provimi Ltd*)
DR P. WILCOCK (*AB Agri Ltd*)

DR J.M. BRAMELD
DR P.C. GARNSWORTHY (*Secretary*)
DR J.N. HUXLEY
DR T. PARR　　　　　　　　　　　　　　　*University of Nottingham*
DR A.M. SALTER
DR K.D. SINCLAIR
PROF R. WEBB
DR J. WISEMAN (*Chairman*)

The conference was held at the University of Nottingham Sutton Bonington Campus, 2-4 September 2008. The following persons registered for the meeting.

Abrahamse, Mr S	Provimi BV, Veerlan 17-23, Rotterdam 521602, The Netherlands
Adsett, Mr B	Perendale Publishers Ltd, 7 St George's Terrace, Cheltenham, Glos GL50 3PT, UK
Ainscough, Mr T	Buchi UK Ltd, 5 Whitegates Business Centre, Jardine Way, Oldham OL9 9QL, UK
Akhtar, Miss S	Antnano plc, Netpark Incubator, Thomas Wright Way, Sedgefield, Durham TS21 3FO, UK
Alfitour, Mr A	University of Nottingham, Sutton Bonington Campus, Loughborough, Leics LE12 5RD, UK
Altaeb, Mr A	University of Nottingham, Sutton Bonington Campus, Loughborough, Leics LE12 5RD, UK
Aronen, Dr I P	Raisio Feed Ltd, P O Box 101, Raisio 21201, Finland
Aurelien, Mr A	University of Nottingham, Sutton Bonington Campus, Loughborough, Leics LE12 5RD, UK
Bartram, Dr C	Mole Valley Feed Solutions, Head Office, Station Rd, South Molton Devon, EX36 4BH
Beardsmore, Dr A J	Ecosyl Products Ltd, Roseberry Court, Ellerbeck Way, Stokesley, N Yorks TS9 5QT, UK
Bedford, Dr M	AB - Vista Feed Ingredients, Woodstock Court, Blenheim Rd, Marlborough SN8 4AN, UK
Bennett, Mr R	Adisseo, 42 Avenue Aristiole Briand, Antony 92160, France
Berry, Dr D	TEAGASC, Moorepark Dairy Prod Research Centre, Fermoy, Co Cork, Ireland

Bird, Miss K	BQP, 1 Stradbroke Business Centre, New St, Stradbroke, Suffolk IP21 5JJ, UK
Booth, Ms A	ABN, Guild House, Oundle Road, Peterborough PE2 9PW, UK
Brameld, Dr J M	University of Nottingham, Sutton Bonington Campus, Loughborough, Leics LE12 5RD, UK
Bruyer, Mr D	Beldem, Rue Bourrie 12 Zl de Seilles, Andenne 5300, Belgium
Chaosap, Miss C	University of Nottingham, Sutton Bonington Campus, Loughborough, Leics LE12 5RD, UK
Chown, Mr M	James & Son (GM) Ltd, Olmar Court, 3 Regent Park, Booth Drive, Wellingborough NN8 6ER, UK
Clarke, Dr E	Nottingham Trent University, Brackenhurst Campus, Southwell, Notts NG25 0QF, UK
Cockshott, Mr I	Kiotechagil, Hercules 2, Calleva Park, Aldermaston, Reading RG7 8DN, UK
Cole, Mr J	BFI Innovations Ltd, 1 Telford Court, Chester Gate, Dunkirk Lea, Chester CH1 6LT, UK
Davies, Miss H	University of Nottingham, Sutton Bonington Campus, Loughborough, Leics LE12 5RD, UK
Davies, Dr Z	National Pig Association, Agriculture House, Stoneleigh Park, Warwickshire CV8 2TZ, UK
De Vos, Mr S	Inve Technologies NV, Hoogveld 93, Dendermonde 9200, Belgium
Deswysen, Mr D	Provimi Research & Innovation Centre, Lenneke Marelaan 2, Brussels 1932, Belgium
Downey, Mr N	SCA Nutec, SCA Mill, Dalton Airfield Ind Est, Dalton, Thirsk, N Yorks YO7 3HE, UK
Farquharson, Miss K	Norvite, Wardhouse, Insch, Aberdeenshire AB52 6YD, UK
Faulks, Miss R	Hi Peak Feeds Ltd, Hi Peak Feeds Mill, Sheffield Rd, Killamarsh, Sheffield S21 1ED, UK
Fowers, Miss R	Frank Wright Trouw Nutrition Int, Blenheim House, Blenheim Rd, Ashbourne, Derbyshire DE6 1HA, UK
Freeston-Smith, Mrs C	Premier Nutrition, The Levels, Rugeley WS15 1RD, UK
Garnsworthy, Dr P C	University of Nottingham, Sutton Bonington Campus, Loughborough, Leics LE12 5RD, UK
Gilbert, Mr R	IFIF, 7 St George's Terrace, Cheltenham GL50 3PT, UK
Golds, Mrs S	University of Nottingham, Sutton Bonington Campus, Loughborough, Leics LE12 5RD, UK
Gould, Ms M	Volac International Limited, 50 Fishers Lane, Orwell, Hertfordshire SG8 5QX, UK
Graham, Mr M R	CMD Agribusiness, Tremywawr, Brezdden Ave, Arddleen, Llanymynech SY22 65P, UK
Green, Dr S	Adisseo, Berkhamsted House, 121 High St, Berkhamsted HP4 2DJ, UK

Gregson, Miss E	University of Nottingham, Sutton Bonington Campus, Loughborough, Leics LE12 5RD, UK
Griffin, Mr P	Hi Peak Feeds Ltd, Hi Peak Feeds Mill, Sheffield Rd, Killamarsh, Sheffield S21 1ED, UK
Hall, Miss C	BOCM Pauls, First Avenue, Royal Portbury Docks, Bristol BS20 7XS, UK
Hall, Mr T	James & Son, Olmar Court, 3 Regent Park, Booth Drive, Park Fm, Wellingborough NN8 6GR, UK
Halls, Mr R	Roquette UK Ltd, Sallow Road, Corby NN17 5JX, UK
Hazzledine, Mr M	Premier Nutrition, The Nutrition Centre, The Levels, Rugeley, Staffs WS15 1RD, UK
Hernandez Medrano, Mr J	University of Nottingham, Sutton Bonington Campus, Loughborough, Leics LE12 5RD, UK
Hooley, Mrs E	University of Nottingham, Sutton Bonington Campus, Loughborough, Leics LE12 5RD, UK
Hough, Mr T	NWF Ag Ltd, Wardle, Nantwich, Cheshire CW5 6AQ, UK
Houseman, Dr R	T C S I Ltd, 18 Melrose Road, Bishop Monkton, Harrogate HG3 3RH, UK
Hughes, Mr J	University of Nottingham, Sutton Bonington Campus, Loughborough, Leics LE12 5RD, UK
Humblot, Dr P	UNCEIA R&D, 13 rue Jouet, 94704, Maisons Alfort Cedex , France
Husband, Mr J	EBVC Ltd, 68 Arthur St, Penrith CA11 7TX, UK
Huxley, Dr J N	University of Nottingham, Sutton Bonington Campus, Loughborough, Leics LE12 5RD, UK
Ingham, Mr R	Yara Phosphates, Animal Nutrition, The Homestead, Troutbeck Bridge, Windermere LA23 1HF, UK
Isaac, Mr P	Mole Valley Feed Solutions, Head Office, Station Rd, South Molton, Devon EX36 4BH, UK
Johnson, Dr R	Farmland Foods, 800 Industrial Drive, P O Box 490, Denison, IA 51442, USA
Jones, Dr G	Aponi2b, Wrens Nest, Pauntley Court, Redmarley GL19 3JA, UK
Keeling, Mrs S	Nottingham University Press, Manor Farm, Church Lane, Thrumpton, Notts NG11 0AX, UK
Keller, Dr H	Buchi Labortechnik AG, Meierseggstrasse 40, Postbox CH-9230, Flawili CH-9230, Switzerland
Kirkland, Dr R	Volac International Limited, 50 Fishers Lane, Orwell, Hertfordshire SG8 5QX, UK
Knudsen, Dr K E B	University of Aarhus, Faculty of Agric. Sciences, Blichers Alle 20, Tjele 8830, Denmark
Krizova, Dr L	Research Inst for Cattle Breeding Ltd, Vyzkumniku 267, Rapotin, Vikyrovice 788 13, Czech Republic
Krogedal, Mr P	FKRA, Sandvikveien 21, Stavanger 4001, Norway

Lahaye, Dr L	Yara Helsingborg AB, P O Box 902 - Industratan 70, Helsingborg 25109, Sweden
Linden, Miss J E	5M Publishing, 4 Haywood House, Hydra Bus. Park, Nether Lane, Sheffield S35 92X, UK
Loughmiller, Dr J	SCA - Nutrition USA, 207 Sisseton Dr, Fairmont MN 56031, USA
Lovendahl, Dr P	Aarhus University, Faculty of Agricultural Science, Dept Genetics & Biotech, Tjele DK 8830, Denmark
Lowe, Dr J	Dodson & Horrell, Kettering Rd, Islip, Northants NN14 3JW, UK
Lucey, Mr P	Dairygold Co-op Ltd, Lambardstown, Co Cork Ireland,
Ludger, Miss A K	Nutreco IRC, Veerstraat 38, Boxmeer 5831 JN, The Netherlands
Magowan, Dr E	Agri-Food and Biosciences Institute, Large Park, Hillsborough, N Ireland BT26 6DR, UK
Malandra, Mr F	Cargill SRL, Via Gibardo Patecchio, Milano 20161, Italy
Marsden, Dr M	AB Agri Ltd, Oundle Rd, Peterborough PE2 9PW, UK
McConnell, Mr P F M	Nutrition Services/Vistavet, 211 Castle Road, Randalstown, Co Antrim BT41 2EB, UK
Mitchell, Mr P P	Crown Chicken Ltd, Green Farm, Edge Green, Kenninghall, Norwich NR16 2DR, UK
Mombaerts, Mr R	Agrimex NV, Achterstenhoek 5, 2275 Lille, Belgium
Moorby, Dr J	IBERS, Aberystwyth University, Gogerddan, Aberystwyth SY23 3EB, UK
Morris, Dr V	University of Bristol, Langford, Somerset BS40 5DU, UK
Morris, Mr W	BOCM Pauls, First Ave, Royal Portbury Docks, Portbury, Bristol BS20 7XS, UK
Mul, Mr A	CCL-BV; CCL-Research, P O Box 107, Veghel 5460 AC, Netherlands
Mulder, Dr I	Rowett Research Institute, Greenburn Rd, Aberdeen AB21 9SB, UK
Northover, Mrs S	University of Nottingham, Sutton Bonington Campus, Loughborough, Leics LE12 5RD, UK
Papasolomontos, Dr S	Kego S.A., 1st km nea Artaki - Psachna, Nea Artaki GR 34600, Greece
Parker, Dr D	Novus Europe, 200 Avenue Marcel Thiry, B-1200 , Brussels
Parr, Dr T	University of Nottingham, Sutton Bonington Campus, Loughborough, Leics LE12 5RD, UK
Peron, Dr A	Danisco, P O Box 777, Marlborough SN8 1XN, UK
Pickering, Miss K	University of Nottingham, Sutton Bonington Campus, Loughborough, Leics LE12 5RD, UK
Pinkney, Mr J	Ensus Biofuels, The Granary, 17a High St, Yarm TS15 9BW, UK
Piva, Dr A	Vetagro Spa, Via Colletta 12, Reggio Emilia 42100, Italy
Piva, Prof G	Universita Cattolica Del Sacro Cuore, Faculty of Agriculture, Via Emilia Parmense 84, Piacenza 29100, Italy
Pope, Mr B	BASF PLC, P O Box 4, Earl Road, Cheadle Hulme, Cheadle, Cheshire SK8 6QG, UK

Potterton, Miss S	University of Nottingham, Sutton Bonington Campus, Loughborough, Leics LE12 5RD, UK
Pritchard, Mr R	M E Waterhouse Limited, Station Mills, Malpas, Cheshire SY14 8JQ, UK
Richards, Dr S	James & Son (GM Ltd), Olmar Court, 3 Regent Park, Booth Drive, Wellingborough NN8 6ER, UK
Riley, Mr A	Danisco Animal Nutrition, 88 Mill Drove, Bourne, Lincs PE10 9BZ, UK
Roele, Mr D J	Perstorp Performance Additives, Industrieweg 8, Waspik 5165 NH, The Netherlands
Rogers, Mr M	Volac International Ltd, Volac House, Orwell, Royston SG8 5QX, UK
Rose, Mr D	Carrs-Billington Agriculture, Lansil Industrial Estate, Lansil Rd, Lancaster LA1 3QY, UK
Salter, Prof A	University of Nottingham, Sutton Bonington Campus, Loughborough, Leics LE12 5RD, UK
Sas, Mr A H	Provimi BV, Veerlaan 17-23, Rotterdam 521602, The Netherlands
Serra, Mr D	Hydronix, 7 Riverside Business Centre, Walnut Tree Close, Guildford GU1 4UG, UK
Setta, Mr S	University of Nottingham, Sutton Bonington Campus, Loughborough, Leics LE12 5RD, UK
Sinclair, Dr K	University of Nottingham, Sutton Bonington Campus, Loughborough, Leics LE12 5RD, UK
Smith, Mr A	Biotal Ltd, Collivaud House, Ocean Way, Cardiff CF24 5PD, UK
Swart, Miss C	NWF Ag Ltd, Wardle, Nantwich, Cheshire CW5 6AQ, UK
Tan, Mrs T	Perendale Publishers Ltd, 7 St George's Terrace, Cheltenham, Glos GL503PT, UK
Terrier, Mrs S	ABN, ABN House, Oundle Rd, Peterborough PE2 9PW, UK
Thompson, Dr J	Scottish Agricultural College, Veterinary Services, Bush Estate, Penicuik, Midlothian EH26 OQE, UK
Thornber, Miss V	Premier Nutrition, The Levels, Rugeley WS15 1RD, UK
Thurman, Mr K	Beneo-Animal Nutrition, Aandorenstraat 1, Tienen 3300, Belgium
Timms, Dr A	University of Nottingham, Sutton Bonington Campus, Loughborough, Leics LE12 5RD, UK
Toplis, Mr P	ABN, ABN House, Oundle Road, Peterborough PE2 9PW, UK
Trinacty, Dr J	Research Inst for Cattle Breeding Ltd, Vyzkumniku 267, Rapotin, Vikyrovice 788 13, Czech Republic
Upton, Miss E	Yara, Industrigatian 70, Helsingborg 25109, Sweden
van Ginderachter, Mr J	Agrimex NV, Achterstenhoek 5, 2275 Lille , Belgium
van Helvoirt, Miss G	Perstorp Performance Additives, Industrieweg 8, Waspik 5165 NH, The Netherlands
van Milgen, Dr J	INRA, UMR SENAH, Domaine del la Prise, Saint-Gilles F-35590, France

van Straalen, Dr W	Schothorst Feed Research, P O Box 533, Lelystad 8200AM, The Netherlands
Vande Ginste, Dr J	Vitamex/Nutrition Sciences, Booiebos 5, Drongen 9031 , Belgium
Vandi, Dr L	Vetagro, Spa, Via Colletta, 12, Reggio Emilia 42100, Italy
Varley, Dr M	The Pig Technology Co, Whitegates, Willow Lane, Clifford, Wetherby, W Yorks LS23 6JH, UK
Vecqueray, Mr R	EBVC Ltd, 68 Arthur St, Penrith LA11 7TX, UK
Wagner, Dr H	Dr Eckel GmbH, Im Stiefelfeed 10, Niederzissen 56651, Germany
Waterhouse, Mr A	M E Waterhouse Limited, Station Mills, Malpas, Cheshire SY14 8JQ, UK
Webb, Mrs R	Nottingham University Press, Manor Farm, Church Lane, Thrumpton, Notts NG11 0AX, UK
Webb, Prof R	University of Nottingham, Sutton Bonington Campus, Loughborough, Leics LE12 5RD, UK
Wellock, Dr I	ABN, ABN House, Oundle Rd, Peterborough PE2 9PW,
Whitehead, Mr J	Wyreside Products Ltd, Lune Bank, School Lane, Pilling PR3 6AA, UK
Wilcock, Dr P	ABN, ABN House, Oundle Road, Peterborough PE2 9PW, UK
Wilde, Mr D	Alltech, Alltech House, Ryhall Road, Stamford PE9 1TZ, UK
Williams, Mr E	AB Vista, Marlborough Business Park, Blenheim Rd, Marlborough, Wilts , UK
Williams, Dr P E V	AB Agri, Oundle Rd, Peterborough PE2 9PW, UK
Williams, Mr S	AIC, Confederation House, East of England Showground Peterborough, PE2 6XE, UK
Wills, Miss J	University of Nottingham, Sutton Bonington Campus, Loughborough, Leics LE12 5RD, UK
Wiseman, Prof J	University of Nottingham, Sutton Bonington Campus, Loughborough LE12 5RD, UK
Wonnacott, Miss K	University of Nottingham, Sutton Bonington Campus, Loughborough, Leics LE12 5RD, UK
Wynn, Dr R	KW Trident (AB Agri), Oundle Road, Peterborough PE2 9PW, UK
Zijlstra, R	University of Alberta, 4-10 Agriculture/Forestry Centre, Edmonton, AB T6H 197, Canada

INDEX

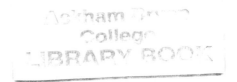